Handbook of
Patient Care in
Vascular Diseases

Handbook of Patient Care in Vascular Diseases

Fourth Edition

John W. Hallett, Jr., M.D.
Professor of Surgery and Associate Dean for Faculty Affairs, Mayo Medical School and Mayo Clinic; Attending Surgeon, Saint Mary's Hospital and Rochester Methodist Hospital, Rochester, Minnesota

David C. Brewster, M.D.
Professor of Surgery, Massachusetts General Hospital and Harvard Medical School, Boston, Massachusetts

Todd E. Rasmussen, M.D.
Instructor in Surgery, Mayo Medical School, Clinical Assistant Professor of Surgery, Uniformed Services Health Science Center, Bethesda, Maryland

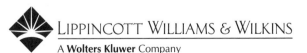

LIPPINCOTT WILLIAMS & WILKINS
A **Wolters Kluwer** Company
Philadelphia · Baltimore · New York · London
Buenos Aires · Hong Kong · Sydney · Tokyo

Acquisitions Editor: Lisa McAllister
Developmental Editor: Brian Brown
Production Editor: Jonathan Geffner
Manufacturing Manager: Benjamin Rivera
Cover Illustrator: Patricia Gast
Compositor: Circle Graphics
Printer: RR Donnelly–Crawfordsville

Printed in the USA

Library of Congress Cataloging-in-Publication Data

ISBN: 0-7817-2614-X

Care has been taken to confirm the accuracy of the information presented
and to describe generally accepted practices. However, the authors and
publisher are not responsible for errors or omissions or for any consequences
from application of the information in this book and make no warranty,
expressed or implied, with respect to the currency, completeness, or accuracy
of the contents of the publication. Application of this information in a
particular situation remains the professional responsibility of the
practitioner.

The authors and publisher have exerted every effort to ensure that drug
selection and dosage set forth in this text are in accordance with current
recommendations and practice at the time of publication. However, in view of
ongoing research, changes in government regulations, and the constant flow
of information relating to drug therapy and drug reactions, the reader is
urged to check the package insert for each drug for any change in indications
and dosage and for added warnings and precautions. This is particularly
important when the recommended agent is a new or infrequently employed
drug.

Some drugs and medical devices presented in this publication have Food
and Drug Administration (FDA) clearance for limited use in restricted
research settings. It is the responsibility of the health care provider to
ascertain the FDA status of each drug or device planned for use in their
clinical practice.

The views expressed in this book are our those of the authors and do not
necessarily represent the opinions of the entire staff at the Mayo Clinic or
Massachusetts General Hospital.

10 9 8 7 6 5 4 3 2 1

Dedication

R. Clement Darling, Jr., M.D.
(1927–1999)

In 1979, David Brewster and I approached Clem Darling with the idea of a handbook of patient care in vascular surgery. At the time, there was no published handbook written specifically for students, residents, and nurses. Dr. Darling understood the value that such a handbook would add to the learning and practice of vascular trainees and practitioners. His enthusiasm for the project was prompt and unwavering through the three previous editions.

As Senior Vascular Surgeon at the Massachusetts General Hospital (MGH), Clem Darling understood the key concepts that culminate in excellent outcome for vascular patients. The original and subsequent handbooks have embodied these concepts that he and his colleagues at the MGH knew would result in good outcomes.

What were the key concepts that he stressed? There are many, but three stand out. First, he believed that protocols and methods could be used to consistently give excellent surgical results irrespective of the initial skills of the trainee. Second, he emphasized the development of noninvasive technologies that could measure the preoperative physiology of the vascular patient and could document the postoperative and long-term results. Third, he stressed clinical research that focused on pragmatic questions that examined the durability of surgical procedures.

When he died unexpectedly on June 26, 1999, at age 71, we lost a unique colleague and friend. Those who knew him remember his special wit and inquisitive mind. When a good idea arose, his support could be avid. When he did not agree with some statement or action, his criticism could also be prompt and sharply perceptive. The bottom line for him was dedication to excellence in surgical outcome and clinical research. That is not always an easy dedication for any of us to sustain. Despite the challenges of his personal and professional life, Clem Darling knew that his legacy would be sustained by his students, residents, and fellows. He loved and admired them. Those of us who were fortunate enough to know and work with him will not soon forget his influence.

J.W.H.

Contents

Preface

In 1982, we introduced the practical *Manual of Patient Care in Vascular Surgery*. This new *Handbook of Patient Care in Vascular Diseases* moves from a primary emphasis on vascular surgery to the multidisciplinary trends in patient care. The enduring principles of the first edition remain. However, we emphasize the numerous developments in pathophysiology, diagnosis, and treatment that have arrived in the past several years, not least in the new area of endovascular therapy. Above all, we continue to focus on fundamentals that guide students, residents, technicians, and nurses who work on the front lines of patient care.

This edition also introduces a new collaborative author, Dr. Todd Rasmussen. Dr. Rasmussen is of the "new generation" of vascular specialists. He brings the latest perspective of students, residents, and fellows who are currently completing their training. His fresh insight, added to the experience of the senior authors, provides a unique balance to this new edition.

Each chapter has been revised to reflect the latest advances. References emphasize evidence-based medicine. In particular, we have included as many randomized clinical trials as possible. Also, selected reviews by experts in the field provide a quick overview to the busy learner. Many more articles and books are obviously available and must be consulted for second opinions and additional details on topics.

A number of new illustrations add to several of the topics that are under dynamic change, e.g., aneurysm disease and new stent grafts. Also, a new chapter on coagulation problems emphasizes the expansion of new knowledge in this important area.

All of you who have used previous editions have offered many suggestions that enhance the new *Handbook of Patient Care in Vascular Diseases*. We thank you for your valuable input over the years. We hope that those who use the new edition will take time again to let us know how future editions might be improved.

J.W.H.
D.C.B.

Acknowledgments

We gratefully acknowledge the contributions of the following individuals, whose efforts were essential to the development and completion of this handbook: Lisa McAllister and Jonathan Geffner of Lippincott Williams & Wilkins; David Factor, in the Department of Medical Illustrations at the Mayo Clinic, for his new contributions; and Renee Brandt for her help in manuscript preparation.

We also extend special thanks to the following colleagues for their thoughtful review and suggestions: Anthony W. Stanson, M.D. (Vascular Radiology) and John A. Heit, M.D. (Vascular Medicine). Their experience and insights have enhanced these special sections of the handbook.

Finally, we acknowledge the input that so many students, residents, fellows, and colleagues have given us over the past several years. These suggestions have strengthened each and every edition of the handbook.

Handbook of
Patient Care in
Vascular Diseases

Basic Concepts

A limited number of basic principles guide the management of most vascular problems. Following these principles, one can consistently provide logical and appropriate patient care. In the first two chapters, we outline and emphasize these basic concepts. Since the scope of this handbook covers primarily atherosclerotic arterial disease and acquired venous disease, we have organized the basic concepts around these two broad disease groups. Each chapter is further subdivided under the headings "magnitude of the problem," "anatomy," "etiology," "pathophysiology," and "natural history."

Arterial Disease

I. Magnitude of the problem. Arterial diseases are a leading cause of death in the United States and many other countries. Perhaps more important than mortality is the disability that cardiovascular disease causes in so many people. For example, approximately 500,000 Americans have strokes each year. Many of these people are left with a permanent neurologic deficit. The social and economic impact of a stroke can be devastating to both the patient and his or her family. Others are incapacitated by angina pectoris, leg claudication, and ischemic foot lesions.

Advances in the accurate diagnosis and successful treatment of these arterial problems have been rapid. However, significant progress in prevention has been much slower and may improve with better control of specific risk factors. Currently, many patients are reluctant to modify their diets, to stop smoking, and to take medications regularly. Thus, arterial disease will remain a leading health problem during the entire career of most physicians alive today.

II. Arterial anatomy. The arterial system is a complex, highly structured organ system. Like the heart, arteries must withstand the stress of pulsatile blood flow for many years. Three distinct layers of large- and medium-sized arteries must remain intact for normal function. These layers are the intima, media, and adventitia (Fig. 1.1).

A. The intima, the innermost layer, is a monolayer of endothelial cells with a thin underlying matrix of collagen and elastic fibers. An **internal elastic membrane** separates the intima from the media.

B. The media is a relatively thick middle layer of varying amounts of smooth muscle, collagen, and elastic fibers. The amount of elastic tissue decreases progressively from the thoracic aorta (elastic artery) to the distal medium-sized arteries, such as the femoral or carotid (muscular arteries). In contrast to the intima, the media has a dual source of nourishment. The innermost portion receives its nutrients by diffusion from the circulating blood. The outer regions are nourished by small vessels that penetrate the outer arterial wall. These **vasa vasorum** may be affected by the arteriosclerotic process, leading to degeneration of wall strength. An **external elastic membrane** encloses the outer border of the media and separates it from the adventitia.

C. The adventitia, the outermost layer of an artery, may appear thin and weak. However, its collagenous and elastic structure make it a key element in the total strength of the arterial wall. In muscular arteries, it may be as thick as the media. Primary surgical closure of the arterial wall or anastomosis of a synthetic graft to the vessel must incorporate the adventitia. Failure to include the adventitia may result in a weakened spot and eventual pseudoaneurysm formation.

III. Etiology. The basis of most arterial diseases today can be considered atherosclerosis. There is some confusion about the

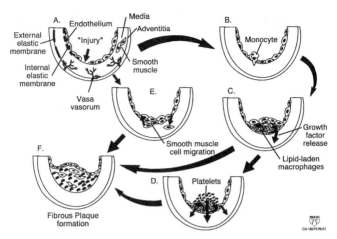

Figure 1.1.   Pathogenesis of atherosclerosis. Inflammation is now considered central to atherosclerosis. Endothelial "injury" or dysfunction can be initiated by a variety of forces: hyperlipidemia; free radicals caused by cigarette smoking, hypertension, and diabetes mellitus; genetic alterations; elevated plasma homocysteine; infectious microorganisms such as *Chlamydia pneumoniae*; and combinations of these and other factors. *A*: Monocytes attach to injured endothelium (*B*), secrete growth factors (*C*), and finally migrate into the subendothelial layer. Lipid-laden macrophages become part of the fatty streak. Endothelial disruption attracts platelets (*D*) that secrete platelet-derived growth factor (PDGF). Smooth muscle cells in the proliferative atheromatous lesion may also secrete growth factors such as PDGF. Increased endothelial turnover results in enhanced growth factor production. Smooth muscle cells are stimulated to migrate into the intimal layer (*E*). Smooth muscle and "injured" endothelial cells turn up their growth factor production. Fibrous plaques (*F*) evolve from fatty streaks. Atheroma develop from fatty streaks to fibrous plaques that can degenerate eventually into complicated plaques with surface ulceration, hemorrhage, and embolization. This fibrous plaque rupture and ulceration appears to be related to macrophages releasing proteolytic enzymes. (Adapted from Ross R. Atherosclerosis—an inflammatory disease. *N Engl J Med* 1999;340:115–126.)

terms **atherosclerosis** and **arteriosclerosis.** Arteriosclerosis was introduced originally to describe any arterial disease that caused wall thickening. Atheroma was applied to plaques that contained soft fatty contents. Finally, atherosclerosis was defined by the World Health Organization as a combination of changes in the intima and media. These changes include focal accumulation of lipids, hemorrhage, fibrous tissue, and calcium deposits. The development of atherosclerotic lesions is a complex immune-related process involving hemodynamic shear stress as well as environmental and genetic factors. A detailed discussion of atherosclerosis is beyond the scope of this handbook; however, the gross appearance and developmental sequence may be divided into three major stages.

A. **Early lesions** usually appear as fatty streaks in childhood or young adult life. Their content is primarily lipid—specifically, lipid-laden macrophages called "foam cells." Cholesterol or low-density lipoproteins are the main lipid components. Cigarette smoking accelerates formation of these early lesions by increasing the oxidation of low-density lipoproteins and their phagocytosis by macrophages. Evidence suggests that, with exercise and risk factor modification, these early lesions can regress.

B. **Fibrous plaques** appear in later life. They represent a more permanent lesion and follow the development of symptomatic atherosclerosis. Located mainly at arterial bifurcations, fibrous plaques have a lipid core surrounded by a capsule of elastic and collagenous tissue.

C. **Complicated lesions** develop from the fibrous plaque. Specifically, necrosis of the plaque leads to surface ulceration and creation of a thrombogenic surface, which leads to platelet aggregation and formation of thrombus. Intramural hemorrhage also may occur, with or without ulceration. The elasticity of the arterial wall is lost and the process may narrow the vessel lumen, or the wall may degenerate and dilate, to form an aneurysm.

D. **The development of atherosclerosis** follows a variable course. In the same patient, one may find a spectrum of early and complicated lesions. Intimal thickening and calcification of arteries apparently are a normal aging process. However, complicated atherosclerosis is a disease process whose course is influenced by a number of risk factors. The primary ones appear to be smoking, hypertension, hyperlipidemia, and diabetes mellitus. Failure to control these factors usually leads to accelerated atherogenesis.

IV. **Pathophysiology.** Basic principles of fluid dynamics (Table 1.1) explain the physiologic consequences of arterial occlusive and aneurysmal disease. In some patients, both processes coexist.

A. **Occlusive disease.** Atherosclerosis becomes symptomatic by gradual occlusion of blood flow to the involved extremity or organ. Symptoms finally occur when a **critical arterial stenosis** is reached. Blood flow and pressure are not significantly diminished until at least 75% of the cross-sectional area of the vessel is obliterated (Fig. 1.2). This figure for cross-sectional area can be equated with a 50% reduction in lumen diameter. The formula for the area of a circle (area = $3.14 \times radius^2$) explains the relationship between vessel diameter and cross-sectional area.

Factors other than radius influence critical stenosis but to a lesser extent. These include the length of the stenosis, blood viscosity, and peripheral resistance. Longer stenotic segments reach a critical stenosis earlier. Likewise, flow and pressure across a stenosis diminish sharply when the blood becomes more viscous. In low-resistance situations, flow is increased, but turbulence at a stenosis is also worsened and pressure across the lesion may decrease.

Evidence also suggests that a series of subcritical stenoses can have an additive effect that is similar to a single critical stenosis. This cumulative effect, however, is not linear. Thus, three subcritical stenoses (30%, 40%, and 10%) may not have the same effect as a single 80% narrowing of a vessel.

Table 1.1. Basic principles of fluid dynamics

Principle	Definition	Equation	Terms of Equation
Bernoulli's	Relationship between pressure, gravitational (potential) energy, and kinetic energy in an idealized fluid system. In moving blood through arteries, the portion of total fluid energy lost is dissipated in the form of heat.	$P_1 + \rho g h_1 + \frac{1}{2}\rho v_1^2 =$ $P_2 + \rho g h_2 + \frac{1}{2}\rho v_2^2 + \text{heat}$	P = pressure $\rho g h$ = gravitational potential energy $\frac{1}{2}\rho v_2^2$ = kinetic energy
Poiseuille's	Relationship between flow and the pressure difference across the length of a tube, its radius, and the fluid viscosity. The most important determinant of flow is radius.	$Q = \pi r^4 (P_1 - P_2)/8L\eta$	Q = flow r = radius of vessel $P_1 - P_2$ = potential energy between 2 points L = distance between 2 points η = viscosity coefficient
Reynolds number	A dimensionless quantity that defines the point at which flow changes from laminar (streamlined) to turbulent (disorganized). If Re > 2,000, disturbances in laminar flow will result in fully developed turbulence. In normal arterial circulation, Re is usually < 2,000.	$\text{Re} = \rho v d/\eta$	Re = Reynolds number d = tube diameter v = velocity ρ = specific gravity η = viscosity
Resistance (rearranged Poiseuille's law)	Analogous to Ohm's equation of electrical circuits (resistance = pressure/flow)	$R = P_1 - P_2/Q = 8\eta L/\pi r^4$	R = resistance $P_1 - P_2$ = pressure drop Q = flow η = viscosity L = length of tube r = radius of tube

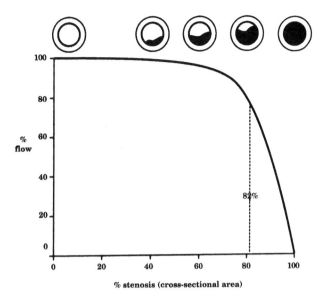

Figure 1.2. **Critical arterial stenosis. Blood flow remains relatively
normal across an arterial stenosis until at least 75% of the cross-
sectional area is obliterated (50% diameter reduction).**

Turbulence has been identified as the most important cause of
blood flow and pressure drop across a stenosis. The turbulence
occurs in the poststenotic section of the vessel, where kinetic
energy is dissipated by these turbulent eddies. The influence of
blood flow on the degree of narrowing of a vessel necessary to
cause a critical stenosis explains why ankle pressures may be
normal at rest but fall sharply with exercise. Exercise increases
extremity blood flow. Because increased blood flow across a
stenosis causes more turbulence, flow and pressure eventually
will decrease. The patient who may have no complaints at rest
will experience claudication with exercise. Hence, a stenosis may
be noncritical at rest but critical with exercise.

Experimental and clinical observations indicate that atherosclerotic lesions form near areas of blood flow separation and low
shear stress (Fig. 1.3). The layer of blood adjacent to an arterial
wall, as blood flows through an artery, is referred to as the
boundary layer. Although flow in the center of the arterial
lumen is laminar, the area of boundary layer separation has
slower, more disturbed currents. These areas of boundary layer
separation and low shear force (<4 dyne/cm^2) induce endothelial
dysfunction and generally occur at the outer wall of arterial
bifurcations, where atherosclerosis is more pronounced.

B. Aneurysmal disease. Aneurysms are the result of degeneration and weakening of the network of structural proteins
(e.g., elastin and collagen) in the arterial wall. The mechanisms
that result in aneurysm formation are multifactorial (Fig. 1.4)
(see Chap. 16). Rupture occurs if the intraluminal pressure

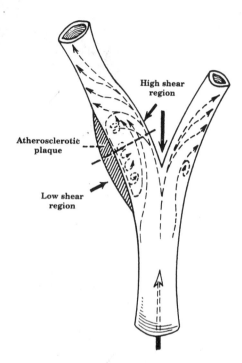

Figure 1.3.   Patterns of low and high shear stress. Atherosclerotic plaques, which usually localize to the outer wall at arterial bifurcations, tend to develop at areas of boundary layer separation and low shear stress. (Adapted from Malek AD, Alper SL, Izumo S. Hemodynamic shear stress and its role in atherosclerosis. *JAMA* 1999;282:2035–2042.)

exceeds the tensile strength of the wall. The etiology of this wall degeneration and the mechanisms of its dilation and rupture are not fully understood. In recent years, the role of local inflammation and destructive proteolytic enzymes (e.g., metalloproteinases) have been emphasized. Certain observations and hemodynamic principles also provide a reasonable explanation for why aneurysms localize to some aortic segments more than other areas.

When a pulse wave arrives at a vessel bifurcation, a portion of the pressure is reflected against the arterial wall proximal to the bifurcation. Minimal reflections occur when the sum of the cross-sectional areas of the daughter arteries (e.g., iliacs) to the parent artery (aorta) is 1.15 or greater. With advancing age, this ratio decreases, even in aortas without atheromatous change, and so more oscillating pressure is reflected. The result is a partial standing wave in the abdominal aorta. These reflective pressure waves at major bifurcations may determine the increased incidence of aneurysms at these locations.

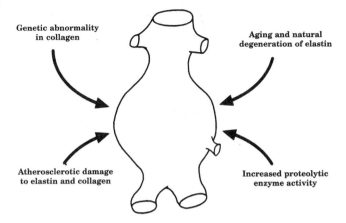

Figure 1.4.   Factors contributory to the multifactorial pathogenesis of arterial aneurysms.

In addition to reflected pressure waves, the paucity of vasa vasorum in the abdominal aorta also may contribute to its susceptibility to aneurysm formation. When arteriosclerosis obliterates vasa vasorum, necrosis of the media results in weakening and vessel dilation. Vasa vasorum are more plentiful in the thoracic aorta, where aneurysms are less common.

Defects in the structural integrity of the vessel collagen and elastic content are found in certain congenital conditions, such as Marfan's syndrome. Whether normal adults who develop aneurysms have an inherited predisposition to arterial dilatation has not been proved but has been clinically observed in some families. The collagen content of an atherosclerotic aneurysm is reduced. Collagen fibers constitute about 25% of an atherosclerotic arterial wall but only 6% to 18% of an aneurysmal wall.

The risk of aneurysm rupture increases with increased aneurysm size. The stress in the vessel wall increases as the vessel diameter (d) enlarges and its wall thickness (t) decreases. Wall stress is also proportional to intraluminal pressure (P):

Stress $= P \times d/t$

The importance of blood pressure control becomes obvious when this **Laplace relationship** is examined. In addition, a layer of thrombus frequently lines the interior of aneurysms, but does not protect against rupture.

V.   Natural history. For most patients, atherosclerosis is diffuse and slowly progressive. During early adult life, it usually remains asymptomatic. However, when it becomes symptomatic in one part of the body, a careful history and physical examination will often reveal evidence of significant disease at other sites. Sometimes, the asymptomatic disease is more life threatening. For example, a patient may present with calf claudication but have an unknown abdominal aortic aneurysm palpable on routine physical examination. The diffuse nature of atherosclerosis requires that the initial patient evaluation include a baseline examination of the entire vascular system.

The natural history of atherosclerosis is variable. Some patients are minimally bothered by its presence, while others are incapacitated. Although atherosclerosis, like cancer, may follow a malignant course despite therapeutic intervention, the natural history can be altered satisfactorily in most cases by appropriate treatment. Although not curative, properly selected arterial interventions can offer excellent palliation of the atherosclerotic process. Subsequent chapters will emphasize specific aspects of the natural history of atherosclerosis so that clinicians can select patients who are most likely to benefit from medical, radiologic, and surgical intervention.

SELECTED READING

Akbari CM, LoGerfo FW. Diabetes and peripheral vascular disease. *J Vasc Surg* 1999;30:373–384.

Allaire E, Clowes AW. Endothelial cell injury in cardiovascular surgery: the intimal hyperplastic response. *Ann Thorac Surg* 1997; 63:582–591.

Brophy CM. The dynamic regulation of blood vessel caliber. *J Vasc Surg* 2000;31:391–395.

Frangos SG, Chen AH, Sumpio B. Vascular drugs in the new millennium. *J Am Coll Surg* 2000;191:76–92.

Malek AM, Alper SL, Izumo S. Hemodynamic shear stress and its role in atherosclerosis. *JAMA* 1999;282:2035–2042.

Rehm JP, Grange JJ, Baxter BT. The formation of aneurysms. *Semin Vasc Surg* 1998;11:193–202.

Ross R. Atherosclerosis—an inflammatory disease. *N Engl J Med* 1999;340:115–126.

Sumner DS. Essential hemodynamic principles. In: Rutherford RB, ed. *Vascular surgery,* 5th ed. Philadelphia: WB Saunders, 2000: 73–120.

Venous Disease

The most common venous disorders are varicose veins, superficial and deep venous thrombosis, pulmonary embolism, postphlebitic syndrome, and chronic deep venous insufficiency. As in arterial disease, a limited number of basic principles can explain the physiologic consequences of these different conditions. Proper treatment is based on these concepts.

I. Magnitude and Classification. Simple varicose veins affect about 15% of the adult population and rarely cause significant morbidity. In contrast, acquired deep venous thrombosis and its complications debilitate or kill thousands of patients each year. Pulmonary embolism is the most common lethal pulmonary disease in the United States, and, of those who survive deep venous thrombosis and pulmonary embolism, the majority develop postphlebitic syndrome. Others have chronic deep valvular incompetence and reflux unrelated to postphlebitic syndrome. The incidence of serious venous problems in the United States is increasing.

To standardize the classification of chronic venous insufficiency, a system has been developed based on the clinical symptoms, etiology, anatomic distribution and pathology of a given venous problem. This system is referred to as the **CEAP grading system.** Clinical signs range from spider veins (C1) to an active venous ulcer (C6). The etiology is classified as congenital (E_C), primary (E_P), or secondary (E_S). The anatomic classification is superficial (A_S), deep (A_D) or perforator (A_P) in location. Finally, the pathology is reflux (P_R), obstruction (P_O), or both ($P_{R,O}$).

II. Anatomy

A. Valves. Of all the anatomic features of veins, the valves play the central role in most venous disorders. Normal venous valves are bicuspid, opening so that blood flows toward the heart and closing so as to prevent reflux. The greatest number of valves are located in the lower leg. The number decreases as the veins approach the inguinal ligament. A single valve usually is found in the external iliac or common femoral vein, and it is the only valve preventing reflux into the superficial saphenous vein. In approximately one-third of the population, no external iliac or common femoral valves exist. The inferior vena cava is always valveless.

B. Layers. Although veins have the same three layers comprising their wall as arteries, the composition and function of these layers differ from those in an artery. These differences include (a) a thin wall that is one-tenth to one-third as thick as the artery; (b) less elastic tissue; (c) a media that is predominantly smooth muscle; (d) venules that lack a media and smooth muscle; and (e) an adventitia composed of collagen and elastin that forms the major portion of large veins. Although veins have vasa vasorum, they do not completely penetrate the vein wall, which receives most of its nourishment by diffusion from the bloodstream.

C. Veins can be divided into a **superficial** and a **deep system.** The superficial system has relatively thick-walled and muscular veins. The superficial vein most commonly diseased is the greater saphenous vein. Deep veins are thinner and accompany arteries. Some deep veins are large and form sinusoids within skeletal muscle. The soleus sinusoids, for example, empty into the posterior tibial vein and are a common site for early deep venous thrombosis. Communicating veins perforate the muscle fascia to connect the deep and superficial systems, and, normally, blood flows from the superficial to the deep system. Normally, one-way valves in the communicating veins resist reflux of blood from the deep to the superficial system.

D.   Musculovenous pump mechanism. When leg muscles contract around intramuscular and surrounding veins, blood is propelled toward the heart. The major reservoirs of this pump are the soleus and gastrocnemius sinusoids. Pressures in excess of 200 mm Hg occur when these calf muscles contract. This mechanism may provide as much as 30% of the energy to circulate blood during strenuous exercise.

III.   Etiology

A.   Varicose veins. Varicose veins occur when the valve cusps of the saphenous system fail to close properly and the structural integrity of the vein weakens. The result is downward reflux of blood and chronic vein dilation. Many patients with varicose veins appear to have a familial predisposition. It usually is a progressive, functional failure of the valves rather than the absence of valves. In other cases, valvular incompetence is acquired after venous thrombosis has damaged the valves. Fibrous contracture of the valve cusps leads to valvular incompetency.

B.   Venous thrombosis. Several factors contribute to the etiology of **superficial** and **deep venous thrombosis.** Most physicians recall Virchow's triad: venous stasis, intimal injury, and blood hypercoagulability.

1.   Although **venous stasis** in an immobile extremity has been associated with deep venous thrombosis, the mechanism of clot formation is less clear. Evidence suggests that flow patterns through venous valves create a slow, disturbed movement in the deepest part of valve cusps. Stasis in venous valve cusps has been associated with local hypoxia that may lead to endothelial injury and thrombosis.

2.   Other studies confirm the role of focal **endothelial injury.** Characteristic endothelial injury most frequently occurs at the confluence of side branches with main veins. Leukocytes are the predominant cellular element to initially attach to sites of endothelial injury and are followed by attachment of fibrin and platelets. In most patients, the normal fibrinolytic system prevents extensive thrombosis; however, fibrinolytic activity may be reduced in patients with recurrent deep venous thrombosis.

3.   Understanding **hypercoagulability** leading to venous thrombosis has improved with description of the factor V Leiden mutation that results in activated protein C resistance (see Chap. 25). Other genetic abnormalities associated with thrombophilia are being investigated that will also increase our understanding of this process. Hypercoagulability results also from deficiency of protein C and its cofactor protein S (see Chap. 25). A hypercoagulable situation is present in the post-

Table 2.1. Postphlebitic syndrome

Years after deep venous thrombosis	Percentage of patients with lower leg swelling	Percentage of patients with leg ulcers
5	45	20
10	72	52
>10	91	79

Adapted from Dodd H, Crockett FB. The post-thrombotic syndrome and venous ulceration. In: Dodd H, Crockett FB, eds. *The pathology and surgery of the veins and lower limb*. Edinburgh: Churchill Livingstone, 1976.

operative patient and is particularly important as venous stasis and or endothelial injury may also exist to increase the risk of venous thrombosis. In addition, women using oral contraceptives have an increased incidence of thromboembolism thought to be associated with decreased levels of antithrombin III.

C. Pulmonary embolism from lower-extremity clots is the most common cause of **pulmonary thrombi.** In rare cases, the pulmonary thrombi may form *in situ*. Occasionally, they will embolize from other sites, such as the arms or pelvic venous plexus.

D. Postphlebitic syndrome eventually follows most severe cases of deep venous thrombosis of the leg (Table 2.1). Edema, subdermal scarring (lipodermatosclerosis), and chronic venous ulceration are related to chronic venous hypertension and are most commonly located on the medial and lateral aspects of the leg just above the ankle. Venous hypertension is the result of incompetent deep venous valves in the popliteal segment and incompetent communicating veins that perforate the fascia of the calf. The location of the chronic venous ulceration often matches the location of the incompetent perforating veins. Postphlebitic complications are time-related, often becoming manifest years after the initial phlebitis.

IV. Pathophysiology. The physiologic consequences of venous disease relate to two factors: valve insufficiency and vein obstruction (Fig. 2.1).

A. Normal physiology. Standing still, the normal individual will have a venous pressure at the ankle equal to a column of blood rising to the right heart. This pressure approximates arterial pressure. With calf exercise, the musculovenous pump moves blood from the superficial system through the communicating veins and propels it via the deep system toward the heart. Normally, baseline pressure in the foot veins **decreases** by approximately 70%.

B. Varicose veins. When patients with varicose veins exercise their legs, foot vein pressures drop only 30% to 40%. As much as one-fifth to one-fourth of the total femoral outflow is refluxed into the varicose saphenous system and back down the leg in "circus" motion. Patients with acquired varicosities after deep venous thrombosis also have incompetent deep or communicating veins. Consequently, these patients suffer from

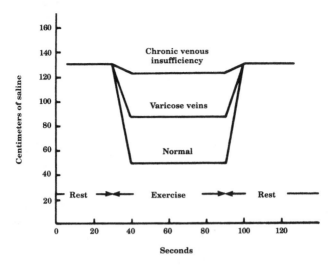

Figure 2.1.   Ambulatory venous pressures. Normally, leg exercises cause lower-extremity venous pressure to drop approximately 70% because the musculovenous pump propels blood toward the heart and competent venous valves prevent reflux. Varicose veins are associated with a 30% to 40% venous pressure reduction with exercise, because a portion of deep venous return is refluxed down the incompetent saphenous vein. Deep venous valve incompetence results in a minimal fall in venous pressure when chronic venous insufficiency (postphlebitic syndrome) is present.

ambulatory venous hypertension. With exercise, their foot vein pressures drop less than 20% of baseline values.

C.   Venous thrombosis results in obstruction of venous outflow. In the supine position, venous pressure in acute thrombosis is about twice normal at the foot. The extent of the thrombus and the adequacy of collateral channels determine severity of limb swelling. If the patient is standing, the venous pressure is only mildly elevated, but it changes minimally with exercise.

D.   Pulmonary embolism. The main physiologic consequence of acute pulmonary embolism is hypoxemia, which appears to be primarily the result of mechanical blockage of the pulmonary arteries. Some evidence indicates that humoral factors also may contribute to the hypoxic state. The chronic physiologic result can be pulmonary hypertension, chronic hypoxemia, and right heart failure.

E.   Postphlebitic syndrome. Two main physiologic abnormalities occur in patients experiencing postphlebitic syndrome: venous outflow obstruction and valve incompetence. The venous obstruction tends to be less important and to decrease with time, as the deep veins often recanalize over a 3- to 6-month period. Valve incompetence resulting from damage to the valve cusps by the thrombotic process is the most important physiologic abnormality. It results in a minimal drop in venous pressure with exercise in the postphlebitic limb, because the musculovenous pump functions poorly when the deep vein valves are incompetent. Chronic edema is the primary manifestation of the high venous pressures. Heavy (40 mm Hg) below-the-knee support hose can assist the limb with venous emptying and help to minimize elevated venous pressure.

V. Natural history. Although venous diseases can acutely threaten life, they frequently are chronic problems. It is important that both the patient and physician understand this chronicity. In most cases, the natural history can be altered so that the patient remains productive and comfortable.

A. Varicose veins. Varicose veins usually follow a chronic and benign course, and, for many, the main annoyance is their unsightly appearance. They become worse during pregnancy and with obesity. Occasionally, superficial thrombophlebitis occurs but is seldom complicated by deep venous extension or embolism. Hemorrhage is rare but can lead to bleeding, especially in elderly debilitated people. For most patients, varicose veins cause a tired, heavy feeling of the legs after prolonged standing.

B. Venous thrombosis. The most serious consequence of deep venous thrombosis is thromboembolism to the lung. Pulmonary embolism seldom occurs when the thrombus is located below the knees and is more common with iliofemoral thrombosis. The natural course for many patients with simple deep venous thrombosis, even without anticoagulation, is resolution of the acute tenderness and swelling. Over a period of several months, the deep veins usually recanalize. Without appropriate anticoagulation, about 30% of untreated patients have recurrent thrombosis or pulmonary embolism with a high mortality. Most limbs with acute venous thrombosis are normal in color or have a cyanotic appearance. In contrast, **phlegmasia alba dolens** (turgid, white, painful leg) is a swollen, white extremity in moderate pain. A more severe manifestation of major venous thrombosis is **phlegmasia cerulea dolens** (turgid, blue, painful leg), which can cause gangrene and has a poor prognosis.

C. Pulmonary embolism. Because many episodes of deep venous thrombosis probably go undetected, the incidence of thromboembolism to the lungs is difficult to ascertain. Estimates indicate a pulmonary embolism rate of about 25% in untreated deep venous thrombosis of the lower limb and 5% in adequately treated patients. Approximately one patient in 10 with a symptomatic pulmonary embolus dies within an hour. The remaining patients who are adequately treated with anticoagulants usually follow a course of complete resolution and return to good cardiopulmonary function within several weeks. The most important factor predicting a poor prognosis is preexisting heart disease. A minority of patients develop recurrent emboli and pulmonary hypertension with cor pulmonale (right heart failure).

D. Postphlebitic syndrome. To delineate the natural history of chronic venous insufficiency and postphlebitic syndrome, patients must be followed for a long period of time (5 to 10 years). Within 5 years, approximately 50% of patients with a previous deep venous thrombosis have developed chronic induration and stasis dermatitis at the ankle. Nearly 20% have had a venous ulcer. The natural history of postphlebitic syndrome can be altered, most commonly by compression therapy using leg support hose and less frequently with surgery in select patients.

SELECTED READING

Belcaro G, Christopoulos D, Nicolaides AN. Lower extremity venous hemodynamics. *Ann Vasc Surg* 1991;5:305–310.

Gloviczki P, Yao JST, eds. *Handbook of venous disorders. Guidelines of the American Venous Forum.* London: Chapman & Hall Medical, 1996.

Moneta GL, Dorfman GS. Acute and chronic venous disorders. In: Standness DE Jr, van Breda A, eds. *Vascular diseases: surgical and interventional therapy.* New York: Churchill Livingstone, 1994.

Nicolaides AN, Hussein MK, Szendro G, et al. The relation of venous ulceration with ambulatory venous pressure measurements. *J Vasc Surg* 1993;17:414–419.

Padberg FT Jr, Hobson RW. Impact of superficial venous reflux in chronic venous insufficiency. In: Yao JST, Pearce WH, eds. *Practical vascular surgery.* Stamford: Appleton and Lange, 1999:491–505.

Initial Patient Evaluation

The initial patient interview and physical examination provide information that directs subsequent diagnostic tests and treatment. Noninvasive vascular testing and imaging technology tend to divert attention from the importance of talking to and examining the patient. These diagnostic tests add valuable hemodynamic and anatomic data to the patient evaluation but **do not replace the need for a careful history and physical examination as the first step in optimum patient care.**

The initial history and physical examination serve several purposes. First, they enable the clinician to establish a **clinical impression** or preliminary diagnosis. Vascular diseases result in physical changes that are apparent by inspection, palpation, and auscultation. Interviewing and examining the patient often provide enough information for an accurate clinical impression. Additional diagnostic tests can then be selected to confirm and further define clinical impressions.

Second, the history and physical exam allow the clinician to determine the **urgency for treatment.** Although some arterial and venous problems require emergency care, the majority require elective evaluation and treatment. This important distinction must be made on the basis of patient history and physical examination.

Third, the initial clinical encounter provides an opportunity to assess the **physiologic age** and **comorbidities** of the patient. These factors impact the risk of intervention and the likelihood of a good recovery. Experienced clinicians never underestimate the value of the "eye ball test" as they perform a review of organ systems and consider the most appropriate treatment plan for the patient. An astute clinician also will keep in mind the possibility that the vascular patient may harbor an occult nonvascular disease such as gastrointestinal or pulmonary malignancy.

Finally, the initial interview defines a rapport or **relationship** between the patient and physician through which the physician hopes to gain the trust, to reassure the patient, and to obtain insight into the patient's socioeconomic situation. All subsequent interactions are influenced by the rapport developed at the initial evaluation.

This section outlines the basic techniques of the initial vascular examination. The equipment needed is simple: a stethoscope, blood pressure cuff, tape measure, and funduscope. A portable Doppler unit also is helpful and allows measurement of arterial pressures and evaluation of arterial and venous sounds. With this modest amount of equipment, the clinician can make an accurate diagnosis at the bedside of most patients. The examinations of the arterial and venous systems are discussed individually, although some patients will have combined arterial and venous problems. The discussion is further subdivided into body regions, since the patient's symptoms usually are localized to one area of the body.

Examination of the Arterial System

I. General examination. Atherosclerotic arterial disease often is diffuse. Therefore, the initial patient evaluation, regardless of the complaint, should include the entire arterial system in order to identify signs of other previously undiagnosed atherosclerotic disease. This comprehensive exam provides an impression of the patient's general cardiovascular condition, especially the cardiac status. Such an evaluation should include the following:

A. Checking of heart rate and rhythm.

B. Checking of bilateral arm blood pressures.

C. Neck auscultation for carotid bruits.

D. Cardiac auscultation for arrhythmias, gallops, and murmurs.

E. Abdominal palpation for an aortic aneurysm.

F. Abdominal auscultation for bruits.

G. Palpations of peripheral pulses.

H. Auscultation of the femoral region for bruits.

I. Inspection of the legs and feet for ulcers, gangrene, and microembolic phenomena.

II. Head and neck. This includes, most commonly, carotid bruits, transient neurologic attacks, and an enlarged carotid pulsation, suggesting an aneurysm or carotid body tumor.

A. Inspection. Normally, the carotid pulsation is not visible. However, it may become prominent at the base of the right neck in patients with long-standing hypertension. Such patients often are referred with the clinical diagnosis of carotid aneurysm, when in fact they have a tortuous carotid artery. Carotid artery aneurysms generally occur near the carotid bifurcation and consequently are located at the middle or upper anterior neck area. Carotid body tumors also originate at the carotid bifurcation. Unless an aneurysm or tumor is fairly large, it may not be visible on simple inspection of the neck.

If the patient complains of transient monocular blindness (amaurosis fugax), funduscopic exam may reveal bright, reflective spots in the retinal arteries. These arterial defects, called **Hollenhorst plaques,** represent cholesterol emboli from atherosclerotic disease of the carotid or innominate arteries.

B. Palpation. The common carotid pulse is palpable low in the neck between the midline trachea and the anterior border of the sternocleidomastoid muscle. It is difficult to distinguish separate internal and external carotid pulses in the mid-neck, where the common carotid artery bifurcates. The internal carotid artery may be occluded and the carotid pulse normal, as long as the external carotid artery remains patent. A strong temporal artery pulse anterior to the ear usually indicates a patent common and external carotid artery. Palpation often cannot distinguish a carotid aneurysm or carotid body tumor from benign conditions such as an enlarged lymph node or tortuous artery.

This differentiation requires ultrasonography, computed tomography (CT), or magnetic resonance imaging (MRI).

The vertebral artery is not readily accessible to palpation since it lies deep at the posterior base of the neck and is surrounded by cervical bone for most of its course. Pulsatile masses at the base of the neck or in the supraclavicular fossa generally originate from the thyrocervical trunk or subclavian artery.

C.   Auscultation. Normally, the stethoscope can detect heart sounds over the carotid artery. Pulsatile cervical bruits are an abnormal physical finding and may originate from carotid stenosis or from lesions of the aortic valve or arch vessels. A bruit from a carotid stenosis is usually loudest at the midneck over the carotid bifurcation. Transmitted bruits tend to be loudest over the upper chest and at the base of the neck. A duplex ultrasound may help localize the source of the bruit.

The significance of a cervical bruit depends on the presence of associated cerebrovascular symptoms and the results of diagnostic tests. The severity of the stenosis cannot be determined by the loudness of the bruit, as a tight carotid stenosis may have low flow and a faint bruit. Approximately one-half of patients with asymptomatic carotid bruits will have carotid stenoses of 30% or more, and one-fourth will have stenoses of greater than 75%. Noninvasive vascular testing is standard practice in determining the presence and hemodynamic significance of carotid artery stenoses. Although not routine, arteriograms are indicated when duplex ultrasound does not clearly delineate a carotid stenosis, or when the patient's symptoms are suspected to originate from the brachiocephalic or intracranial arteries.

III.   Upper extremity. The most common symptoms suggesting upper-extremity arterial insufficiency are pain, coldness, and exertional muscle fatigue.

A.   Acute arterial ischemia is characterized by the sudden onset of pain, pallor, paresthesias, and finally paralysis. The etiology usually is embolic, although occasionally the problem is thrombosis of a subclavian-axillary aneurysm or stenosis.

B.   Chronic exertional muscle fatigue or arm claudication suggests a **severe occlusive lesion** of a more proximal upper-extremity artery, such as a left subclavian occlusion. Patients with thoracic outlet syndrome also may complain of arm pain or numbness with activity. These symptoms generally are initiated by elevation or hyperabduction of the arm and are more the result of brachial plexus nerve compression than of arterial occlusion. However, thoracic outlet syndrome may be associated with acute arterial ischemia from thrombosis of or embolization from the subclavian artery.

C.   Intermittent hand coldness, pain, and numbness, especially associated with cold exposure, suggest **small vessel vasospasm or Raynaud's syndrome.** The etiology may be idiopathic (Raynaud's disease) or associated with other systemic collagen vascular diseases or prior frostbite (Raynaud's phenomenon).

D.   Physical examination

1.   Inspection. Inspection of the upper extremity provides a considerable amount of information about arterial perfusion. Pink fingertips with a capillary refill time of less than

3 seconds are a reliable sign of adequate perfusion. In contrast, the acutely ischemic upper extremity is pallid, and its motor function may be diminished. The main change in appearance of the extremity with chronic arterial ischemia is muscle atrophy, especially in the forearm and proximal hand. Recurrent microemboli or severe small-vessel disease may be recognized by fingertip lesions, such as painful mottled areas, skin ulcerations, or gangrene. **Raynaud's phenomenon** is associated with a triphasic color change that the fingers undergo after cold exposure or emotional stress. The fingers appear pallid (white), then cyanotic (blue), and finally hyperemic (red) as circulation is restored.

2. Palpation. Normally, the upper-extremity arterial pulse can be palpated at three locations: the upper medial arm just distal to the axilla and in the groove between the biceps and triceps muscles (axillary and proximal brachial); the antecubital fossa just medial to the biceps tendon (brachial); and the wrist over the distal radius (radial) or distal ulna (ulnar).

Skin temperature also can be assessed by palpation, especially using the more sensitive back of the examining hand or fingers. The level of skin temperature demarcation in the acutely ischemic arm is just distal to the level of occlusion. For example, if the extremity is cold to the midforearm, the occlusion is likely in the brachial artery at the elbow.

Aneurysms of the upper-extremity arteries generally are detectable if they occur in regions where the pulse normally is accessible to palpation. Large subclavian aneurysms may be palpable in the supraclavicular fossa. Axillary aneurysms may be detected high in the axilla. However, small aneurysms in these locations may be missed by palpation.

3. Auscultation. Auscultation of upper-extremity arteries should include measurement of bilateral brachial blood pressures and examination of the supraclavicular fossa for bruits. A difference of more than 10 mm Hg between arm blood pressures indicates a hemodynamically significant innominate, subclavian, axillary, or proximal brachial stenosis on the side with the lower blood pressure. Because collateral blood flow to the arm is extensive, a proximal subclavian stenosis may be asymptomatic.

When pulses are not palpable, the Doppler unit can be used to assess arterial signals and measure arm and forearm blood pressures. If the patient has symptoms suggesting arm claudication, the arm should be exercised for 2 to 5 minutes and the brachial pressures rechecked. Brachial pressures should fall if significant arterial occlusive disease exists. Digital perfusion in patients with vasospastic symptoms can be assessed by digital plethysmography.

IV. Abdomen. The retroperitoneal position of the abdominal aorta and its branches limits the amount of information obtained by physical examination. However, certain abnormalities can be recognized by inspection, palpation, and auscultation of the major abdominal arteries. In most cases, the abdominal vascular anatomy must be defined by further tests such as ultrasonography, CT scans, MRI scanning, and contrast arteriography.

A.   Symptoms. Certain clinical syndromes suggest both the presence and location of significant abdominal arterial disease. The most common symptom patterns include the following:

1.   Bilateral leg claudication and impotence (chronic aorto-iliac occlusive disease).

2.   Mottled, painful "blue toe" syndrome and abdominal bruits (atheroembolism from ulcerated aortoiliac atherosclerosis).

3.   Sudden, severe bilateral leg pain, coldness, paresthesias, and paralysis (acute distal aortic occlusion).

4.   Severe abdominal pain following meals (chronic mesenteric arterial disease).

5.   Sudden, severe general abdominal pain with minimal abnormal physical findings (acute mesenteric arterial occlusion).

6.   Acute progressive back pain and pulsatile abdominal mass (aortic aneurysm rupture).

7.   Severe hypertension in a child or young adult (renovascular stenosis).

Later chapters discuss the details of these clinical syndromes.

B.   Physical examination

1.   Inspection of the abdomen is the most limited part of the examination of the abdominal aorta and its branches. The normal aortic pulsation usually is not visible. However, a large abdominal aortic aneurysm may be seen pulsating against the anterior abdominal wall, especially in thin patients.

2.   Palpation remains the simplest technique of detecting an abdominal aortic aneurysm and should be a part of the routine physical examination of any adult over 40 years of age. Most aneurysms are asymptomatic and are recognized incidentally by palpation of the abdomen. In addition, palpation for diminished or absent femoral pulses is the quickest way to confirm a clinical history suggesting aortoiliac occlusive disease.

Certain anatomic features of the aorta should be remembered when one palpates the abdomen. The aorta bifurcates at about the level of the umbilicus, and unless the patient is obese, the aortic pulse is palpable, especially if the abdominal wall is relaxed. Having the patient bend his or her knees, flexing the hips, and relaxing the abdominal musculature can facilitate the exam. The normal aorta is approximately the width of the patient's thumb.

An aortic aneurysm should be suspected when the aortic pulse feels expansile and larger than 4 to 5 cm. Elderly patients with kyphoscoliosis of the lumbar spine may have a tortuous, anteriorly displaced aorta that is easily mistaken for an aneurysm. An incorrect diagnosis of aortic aneurysm also may be made if one palpates too low in the abdomen and mistakes the outer limits of the iliac arteries for an aortic aneurysm.

In addition to size, other characteristics of an aneurysm may be identified by palpation. If the expansile mass extends to the xiphoid or costal margins, a suprarenal or thoracoabdominal aneurysm should be suspected. Aneurysm tenderness or referred pain with palpation are important signs which may indicate pending rupture, perianeurysmal leak, or the presence of an inflammatory aneurysm. In general, iliac aneurysms cannot be palpated unless they are large. Occasionally an internal iliac artery aneurysm is palpable by digital rectal examination.

3. Auscultation with a stethoscope commonly reveals bruits when significant occlusive disease of the aorta or its branches is present. Aortoiliac disease causes bruits in the middle and lower abdomen and the femoral region. Bruits secondary to isolated renal artery stenosis are faint and localized in the upper abdominal quadrants lateral to the midline. Mesenteric artery occlusive disease may be associated with epigastric bruits.

Asymptomatic abdominal bruits are an occasional incidental finding on abdominal examination of young adults, especially thin women. If the patient is not hypertensive and does not have intestinal angina or leg claudication, these bruits may be considered benign. The bruits may originate from impingement of the diaphragmatic crura on the celiac axis.

V. Lower extremities. Physical examination is especially helpful in the initial evaluation of arterial problems of the lower extremities. Chronic and acute arterial insufficiency produce changes that can be recognized by inspection, palpation, and auscultation. The physical examination is more revealing in the lower extremities than in any other body region where arterial problems occur.

A. Symptoms. Lower-extremity arterial problems present in one of three clinical patterns. The most common is chronic intermittent **claudication.** The natural history of this arterial disease is important to consider when talking to patients and their families. With risk factor modification and exercise programs, claudication is stable or improved in one-half of patients. Only 25% ever require surgery or have tissue loss, and fewer than 5% require an amputation. If the disease process does progress, **threatened limb loss** may develop. The manifestations of severe ischemia are rest pain, nonhealing ulcers, or gangrene (tissue loss). The third general presentation is **acute arterial ischemia.** Its classic findings are referred to as the five P's: pain, pallor, paresthesias, paralysis, and pulselessness. When a patient presents with any of these clinical scenarios, examination of the leg is the best method to assess the severity of ischemia and to determine the urgent need for further tests and treatment.

B. Physical examination

1. Inspection of the leg and foot will reveal most of the important signs of chronic or acute arterial insufficiency. Early chronic arterial disease may cause no change in the appearance of the lower extremity. Eventually, muscle atrophy may become apparent. Hair loss on the foot also has been associated with poor peripheral circulation but is not a consistent sign. A reliable indicator of chronic severe ischemia is elevation pallor and dependent rubor of the forefoot. Finally, tissue necrosis may occur and nonhealing ulcers or gangrene will appear.

Likewise, acute arterial insufficiency will produce definite changes in the appearance of the extremity. The color change of marked pallor is unmistakable in such patients and with time, cyanosis or skin mottling may become predominant. In addition, muscle weakness or paralysis, especially of the foot dorsiflexors (anterior compartment), becomes obvious. After approximately 24 hours of severe ischemia, the leg usually is swollen and the skin may blister. Black gangrene of the skin is the final change in appearance but may not occur for several days.

2.   Palpation. Four lower-extremity pulses normally are palpable. The common femoral pulse is best felt just below the inguinal ligament and approximately one and one-half, to two fingerbreadths lateral to the public tubercle. In obese patients, external rotation of the hip may facilitate palpation of the artery. The popliteal pulse is more difficult to palpate as it lies deep in the popliteal space. With the patient supine and the knee slightly flexed, the examiner should hook the fingertips of both hands around the medial and lateral knee tendons and press the fingertips into the popliteal space. The popliteal pulse usually lies just lateral of midline. The dorsalis pedis artery is a terminal branch of the anterior tibial artery and is normally is found in the mid-dorsum of the foot, between the first and second metatarsals. The posterior tibial artery is found in the groove behind the medial malleolus of the tibia. The peroneal pulse is not usually palpable.

Grading of pulses is subjective but a simple distinction is either their presence or absence. Some physicians use a graded system: 0, absent; 1+, barely palpable; 2+, palpable but diminished; 3+, normal; 4+, prominent, suggesting local aneurysm.

Palpation also is helpful in the assessment of the acutely ischemic leg. Extremity skin coldness and the level of temperature demarcation can be detected by palpation of the ischemic limb with the back of the examiner's hand and fingers, which are most sensitive to temperature differences. Acute ischemia also may be associated with tenderness and tenseness of the ischemic calf muscles, especially the anterior compartment. In addition, acute arterial insufficiency may cause sensory nerve damage, detectable by simple pinprick sensory examination.

3.   Auscultation of lower-extremity arteries is most useful in the femoral area, where bruits indicate local femoral artery disease or more proximal aortoiliac disease with bruits transmitted to the groin. If the femoral bruits is questionable, walking the patient for 25 to 50 quick steps at the bedside often will increase lower-extremity blood flow enough to make the bruit louder and easier to auscultate. Auscultation also is important when an arteriovenous fistula is suspected, which generally has a characteristic continuous to-and-fro bruit.

Examination of the Venous System

Venous disease usually is localized to one anatomic area, unlike arterial disease, which is more diffuse. The lower extremities are most commonly involved, although venous problems can impair function of the upper extremities.

I. Upper extremities. Acute or chronic obstruction of the axillary or subclavian veins constitutes a serious venous disorder of the arms. The chief complaint in most cases is arm swelling. Diffuse aching pain frequently accompanies the swelling and is worse with prolonged use or dependency of the arm.

Acute axillary or subclavian vein thrombosis, also called "Paget–Schroetter syndrome," occurs in one of two clinical settings. The first is chronic subclavian vein catheterization, and the second is thoracic outlet syndrome. In thoracic outlet syndrome, extrinsic compression causes venous stasis and endothelial injury with resultant thrombosis. The term **effort thrombosis** is used if acute thrombosis follows vigorous upper extremity exercise.

Chronic arm swelling may be the result of venous or lymphatic obstruction. Venous obstruction may follow acute thrombosis or result from partial extrinsic compression of the subclavian vein by a thoracic outlet syndrome. Lymphatic obstruction generally is associated with an operation (e.g., mastectomy), infection, or irradiation that involved the axillary lymph nodes.

A. Inspection. Subclavian vein thrombosis causes swelling of the entire arm and hand. Acutely, the arm may appear bluish or cyanotic. Rarely, extensive subclavian-axillary venous thrombosis results in venous gangrene. These patients often have underlying malignant disease or a coagulopathy such as heparin-induced thrombocytopenia and thrombosis. Characteristically, they have palpable arterial pulses despite cutaneous gangrene. Around the shoulder region, numerous super-ficial venous collateral channels may become visible, especially compared to the opposite normal arm.

The upper extremity generally does not develop the stasis dermatitis appearance that accompanies postphlebitic syndrome of the legs. However, upper-extremity chronic venous swelling, hyperpigmentation, and ulceration may occur after construction of an arteriovenous fistula for hemodialysis. Distinguishing between venous obstruction and lymphedema may be difficult, although the clinical setting suggests the most likely etiology.

B. Palpation offers limited information about venous problems of the arm. The axillary and subclavian veins are not palpable because they lie deep to the clavicle. In contrast, phlebitis of a superficial arm vein classically is recognized by a warm, tender cord with erythema.

C. Auscultation. Normally, venous sounds are not audible with a stethoscope. If arm swelling follows a penetrating injury or operation of the arm, listening over the scar may reveal a bruit caused by an arteriovenous fistula. A continuous-wave Doppler unit can be used to listen to deep venous sounds.

II.   Lower extremities. The most common venous problems of the legs are varicose veins, deep venous thrombosis, and post-phlebitic syndrome. Although these conditions may be asymptomatic, they usually are associated with some degree of leg pain and swelling. Physical examination is the primary method of evaluating varicose veins and postphlebitic syndrome, since these conditions cause visible changes on the surface of the leg. In contrast, the patient history and physical examination often are unreliable in making an accurate diagnosis of deep venous thrombosis. In fact, only about 50% of patients who are initially thought to have deep venous thrombosis by history and physical examination will have an abnormal duplex ultrasound or venogram. This latter finding should not be surprising, since acute leg pain and tenderness may have many etiologies. Gastrocnemius musculotendinous rupture is one condition that may mimic acute venous thrombosis.

It is important to keep in mind that the severity of symptoms associated with varicose veins does not necessarily correlate with their appearance. In addition, acute deep venous thrombosis may not cause typical calf pain and tenderness. The presenting sign may be nothing more than leg swelling. Rarely, the patient's first sign of lower-extremity deep venous thrombosis may be a pulmonary embolus. Finally, postphlebitic syndrome usually does not present until months or years after the acute thrombotic episode. Some patients with postphlebitic problems may not have a history of previous deep venous thrombosis. Acute venous thrombosis may have been silent or misdiagnosed.

A.   Inspection should be done with both legs completely exposed from the groin to the feet. Important findings may be recognized by comparing the abnormal and normal extremities. When possible, the patient should stand so that superficial veins fill. We prefer that the patient stand on a short stool while the examiner sits on a chair or stool. If good overhead lighting or sunlight is not available for illumination of all aspects of the leg, an adjustable bedside examining lamp is useful. The entire leg should be examined as the patient turns 360 degrees.

1.   Varicosities most commonly involve the greater saphenous vein on the medial side of the leg. Varicose branches of the greater saphenous often course around the upper calf to appear on the posteromedial aspect of the midcalf. Lesser saphenous varicosities appear on the posterior calf from the knee to the ankle. The location of the varicosities may suggest the etiology. For example, a dilated greater saphenous vein from the groin to the ankle is typical of familial valvular incompetence. In contrast, varicosities that begin at or below the knee may be secondary to incompetent communicating veins from the deep venous system.

A rare congenital pattern of varicosities is present in **Klippel–Trenaunay syndrome.** This syndrome includes the triad of capillary malformations (port-wine stains), atypical varicosities, and bony or soft tissue hypertrophy. Importantly, these patients may have persistent lateral embryologic veins and an absent or abnormal deep venous system.

In most cases of simple varicosities, two bedside tests help identify whether the greater saphenous valves or the communicating (perforating) veins are competent.

   a.   Trendelenburg's test (modified). In the modified Trendelenburg's test, the patient lies supine, and the leg is elevated to empty all varicosities. A soft rubber tourniquet is applied to the leg just below the knee, and the patient stands. If the lower leg varicosities fill slowly with the tourniquet in place but then dilate suddenly when the tourniquet is released, the greater saphenous valves are incompetent. In contrast, incompetent deep and communicating veins will cause immediate filling of the varicosities despite the tourniquet.

   b.   Perthes' test checks the patency and competency of the communicating and deep venous system. While the patient stands, a soft tourniquet is applied around the upper calf. The patient repeatedly plantar flexes the foot, contracting the gastrocnemius and soleus muscles (musculovenous pump). Normally, this exercise causes flow from the superficial to the deep venous system and results in partial emptying of the surface veins. However, if the communicating and deep veins have incompetent valves, the varicosities remain distended.

2.   Acute deep venous thrombosis. Most limbs with acute venous thrombosis are normal in color or have a cyanotic appearance. Extremity swelling is the most common sign and usually is limited to the lower leg, with tibial or popliteal venous thrombosis. **Phlegmasia alba dolens** (turgid, white, painful leg) is a swollen, white extremity in moderate pain and a sign of more progressive thrombosis. If the iliac vein is obstructed, swelling may extend to the groin. The amount of swelling should be documented by measurements of calf and thigh diameters of both legs. Serial examinations will be more accurate if these measurements are made at a given distance above and below a bony landmark such as the tibial tuberosity. With severe iliofemoral thrombosis, **phlegmasia cerulea dolens** may be observed, that is, a severely edematous, cyanotic, and painful leg that progresses to cutaneous gangrene.

   Inspection also helps with the differential diagnosis of acute leg pain and swelling. Superficial thrombophlebitis often is evidenced by a localized erythematous streak along the course of the involved vein, usually the greater saphenous vein. A break in the skin with surrounding erythema and induration suggests cellulitis. A localized ecchymosis over the thigh or calf may indicate that the leg pain is caused by a muscle contusion or hematoma. Diffuse, nonpainful leg edema with a thick "pigskin" appearance (peau d'orange) is typical of lymphedema.

3.   Postphlebitic syndrome is associated with rather specific changes in the appearance of the lower leg. Because of incompetent deep venous valves and venous hypertension, the lower leg becomes chronically swollen, mainly at the ankle. With progression, irregular thickened areas of brownish skin pigmentation (lipodermatosclerosis) appear around the ankle. Stasis dermatitis may be complicated by skin ulceration classically on the medial ankle at the site of the lowest perforating vein (Crocket I). Venous ulcers are usually shallow, with healthy-appearing granulation tissue that bleeds with manipulation.

4. Chronic diffuse lower-limb swelling without post-phlebitic stasis dermatitis may be caused either by iliac vein obstruction, deep valvular incompetence, or lymphedema. Compression of the left common iliac vein by the right common iliac artery (May–Thurner syndrome) can eventually result in venous intimal fibroplasia, partial obstruction, and progressive left leg swelling. In contrast, primary or secondary lymphedema can result in chronic leg swelling that typically has a diffuse pitting "pigskin" appearance and does not resolve with bedrest at night. Venous edema, on the other hand, may resolve with bedrest and worsen with dependency.

B. Palpation provides useful information in the evaluation of varicose veins and acute venous thrombosis but does not add much to initial evaluation of the postphlebitic limb.

1. If the varicosities on the medial leg are palpated, sites of communicating veins often can be recognized by indentations where these veins perforate the fascia of the muscle. It is important to identify these perforating sites when an operation to ligate the incompetent communicating veins is planned (e.g., subfascial endoscopic perforator surgery). Duplex ultrasound can also be used to locate and mark these perforating sites.

2. Deep venous thrombosis may cause tenderness of calf or thigh muscles. Such tenderness is not specific for thrombosis, since muscle strain, contusion, or hematoma may cause similar tenderness. Forceful dorsiflexion of the foot contracts the gastrocnemius muscle and may cause pain when deep vein thrombophlebitis is present (Homans' sign). Again, this sign is suggestive of but not diagnostic for deep venous thrombophlebitis. In contrast, tenderness, heat, and induration over a superficial vein are the primary diagnostic criteria for superficial thrombophlebitis.

3. Palpation may help determine the possible cause of leg swelling associated with venous insufficiency. Occasionally, chronic venous obstruction is secondary to extrinsic compression by a pelvic, femoral, or popliteal mass, and so these regions should also be examined for aneurysms or tumors.

C. Auscultation with a stethoscope does not provide much information about superficial or deep venous flow. However, the Doppler unit is helpful in the examination of lower-extremity veins (see Chap. 5). It allows assessment of both deep vein patency and incompetency of valves. If leg edema or varicosities occur after a penetrating leg injury, the stethoscope or Doppler unit may detect a bruit from an arteriovenous fistula.

Noninvasive Vascular Testing

This chapter summarizes the basic principles of selecting, performing, and interpreting noninvasive hemodynamic studies for both arterial and venous problems. We emphasize that these noninvasive tests do not replace but **supplement** a thorough patient history and physical examination. In some situations, the results of noninvasive studies help the clinician determine the need for an invasive study such as an arteriogram or venogram. In addition, noninvasive tests provide a physiologic baseline before therapy and an objective assessment of outcome after treatment.

The development of clinical vascular laboratories lagged behind the introduction of angiography, synthetic grafts, and modern operative techniques for the treatment of peripheral vascular disease. However, in the past 30 years, noninvasive vascular equipment has become common in medical centers, community hospitals, and office practices. Although experienced clinicians can adequately treat many vascular problems without noninvasive testing, the vascular laboratory provides useful physiologic information that previously was not available from history, physical examination, or angiograms. Of course, such noninvasive testing must be selected carefully to avoid unnecessary studies that add considerably to the cost of patient care. Health care reform is focusing more attention on the use and abuse of the noninvasive vascular laboratory.

I. The vascular laboratory. The laboratory should be in a quiet area and located for convenient use by both inpatients and outpatients. Initial equipment costs will vary and may range from $30,000 to $500,000, depending on the installation of sophisticated duplex ultrasonography. A medical sonographer or registered vascular technologist (RVT) usually performs the tests, which are then reviewed by a physician.

In some situations, a sophisticated vascular laboratory is not feasible. Nonetheless, physicians can use a pocket or portable continuous-wave Doppler unit to auscultate arterial and venous flow and measure extremity pressures. We recommend that physicians, nurses, and other paramedical personnel who care for vascular patients learn to use a portable Doppler unit for arterial monitoring.

II. Instrumentation. Instruments for noninvasive vascular testing should be (a) reliable and reproducible, (b) capable of intrinsic standardization, (c) suitable for use by paramedical personnel, (d) suitable for measurements during and after exercise, and (e) adaptable to current recording devices. Our experience indicates that the following list of equipment is sufficient for most arterial and venous problems:

1. Continous-wave bidirectional Doppler system: 9 MHz for arteries, 5 MHz for veins.
2. Plethysmography (optional for various arterial and venous examinations).

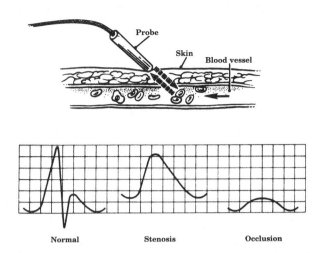

Figure 5.1. Doppler arterial examination. The Doppler probe is coupled to the skin with acoustic gel and angled toward the direction of arterial flow. The normal Doppler arterial signal is triphasic. Stenosis and occlusion cause diminished monophasic signals.

3. A direct method of bruit analysis and imaging (e.g., duplex ultrasonography).
4. Treadmill: speeds of 1.5 and 2.5 mph, 10% to 12.5% grade.
5. Transcutaneous oximetry (optional for documenting cutaneous perfusion).

A. Doppler ultrasound. Low-intensity ultrasound (range, 1 to 10 MHz) has been applied to monitoring arterial and venous blood flow since its introduction over 35 years ago. Simply stated, the Doppler effect shows that flow velocity is proportional to the frequency shift in sound waves that are transmitted toward moving blood cells and reflected back to the Doppler-receiving crystal (Fig. 5.1). A hand-held Doppler probe is placed over the course of the blood vessel being examined and is coupled to the skin with an acoustic gel. Skin lubricants other than an acoustic gel do not have the proper electrolyte content and can damage the probe crystal. Transmitted sound waves strike moving blood cells and are reflected back to the Doppler probe. An amplifier filters the sound and gives a flow signal or tracing that is proportional to the blood flow velocity.

Two types of Doppler instruments are used: **continuous-wave** and **pulsed.** In practice, the continuous-wave Doppler unit is most commonly used for arterial and venous studies. The most useful Doppler instrument for examination of extremity vessels operates at 5 to 10 MHz. Some Doppler units are bidirectional—that is, they can detect direction as well as velocity of flow. Pulsed ultrasound was developed to provide both an image and a velocity profile of an arterial lesion. Unlike the continuous-wave

Doppler, the pulsed Doppler instrument emits bursts of ultra-sound waves. Between each burst, the crystal receives reflected signals. This feature allows the pulsed Doppler to sample a discrete portion of flow within a vessel being examined. Such discrete sampling provides accurate measurement of frequency (velocity) of flow through a focal stenotic lesion. The velocity patterns correlate with the degree of stenosis. Although continuous-wave Dopplers can also analyze velocity patterns, continuous-wave flow detectors may collect other signals from adjacent arteries or veins, making signal interpretation more difficult.

B. Plethysmography. One of the earliest means of measuring extremity blood flow was plethysmography, the measurement of volume change of an organ or body region. This principle has been applied in several forms: volume displacement (air or water), strain gauge (mercury-in-Silastic), mechanical, photoelectric, impedance, and ocular plethysmographs.

1. The pulse volume recorder (PVR), developed by Raines and Darling at the Massachusetts General Hospital, is a segmental plethysmograph that has been used to monitor lower-extremity pulsatility as an indirect reflection of blood flow. The PVR uses air-filled cuffs placed at different levels around the extremity. Momentary volume changes of the limb are detected by pressure changes in the cuffs and recorded on a strip recorder as arterial pulse contours (see Fig. 5.5 on page 36). The PVR contour closely corresponds to direct intra-arterial pressure waveform recordings at that level. The PVR tracings supplement Doppler segmental limb pressures and allow assessment of perfusion of the forefoot and digits where the Doppler unit cannot easily measure pressures.

2. Ocular pneumoplethysmography (OPG) records changes in eye volume caused by pulsatile flow in the ophthalmic artery. This vessel is the first branch of the internal carotid artery, and changes in eyeball pressure are related to significant occlusive disease of the carotid artery.

The OPG-Gee provides direct measurement of the systolic ophthalmic artery pressure, a reflection of internal carotid pressure. An air-filled cup system is applied to the anesthetized sclera of both eyes. A vacuum draws the sclera into the cup, causing intraocular pressure to rise. When the rise in intraocular pressure exceeds systolic ophthalmic artery pressure, the eye pulse trace disappears. As the vacuum is released, pulsations return and an eyeball pressure is recorded. This pressure correlates directly with internal carotid pressure on that side.

3. Impedance plethysmography (IPG) measures volume changes in a limb by changes in electrical resistance. Developed by Wheeler and colleagues, IPG was once a common test for deep venous obstruction due to acute or chronic thrombosis. The rationale for the IPG is based on Ohm's law (voltage = current × resistance). Blood is a good conductor of electricity. Resistance to passage of an electrical current is lower when more blood is present in the extremity. Since deep venous obstruction increases resistance to venous outflow, the IPG can detect deep vein obstruction, although it cannot always determine whether the decreased venous outflow is caused by deep venous thrombosis, peripheral vasoconstriction, congestive heart failure, hypotension, or pulmonary hypertension.

4.   Phleborheography (PRG) uses air-filled cuffs on the thigh, calf, and foot, plus a special thoracic cuff to record volume changes of the leg with respiration. A deep venous thrombus (DVT) attenuates or eliminates the respiratory waves distal to the occlusion, with normal waves seen proximally. With extensive DVT, the respiratory waves are absent at all levels. According to a study by Cranley et al., the PRG is highly accurate (95%) for detecting acute venous occlusion. A relative drawback is that the technique requires significant time to learn and interpret.

5.   Photoplethysmography (PPG) uses a sensor that shines light into the superficial skin layers and a photoelectric detector that measures reflected light. The intensity of reflected light correlates with venous congestion and, consequently, estimates venous limb pressure. A tracing is made at rest, during exercise, and through the recovery phase. The result is defined by the magnitude of the pressure drop during walking and the time required for the pressure to return to baseline. A normal recovery time is over 20 seconds. Recovery times below 20 seconds indicate venous reflux. Since the test is easy to perform and interpret, PPG provides a simple, objective means of assessing chronic venous insufficiency, especially in postphlebitic patients. Unlike the Doppler venous examination that identifies reflux at a given valve level, the PPG indicates the overall effect (recovery response) at the level studied.

C.   Duplex scanning combines the duel utility of real-time brightness-mode (B-mode) ultrasound imaging with a pulsed Doppler analysis of flow velocity. Blood vessels are identified by their B-mode images with prominent wall echoes separated by a dark, sonolucent lumen. Calcified plaques are recognized by bright intraluminal echoes and regions of posterior acoustic shadowing. The operator can place the pulsed Doppler sample in the center of the flow and adjust the Doppler angle to near 60 degrees, which provides the best return signal for spectral analysis and velocity measurements. The Doppler sample is placed near the center stream of the vessel to avoid detection of slower velocities and eddies close to the wall. These disturbances can cause false readings of stenosis in normal arteries.

The spectral analysis allows classification of the degree of stenosis. The parameters used for this classification are (a) spectral width during systole, (b) peak systolic velocity, and (c) diastolic velocity. A normal Doppler spectrum of the carotid artery (Fig. 5.2) consists of a relatively low systolic peak velocity (e.g., less than 125 cm/s in the internal carotid) and a narrow band of frequencies during systole, resulting in a clear region beneath the systolic peak (window). With minimal stenosis, spectral broadening occurs during the deceleration phase of systole. Further stenosis results in increased spectral broadening until the entire window beneath the systolic peak is filled, followed by an increase in peak systolic and diastolic velocities.

Although duplex scanning was applied originally to carotid bifurcation disease, additional applications include examination of lower-extremity arteries, intestinal arteries, veins, and

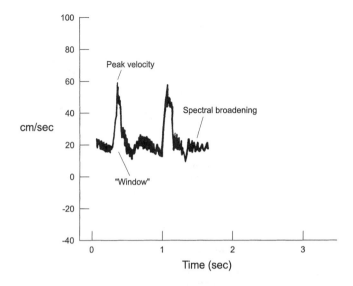

Figure 5.2.   Arterial spectrum analysis. The Doppler spectral analysis allows classification of the degree of stenosis. The most common parameters used for this classification are (a) spectral width (broadening) during systole, (b) peak systolic velocity (normal <120 cm/s), and (c) diastolic velocity.

renal arteries. Two disadvantages of this noninvasive technology are the high cost of the equipment and the extensive operator experience required to obtain good studies.

D.   Transcutaneous oximetry ($TcPO_2$) provides local measurement of skin oxygen tension and can reflect the adequacy of arterial and capillary perfusion. The principle of transcutaneous oxygen determination involves heat application (45°C) to the skin, which produces a localized hyperemia and oxygen excess. Since oxygen diffuses along a concentration gradient from the capillaries to the tissues, it can diffuse across the skin where it is electrochemically reduced and measured by a modified Clark platinum oxygen electrode. It is important to standardize vasodilation since, at skin temperatures above 43°C, the ratio of $TcPO_2$ to arterial PO_2 remains constant and is close to 1.

III.   Lower-extremity arterial occlusive disease. Patients evaluated for lower-extremity arterial occlusive disease fall into two broad groups after preliminary history and physical examination: patients with **intermittent claudication** (discomfort, tiring, or pain in lower-limb muscles with walking) or patients with **severe limb ischemia** (rest pain, nonhealing ulcers, and/or gangrene). Noninvasive vascular testing documents the severity of claudication and provides a baseline for follow-up. Such testing may also be used to confirm more severe ischemia and predict whether ischemic ulcers will heal without arterial revascularization.

A. Intermittent claudication. Patients with lower extremity claudication should undergo Doppler survey of ankle and pedal arterial signals and measurement of resting ankle-brachial pressure indices (ABIs). Some laboratories also record segmental pressures and plethysmographic wave forms (using PVRs). Any of these measurements may also be repeated after exercise on the treadmill.

1. Doppler survey. A normal arterial signal has two, and sometimes three, components (Fig. 5.1). The first part of this crisp, high-pitched sound represents the forward blood flow during systole. The second component is reversed and corresponds to flow in early diastole. As forward flow resumes, a third low-pitched sound may be heard.

When a severe proximal arterial stenosis or occlusion is present, the Doppler signal at rest becomes lower-pitched and monophasic (Fig. 5.1). In the case of a lesser stenosis, the resting Doppler signal may even sound normal. However, after exercise a less intense monophasic sound may be noted. This change in the Doppler sound indicates a stenosis that becomes hemodynamically significant only after exercise.

The initial Doppler survey should note the presence or absence and the quality (biphasic or monophasic) of the femoral, popliteal, posterior tibial, and dorsalis pedis arteries.

2. Segmental leg pressures. The concept that segmental leg pressures (thigh, calf, and ankle) can indicate the level and significance of arterial occlusive disease was introduced more than 35 years ago but was not widely applied to clinical practice until the last 25 years. The test is performed while the patient is at rest in the supine position. Appropriately sized pneumatic cuffs (thigh, 18 to 20 cm in width; calf and ankle, 12 cm in width) are placed as high on the thigh as possible, on the calf immediately below the knee, and on the ankle just above the medial malleolus. A standard blood pressure manometer is used to measure the pressures. Since it is difficult to auscultate ankle pressures with a stethoscope, a Doppler probe or plethysmograph is used. We prefer the Doppler probe and place it over the ankle artery that has the loudest signal (Fig. 5.3). Next, the thigh cuff is inflated until the Doppler signal disappears. As the cuff is slowly deflated, the thigh systolic pressure is recorded when the signal reappears. In a similar fashion, calf and ankle systolic pressures are recorded. All pressures are taken by auscultating the arterial signal **at the ankle level.**

Interpretation of segmental leg pressures is based on the following principles:

a. Normally, systolic ankle pressure should be equal to or greater than systolic arm pressure. In other words, the ankle-brachial pressure ratio should be 1.0 or greater. In limbs with one primary arterial occlusion, the index is usually 0.5 to 0.8. An anklearm ratio of less than 0.5 usually indicates multilevel occlusive disease.

b. A pressure gradient of more than 20 mm Hg between cuff levels strongly suggests a hemodynamically significant occlusive lesion in the intervening arterial segment. Figure 5.4 provides several examples of arterial occlusive disease at various anatomic levels. It must be remembered

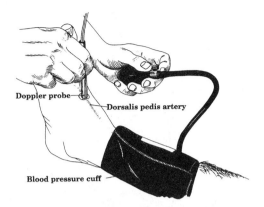

Figure 5.3. Measurement of ankle blood pressure with a standard blood pressure cuff and a hand-held continuous-wave Doppler unit. This ankle pressure can be compared to the brachial (arm) blood pressure to calculate the ankle-brachial index (ABI; normal = 1.0, claudication usually 0.5 to 0.9, rest pain or tissue necrosis usually less than 0.5).

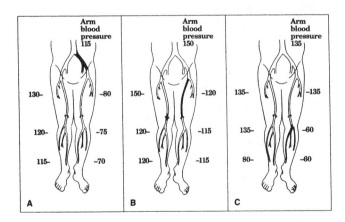

Figure 5.4. Segmental leg pressures. A: Segmental leg pressures in a normal right lower extremity and one with isolated iliac artery occlusion (left). B: Segmental leg pressures in distal, segmental occlusions of the right superficial femoral artery (SFA) compared to proximal occlusion of the left SFA. C: Segmental leg pressures in distal (right) tibial artery occlusions and tibial disease extending into the proximal left popliteal artery.

that the thigh pressure may be falsely elevated if the cuff width is too narrow.

   c. Segmental leg pressures can be misleading in the following situations:

1. Severely calcified vessels (e.g., in diabetics) may not be compressible, so leg pressures will be falsely elevated.
2. Collateral blood flow may be so well developed that a 20-mm gradient not present across a significant occlusive segment.
3. An extensive superficial femoral occlusion may give a thigh to arm ratio that is identical to that seen with an iliac occlusion. Of course, simple palpation for a femoral pulse should differentiate between these two situations. When the femoral pulse strength is equivocal, the hemodynamic significance of proximal aortoiliac arterial disease can be estimated. This can be accomplished by a common femoral artery Doppler blood flow velocity wave form or signal analysis.

   These limitations of segmental leg pressures emphasize that results must be combined with findings on physical exam for accurate location of the occlusive lesions.

   3. Pulse volume recordings supplement the segmental leg pressures and are taken using the same pressure cuffs. Characterized by a sharp upstroke (anacrotic slope), distinct pulse peak, and rapid decline (catacrotic slope), the normal PVR tracing becomes progressively flattened and prolonged with increasing stenosis (Fig. 5.5). Segmental leg PVR tracings normally show an augmentation from thigh to calf

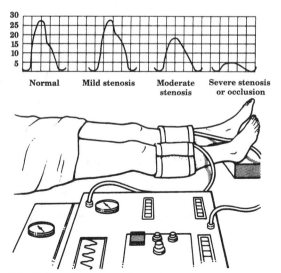

Figure 5.5. Pulse volume recordings. The normal pulse volume recording becomes progressively flattened and prolonged with increasing arterial stenosis.

caused by differences in cuff volume. Therefore, the calf PVR should have greater amplitude than that of the thigh. If it does not, a superficial femoral artery occlusive lesion should be suspected. The PVR also is helpful in evaluating the young patient whose claudication may be due to **popliteal artery entrapment** by the medial head of the gastrocnemius muscle. Such patients usually have normal ankle PVR tracings at rest. With active plantar flexion or passive dorsiflexion of the foot, the gastrocnemius contracts and compresses the popliteal artery, and the ankle PVR tracing flattens.

4.   Exercise testing. Leg exercise normally increases total limb blood flow without significant changes in systolic ankle pressures. However, when arterial occlusive disease is present, ankle pressures decrease after exercise. This decrease in pressure across arterial stenosis occurs for reasons related to basic principles of fluid hemodynamics (Table 1.1). First, increased flow (velocity) occurs across a stenosis resulting in turbulence and decreased pressure distal to the stenosis **(Bernoulli's principle).** Second, blood flow is diverted into smaller higher-resistance collateral beds of the leg muscles **(Poiseuille's law).** If exercise of the limb is not possible, a similar decrease in pressure can be demonstrated by the reactive hyperemia test: inflation of a high thigh cuff to 50 mm Hg above arm pressure for 5 minutes. However, we prefer the patient to walk on a treadmill at 2 mph on a 10% incline for 5 minutes, simulating the activity that causes claudication. At the same time, the cardiorespiratory reserve of the patient can be grossly observed.

In addition to the measurement of ankle pressures and PVRs after exercise, the recording of time of onset, location, and severity of claudication is important. This claudication profile objectively defines how much the claudication limits the patient. Treadmill examinations over time can detect disease progression and early anastomotic stenosis after operation. Exercise testing is also helpful if there is confusion about whether the patient's leg complaints are caused by arterial occlusive disease, a musculoskeletal hip or knee disorder, or a neurologic condition such as spinal stenosis.

Since patients with peripheral arterial disease often have significant heart disease, **continual electrocardiogram (ECG) monitoring** during treadmill exercise should be considered if the patient: (a) has suffered previous myocardial infarction, (b) has angina pectoris requiring nitrates, (c) presents with severe chronic obstructive lung disease, (d) exhibits signs of cardiac arrhythmia as seen on the arterial PVR during initial resting examination, (e) is taking antiarrhythmic medications, (f) has undergone previous cardiac surgery, (g) has a permanent pacemaker, or (h) has suffered a recent stroke or transient ischemic attacks (TIAs). Approximately 33% of our patients undergoing lower-extremity arterial testing will have one or more of these indications for ECG monitoring. When ECG monitoring is not available, treadmill exercise should not be performed on patients with (a) a history of angina pectoris with minimal exertion, (b) a myocardial infarction suffered in the past 6 months, or (c) unknown or untreated cardiac arrhythmia noted on initial pulse check. With or without ECG monitoring, exercise should be terminated if the patient complains of (a) chest pain or chest discomfort, (b) dyspnea, (c) dizziness, or (d) severe claudication. With ECG monitoring, additional indications for stopping exercise include (a) a heart rate greater than 120, (b) a new or increased ventricular arrhythmia, or (c) ST segment depression of more than 2 mm.

B.   Severe ischemia. Patients who present with severe ischemic symptoms (rest pain, nonhealing foot lesions, or gangrene) require only resting noninvasive arterial studies. Treadmill exercise usually is not appropriate or feasible for such patients. The Doppler system and PVRs can help in the following ways:

1.   To ascertain that rest pain is ischemic and not neuropathic (Table 5.1). Patient history and physical examination usually are sufficient to diagnose ischemic rest pain. However, diabetics may have foot pain caused by both peripheral neuropathy and arterial occlusive disease. In such cases, rest pain secondary to severe ischemia should be suspected when the systolic ankle pressure is less than 55 mm Hg. In nondiabetics, rest pain is likely when ankle pressures drop below 35 mm Hg but may occur at levels between 35 and 50 mm Hg. The ankle PVR usually is flat or shows minimal deflection (less than 5 mm). The higher ankle pressure criterion for rest pain in diabetics is due to false pressure elevations secondary to decreased arterial compressibility from severe medial calcinosis of the vessel. Another method analogous to ankle pressure is measurement of systolic blood pressure in toe arteries (toe pressures). A small pneumatic cuff is wrapped around the toe and a photoplethysmograph, applied to the terminal phalanx, is used to sense the return of blood flow. A toe pressure less than 30 mm Hg indicates severe ischemia. In addition, we have used $TcPO_2$ of the forefoot to help differentiate ischemic pain from neuropathic discomfort. Forefoot $TcPO_2$ levels greater than 55 mm Hg can be considered normal at any age. Resting supine levels less than 30 mm Hg suggest arterial ischemia, especially if they drop to 0 to 10 mm Hg with leg elevation.

Table 5.1.   Criteria for ischemic rest pain

Noninvasive study	Unlikely	Probable	Likely
Ankle pressure (mm Hg)			
Nondiabetic	>55	35–55	<35
Diabetic	>80	55–80	<55
Ankle PVR category (mm)			
Nondiabetic	>15	5–15	<5 or flat
Diabetic	>15	5–15	<5
Transcutaneous oxygen tension (torr)	>40	10–20	0–10

PVR, pulse volume recorder.

Table 5.2. Criteria for healing ischemic foot lesions

Noninvasive study	Likely	Probable	Unlikely
Ankle pressure (mm Hg)			
Nondiabetic	>65	55–65	<55
Diabetic	>90	80–90	<80
Ankle PVR category (mm)			
Nondiabetic	>15	5–15	<5 or flat
Diabetic	>15	5–15	<5
Transcutaneous oxygen tension (torr)	>50	40–50	<20
Toe blood pressures (mm Hg)	>50	30–40	<30

PVR, pulse volume recorder.

2. To predict healing of leg or foot ulcers (Table 5.2). Ulcers of the foot or leg have multiple etiologies that are not always clear by history and physical examination. These ulcers may be the result of arterial insufficiency, venous disease, diabetic neuropathy, infection, frostbite, or collagen vascular disease. Ulcers have a significant ischemic component and are unlikely to heal if ankle pressures are less than 55 mm Hg in nondiabetics and less than 80 mm Hg in diabetics. A severely attenuated (<5 mm) or flat PVR tracing at the ankle or transmetatarsal level also correlates with poor healing. Our experience with $TcPO_2$ measurements indicates that levels less than 20 to 30 mm Hg are associated with nonhealing. Chronic ischemic ulcers and gangrene are often accompanied by forefoot $TcPO_2$ levels of 0 to 10 mm Hg. These criteria apply only if local infection has been controlled.
3. To predict healing at various amputation levels (see Chap. 15). Vascular laboratory findings alone have not been sufficient to select an appropriate amputation level. Physical examination remains the best method of selecting an amputation level, although noninvasive studies may help. In general, an amputation is unlikely to succeed if the PVR tracing is nonpulsatile at the proposed amputation level. Ankle pressures have not correlated well with healing of below-knee amputations (BKAs). The ability to heal a BKA has been favorably correlated with distal thigh or calf pressures of greater than 65 mm Hg. The presence of a pulsatile PVR tracing at the transmetatarsal or digital level also is encouraging for likely healing of local amputations at these levels. Our data also suggest that a $TcPO_2$ tension value of at least 40 mm Hg measured on the anterior skin flap at the proposed level of amputation is predictive of success. The conversion of absolute values to a $TcPO_2$ tension index by dividing by the corresponding anterior chest value appears to offer a slightly better discrimination, with a threshold value of 0.59.

C.   Postoperative surveillance. Chapter 9 focuses on the importance and methods of detecting intraoperative problems with arterial reconstructions. Several authors have documented improved long-term graft patency when hemodynamically failing grafts are recognized before occlusion. Although the majority of patients with failing grafts will notice recurrent or worsening claudication, some will not become symptomatic until acute graft thrombosis. The simplest office method of detecting hemodynamic failure is the measurement of the ankle-brachial pressure index. A decrease of 0.15 between office visits is considered significant enough to justify further duplex scanning or arteriography. In addition, a progressive fall in resting ankle pressure after treadmill exercise is another noninvasive means to detect a failing graft.

Duplex scanning may be a better method of detecting a problem requiring revision since resting ankle pressures may fail to detect graft problems in some patients. A decrease in peak systolic flow velocity to less than 40 to 45 cm/s generally identifies a femoropopliteal-tibial graft prone to failure. Real-time B-mode imaging of the graft and anastomoses should be attempted when a low velocity is noted. If scanning of the graft locates a stenosis where the ratio of the poststenotic (V_2) to prestenotic (V_1) velocities is greater than 2 **and** the peak graft velocity is less than 40 cm/s (Fig. 5.6), the graft is at higher risk of occlusion. Long-term postoperative surveillance with duplex scanning and flow velocity determination detects anatomic or hemodynamic abnormalities in at least 5% to 10% of vein arterial bypasses. Most experts agree that graft longevity can be enhanced by correcting such stenoses, even if they are asymptomatic. In fact, about 60% of vein grafts with a significant stenosis will not be associated with symptoms at the time of initial recognition on duplex scanning.

IV.   Extracranial cerebrovascular disease. Noninvasive cerebrovascular testing is evolving. The search continues for a noninvasive test that can match the anatomic information and accuracy of contrast arteriography. Although the risk of angiography is low (1% to 2% morbidity) in experienced hands, the technique is invasive and expensive. In addition, the broad or routine use of angiography for evaluating patients with possible extracranial vascular disease reveals many with insignificant disease. Furthermore, the arteriogram does not provide hemodynamic information about physiologic importance of a vascular stenosis. Consequently, various noninvasive tests have been developed to assist with better selection of patients for arteriography and surgery.

A.   Indications for noninvasive cerebrovascular tests. Before describing the common noninvasive tests for extracranial cerebrovascular disease, we must consider the appropriate indications for such testing.

1.   An asymptomatic cervical bruit in an acceptable surgical candidate. (Obviously, an asymptomatic bruit in a patient who is severely debilitated by any medical condition would be more appropriately followed without further testing or surgery.)

2.   Nonspecific neurologic symptoms (e.g., dizziness).

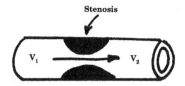

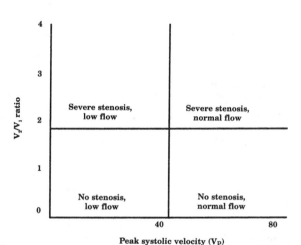

Figure 5.6.   Surveillance of lower-extremity femoropopliteal-tibial vein bypass grafts. This graph categorizes vein graft functional performance into categories based on peak systolic velocity (V_P) measured at the midpoint of the graft and the velocity ratio (V_2/V_1) across a stenosis. The grafts at greatest risk for occlusion have both low velocity ($V_P < 40$ cm/s) and a high velocity ratio across a stenosis ($V_2/V_1 > 2$). (Based on clinical observations by Bandyk et al.).

3.   **Follow-up** of patients after previous carotid endarterectomy to detect restenosis.

4.   **Follow-up** of patients with known mild asymptomatic carotid stenosis (less than 50% diameter).

5.   **Head and neck surgery** in which one carotid artery may require ligation or resection.

6.   **Early postoperative neurologic deficit** after carotid endarterectomy to detect carotid thrombosis.

7.   **Baseline data in symptomatic patients.** The value of noninvasive testing in patients with classic TIAs or strokes

is debatable. Such patients generally require a standard contrast or magnetic resonance cerebral angiogram. However, some surgeons proceed to carotid endarterectomy with only a duplex ultrasound. When the question of brachiocephalic and intracranial disease remains after ultrasound exam, an angiogram remains the best method of imaging the entire extracranial and intracranial vasculature. Either standard contrast or gadolinium-enhanced magnetic resonance arteriography can image the intrathoracic origins of the brachiocephalic arteries, the degree and extent of carotid bifurcation lesions, ulcerative or stenotic lesions of the carotid siphon, and the smaller intracranial arteries where occlusions or aneurysms may cause neurologic symptoms. Spiral CT cerebrovascular reconstruction is also being used in some centers.

Duplex sonography may also provide some useful information about the vertebral arteries in patients with nonlateralizing, posterior cerebral symptoms such as dizziness, vertigo, blurred vision, ataxia, and syncope. In most patients, the proximal vertebral arteries can be identified. Origin stenosis can be detected, and the direction of flow can be ascertained. Direction of flow may be important if proximal innominate or subclavian stenosis or occlusion is present (e.g., subclavian steal). Since the vertebral arteries are surrounded by the vertebral bodies for most of their cervical course, most of their length cannot be seen by ultrasound.

Transcranial Doppler (TCD) may also provide some useful hemodynamic information in patients with symptoms suggesting posterior circulation insufficiency. However, the utility of TCD is still debated.

B.   Noninvasive carotid artery studies are generally classified as indirect or direct. Most early tests (supraorbital Doppler analysis and ocular plethysmography) provided indirect measurement by detecting changes in blood flow and pressure distal to the carotid stenosis or occlusion. Common limitations of **indirect** methods are that they only detect lesions that are sufficiently advanced to reduce mean blood flow and consequently can miss ulcerative lesions that are not associated with severe stenosis. In addition, they cannot differentiate a tight stenosis from an occlusion since the hemodynamic changes in the distal arterial bed are indistinguishable. In contrast, **direct** methods focus on imaging the extracranial carotid arteries (ultrasonic scans) and on determining the degree of stenosis (continuous or pulsed Doppler spectral analysis).

In general, the diagnostic accuracy of noninvasive cerebrovascular testing may be enhanced by performing two complementary procedures. The best combination usually includes one direct method (e.g., duplex scan) to assess the carotid bifurcation with one indirect method (e.g., OPG-Gee) to ascertain the distal hemodynamic significance of any lesion. The selection of tests depends on what equipment is available in a specific lab and on what the accuracies are for the specific techniques used in that lab. Each laboratory must know its limitations if accuracy is to be optimized. The following emphasizes some of the common problems we have encountered in performing and interpreting various tests.

1. Indirect methods. Our experience has been greatest with the ocular pneumoplethysmography (OPG-Gee) and transcranial Doppler.

    a. Ocular pneumoplethysmography (OPG-Gee). Ophthalmic artery pressure correlates reliably with pressure in the distal internal carotid artery. The OPG-Gee can determine ophthalmic artery pressure and identify a hemodynamically significant carotid stenosis (more than 50% diameter) with 85% to 95% accuracy. In our experience, the OPG-Gee has been easier to perform and interpret than other OPG methods. Its main limitations are its inability to detect nonobstructive, ulcerated plaques and to distinguish between severe stenosis and occlusion of the internal carotid artery.

    Since a plastic monitoring eye cup is placed on the lateral sclera after topical anesthesia, the test is not recommended in patients with (a) allergy to topical anesthesia, (b) acute or chronic conjunctivitis, (c) a history of detached retina, (d) eye surgery within the previous 6 months, (e) untreated or unstable glaucoma, (f) recent eye trauma, or (g) an intraocular lens prosthesis, or in an uncooperative or agitated patient.

    Our criteria for an abnormal test include:

1. A difference of 5 mm Hg or more between the two ophthalmic artery pressures.
2. A ratio of ophthalmic artery to brachial artery pressure of less than 0.60 when the eye pressures are equal (i.e., severe bilateral carotid disease).
3. A difference of 1 to 4 mm Hg when the ophthalmic to brachial pressure ration is below 0.66.

One must remember that a low OPG can be caused by one or more occlusive lesions at any point along the carotid pathway, including its intrathoracic origin, carotid bifurcation, carotid siphon, or ophthalmic artery itself.

    b. Transcranial Doppler is a noninvasive method to assess the intracranial circulation. TCD devices emit pulses of ultrasound from a 2-MHz probe. Specific bony "windows" to the intracranial arteries are used. By placing the probe superior to the zygomatic arch, one can insonate the distal internal carotid artery siphon, anterior cerebral artery A1 segment, middle cerebral artery M1 segment, and posterior cerebral artery P1 and P2 segments. The ophthalmic artery and a portion of the internal carotid siphon may be assessed with the transorbital approach. The suboccipital window is used to insonate the distal intracranial segment of the vertebrobasilar system.

    A variety of clinical applications have been established for TCD. These include (a) assessment of intracranial collateral patterns and hemodynamic reserve in occlusive carotid disease, (b) diagnosis of intracranial stenosis and occlusion, (c) diagnosis of vasospasm in the setting of subarachnoid hemorrhage, (d) monitoring the hemodynamic effects of arteriovenous malformation treatment, (e) assessment of intracranial circulation in patients with increased intracranial pressure and cerebral death, and (f) intraoperative and postoperative monitoring. However, the total impact of TCD on the current evaluation of cerebrovascular disease remains relatively small compared to the role of extracranial carotid duplex ultrasonography.

2.   Direct methods. Because it combines the benefit of real-time B-mode ultrasound imaging and pulsed Doppler velocity wave form analysis, duplex scanning has become the direct method of choice for initial evaluation of extracranial cerebrovascular disease. Magnetic resonance imaging and spiral computed tomography are two other methods of imaging that compete with ultrasound in some centers.

Duplex scanning was developed by Strandness and colleagues at the University of Washington to combine the benefits of a real-time B-mode ultrasound image system with a pulsed Doppler detector. The ultrasound image not only shows the vessel and plaque anatomy but also allows precise positioning of the Doppler beam in the center stream of the vessel for optimal study of velocity patterns. The duplex scanner can study calcified lesions since the B-mode scanning allows the examiner to position the Doppler beam distal to the calcification and sample disturbed velocity patterns at this point. Based on flow signal characteristics (Table 5.3, Fig. 5.7), the degree of internal carotid disease is placed in one of six categories: (a) normal, (b) minimal disease (0% to

Table 5.3.   Criteria internal carotid artery disease based on duplex ultrasonography

Grade	Angiogram description (percentage of diameter reduction)	Spectral criteria
A	Normal	Peak systolic velocity < 125 cm/sec; no spectral broadening
B	1–15%	Peak systolic velocity < 125 cm/sec; clear window under peak systole; minimal spectral broadening in deceleration phase of systole
C	16–49%	Peak systolic velocity > 125 cm/sec; spectral broadening throughout systole; no window
D	50–79%	Peak systolic velocity > 125 cm/sec; end diastolic velocity < 140 cm/sec; marked spectral broadening; ICA:CCA ratio > 1.8:1
D+	80–90%	End diastolic velocity > 140 cm/sec; ICA:CCA ratio > 3.5:1
E	Occluded	CCA: Unilateral flow to zero or reversed ICA: no signal

ICA, internal carotid artery; CCA, common carotid artery.

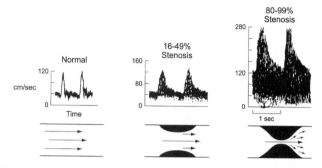

Figure 5.7. Internal carotid artery Doppler spectrum patterns. The criteria for each category are summarized in Table 5.3. The percentages refer to degree of stenosis.

15% diameter reduction), (c) moderate stenosis (16% to 49%), (d) severe stenosis (50% to 79%), (e) critical stenosis (80% to 99%), and (f) occlusion.

Different investigators have demonstrated that the technique is highly accurate, with a sensitivity and specificity over 90%. Of special importance is the high accuracy (95% to 97%) of separating severe stenosis from occlusion. A natural history study of asymptomatic carotid bruits categorized and followed by duplex scanning has documented that stenoses greater than 80% are most commonly associated with subsequent TIAs, strokes, and asymptomatic internal carotid occlusions. This information makes duplex scanning a powerful tool for selecting low-risk patients for possible prophylactic carotid endarterectomy.

Since duplex scanning can provide high-quality ultrasound images of carotid lesions as well as hemodynamic information, some investigators have raised a provocative question: Can selected patients with good quality duplex scans and no signs of proximal brachiocephalic disease (normal proximal carotid pulses, normal arm pressures, and no supraclavicular bruits) and normal brain imaging (computed tomography or magnetic resonance scans) undergo carotid endarterectomy without the risk and expense of carotid arteriography? The answer is no longer so debatable. Advances in the quality and accuracy of duplex scanning have resulted in its sole use without angiography prior to carotid endarterectomy for asymptomatic high-grade stenosis and selected symptomatic patients. However, the reliance on duplex scanning alone depends significantly on the experience and accuracy of the ultrasonographer, a fact that still influences some practices to perform angiography (standard or magnetic resonance) before any carotid surgery.

V. Deep venous thrombosis. Patient history and physical examination are not always reliable in the diagnosis of lower-extremity DVT because leg swelling and tenderness can be caused

by several etiologies. A venogram was once the definitive diagnostic study for deep venous disease but causes discomfort and
sometimes allergic reaction or phlebitis. About 50% of patients
with suspected DVT will have a normal venogram; therefore, noninvasive venous studies (Table 5.4) have replaced venography in
the initial evaluation of acute DVT.

Currently, **duplex ultrasound** is preferred for the initial evaluation of patients with a high risk or suspicion DVT. Other noninvasive venous studies are continuous-wave Doppler examination,
I^{125} fibrinogen scanning, radionuclide phlebography, and various
types of venous plethysmography. Specifically, impedence plethysmography is a low-cost screening test for DVT in low-risk patients.

A. Duplex venous ultrasonography is the noninvasive
test of choice in the detection of venous thrombosis in various
anatomic locations, including the vena cava and the jugular,
portal, renal, and lower-extremity veins. The common femoral
and popliteal veins can be visualized for the presence or absence
of an intraluminal soft-tissue mass, compressibility of the veins,
and response to the Valsalva maneuver. In patients in whom
sonography detects a thrombus in either the common femoral
or popliteal veins, the veins are generally noncompressible.
When the common femoral vein is obstructed, collateral flow
does not respond to the Valsalva maneuver, which normally
stops femoral flow when iliofemoral valves are competent.
Venous duplex ultrasound has both high sensitivity (95%) and
specificity (98%) for proximal lower-extremity DVT. Although
sensitivity is less for detecting thrombus in the calf, accuracy is
improving with experience.

B. Venous plethysmography. The diagnostic accuracy of
venous plethysmography makes it a reasonable screening test.
Although its sensitivity for acute DVT is high, specificity is
lower (60% to 70%), and positive predictive value is only 50%.
Nonetheless, the equipment is portable and can be used at the
bedside. Plethysmography is highly reliable above the knee but
less sensitive for calf thrombosis.

Several types of plethysmography can be used: impedance,
mercury strain gauge, and volume displacement. The accuracy
of each type is comparable. Approximately 80% of the lower-
extremity blood volume is in the veins. The use of plethysmography in detecting deep venous obstruction is based on the
principle that venous occlusion will change deep venous resistance and outflow. These volume changes can be recognized by
a plethysmograph.

A normal venous plethysmograph of the leg shows a gradual
increase after temporary occlusion of venous outflow by a thigh
cuff inflated to 45 to 50 mm Hg for 45 seconds. With cuff
release, the tracing drops rapidly toward the baseline. The
plateau in calf volume after cuff inflation is called the **venous
capacitance (VC)** (Fig. 5.8). The decrease in volume during
the first second after cuff deflation is termed the **maximum venous outflow (MVO).** By plotting VC against MVO, it can be
predicted with 90% accuracy whether the deep veins are normal or obstructed.

Leg position is critical to an accurate examination and the leg
should be slightly elevated to minimize differences in venous

Table 5.4. Noninvasive methods to detect venous disease

Test	Measures	Acute DVT	Chronic occlusion	Valvular reflux
Duplex ultrasound	Venous flow patterns with respiration and muscle compression and valvular incompetence	+	+	+
Impedance plethysmorgraphy	Venous capacity and maximum venous outflow	+	+	–
Phleborrheography	Venous flow patterns with respiration and muscle compression	+	+	–
Photoplethysmography	Response of venous pressure to exercise	–	–	+

DVT, deep venous thrombosis; +, reliable in detection; –, unreliable in detection.

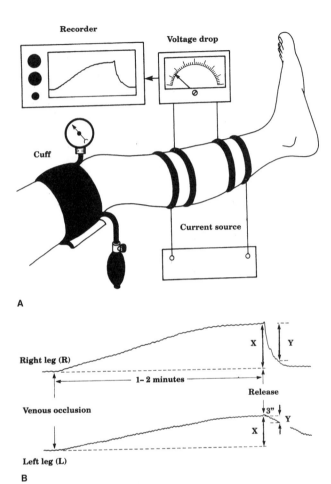

Figure 5.8. A: A high-frequency, low-intensity electrical current is passed between the two outer electrodes, and the voltage change is measured between the two inner electrodes. An inflatable thigh cuff is used to produce venous occlusion. **B:** An IPG tracing from a normal right limb (above) and an obstructed left limb (below). When venous obstruction is present, IPG is typically affected in two ways: (a) The rise in leg volume occurring during venous occlusion is decreased (because the deep venous thrombosis has already occluded venous outflow and thus causes limb distension and a reduction in limb compliance). (b) The decrease in leg volume occurring during the first 3 seconds following cuff deflation is reduced (i.e., the rate of venous outflow is reduced). (From Schlant et al, eds. *The heart*, 8th ed. New York: McGraw–Hill, 1994, with permission.)

pooling. External rotation of the leg enhances muscle relaxation, and slight knee flexion minimizes extrinsic popliteal vein compression.

Certain limitations should be emphasized. Plethysmography is insensitive for detection of calf vein thrombi and small nonocclusive proximal thrombi, which explains the poorer performance in postoperative patients in whom calf vein thrombi are known to occur. Also, plethysmography cannot differentiate between an acute or chronic occlusion. This limitation explains its low positive predictive value. False positive results can also occur in bedridden patients, those suffering from heart failure, and pregnant women. It is also technically difficult to obtain reliable results in patients with altered mental status, with significant obesity, on mechanical ventilation, and after orthopedic procedures or trauma.

If the mentioned noninvasive tests are normal and clinical suspicion for DVT is low, we do not perform venography and pursue other reasons for the symptoms. When the clinical picture suggests thrombosis but noninvasive tests are equivocal, we recommend venography as it remains the best method to visualize calf veins. When calf and thigh swelling are accompanied by abnormal noninvasive tests suggesting iliofemoral venous thrombosis, anticoagulation without venography is reasonable for most patients.

SELECTED READING

Samson RH, Bandyk DF, Showalter DP, et al. Carotid endarterectomy based on duplex ultrasonography: a safe approach associated with long-term stroke prevention. *Vasc Surg* 2000;34:125.

Strandness DE Jr, van Breda A, eds. *Vascular diseases: surgical and interventional therapy.* New York: Churchill Livingstone, 1994.

Sumner DS. Vascular diagnostics. In: Greenfield LJ, ed. *Surgery: scientific principles and practice,* 2nd ed. Philadelphia: Lippincott–Raven Publishers, 1997:1668–1677.

TransAtlantic Inter-Society Consensus Working Group. Management of Peripheral Arterial Disease: TransAtlantic Inter-society Consensus. *J Vasc Surg* 2000;31(Part 2).

Zwiebel WJ, ed. *Introduction to vascular ultrasonography,* 4th ed. Philadelphia: Saunders, 2000.

Vascular Imaging and Endovascular Therapy

In the past, vascular radiologists performed most of the diagnostic vascular imaging and therapy, e.g., angioplasty. In recent years, vascular surgeons and cardiologists have taken more active roles in vascular diagnostic tests and endovascular therapy. These trends are altering the spectrum and format of vascular diagnosis and therapy. The patient benefits when these groups create complementary care teams, which create the foundation for an increasing number of multispecialty vascular centers.

The time-honored imaging techniques of arteriography and venography have been supplemented by ultrasonography, computed tomography (CT), digital subtraction angiography (DSA), magnetic resonance imaging (MRI), and angioscopy. Using the anatomic information provided by these modalities, the vascular interventionalist can use angiographic catheterization to deliver drugs, embolize arteries, dilate/stent occlusive lesions, and deploy aneurysm stent grafts.

The responsibility for ordering either an imaging study or an endovascular therapy remains with the primary physician or surgeon. Therefore, he or she must understand the indications, risks, limitations, and management of any complication associated with both these diagnostic and therapeutic activities.

ARTERIOGRAPHY

Most arteriograms are performed in preparation for an operation or some other therapeutic intervention. Arteriography can also help solve certain diagnostic dilemmas—for example, vasospastic disorders versus occlusive disease of the hands, ergotism, Buerger's disease, temporal arteritis, and periarteritis nodosa. The decision to order an arteriogram must be made with the patient's understanding that the study is invasive, may require hospitalization, and has definite risks. The following guidelines should assist in the preparation and selection of appropriate angiographic views.

   I.   **Preparation.** A member of the vascular surgery or interventional team should perform a history and physical exam on each patient before angiography. This person should explain the study and risks to the patient, record consent, and write appropriate orders. Special attention should be paid to the following:
   A.   Any **allergy to iodinated** contrast material or other complications of prior angiography should be ascertained.
   B.   The patient should be questioned as to his or her **current medications.**
      1.   Care must be exercised in the use of iodinated contrast in patients taking **metformin (Glucophage).** This oral agent used to treat non–insulin-dependent diabetes mellitus can cause a severe lactic acidosis that can be precipitated by contrast agents. The risk is especially high in patients with renal dysfunction. In general, patients should not take metformin

for 48 to 72 hours after the use of iodinated contrast agents. This is especially true in patients who have a creatinine of greater than 1.5 mg/dL prior to the angiogram.

2. Anticoagulants such as warfarin should be stopped before procedures that involve arterial access. This usually means stopping warfarin for 2 to 4 days and allowing the international normalized ratio (INR) to fall below 1.5.

C. The patient should be questioned about **past bleeding problems,** and generally a platelet count and INR are checked.

D. Renal function is assessed by measuring serum creatinine. Contrast material can be nephrotoxic, especially in dehydrated patients and diabetics.

E. Adequate urine output (0.5 mL/kg/h) should be established in dehydrated patients and in diabetics by intravenous hydration. This usually involves the administration of Ringer's lactate solution at 100 to 125 mL/h several hours before the study.

F. All **peripheral pulses** should be noted on physical exam. If pulses are not palpable, noninvasive assessment of extremity perfusion (e.g., ankle-brachial index) should be performed before the intervention.

G. Skin preparation of the puncture site should include cleansing with an antiseptic soap such as chlorhexidine or povidone-iodine.

II.   Risks. The main risks of angiography are hemorrhage from the needle puncture site, allergic reactions to the contrast material, thrombosis of the punctured vessel, and embolization of a clot from the catheter, air, or atheromatous material. In experienced hands, these complications occur in about 1% of all cases. Mortality is less frequent (0.05%) but is a definite risk that the patient must understand.

III.   Methods. Prior to angiography, one must select a contrast agent and a vessel puncture site. Local infiltrative anesthesia is used around the site, and frequently an anxiolytic (e.g., benzodiazepine) is administered to relieve anxiety associated with the procedure. Pain during angiography is rare and is related directly to the osmolarity of the contrast material and the use of angioplasty or stent placement.

A. A variety of **nonionic contrast agents** are used today that are much improved over older ionic contrast agents. Many of these nonionic agents are isoosmolar or only slightly hyperosmolar, which represents the greatest improvement over older agents, which were extremely hyperosmolar and painful during injection. Excreted by the kidneys, contrast agents can induce acute renal dysfunction in patients (with or without renal insufficiency). However, individuals with preexisting renal failure, proteinuria, diabetes mellitus, and dehydration are at higher risk. Postangiographic renal dysfunction peaks at 48 hours and can be minimized by intravenous hydration, limited contrast loads, and, rarely, mannitol infusion. Contrast-induced nephropathy is usually transient and improves within a week's time.

In addition, contrast agents cause allergic reactions in 2% to 5% of patients. These reactions are usually mild, with itching or urticaria. Rarely, more severe anaphylactic reactions occur, manifested by wheezing, bradycardia, and hypotension. Patients with allergies or prior contrast reactions are at higher risk for recurrent allergic complications with repeat angiography. Although the benefits of some type of pretreatment in this high-risk group are controversial, it is generally recommend that steroids and diphenhydramine (Benedryl, Warner–Lambert Consumer, Morris Plains, NJ, U.S.A.) be administered prior to the arteriogram. One such regimen includes 32 mg of methyl-prednisolone (Medrol, Pharmacia & Upjohn Company, Bridge-water, NJ, U.S.A.) by mouth 12 and then 2 hours prior to the pro-cedure. A single dose of 25 to 50 mg of diphenhydramine may also be given 2 hours prior to the administration of contrast.

B. Pain of angiography is usually minimal and transient. Such discomfort is related to vessel puncture, contrast injection, and, occasionally, the use of balloon angioplasty and or stents. Pain accompanying contrast injection has been markedly re-duced with the common use of iso- or only slightly hyperosmolar contrast agents. If an older hyperosmolar contrast agent is used, the patient may experience an intense hot or burning pain that lasts seconds but is remarkably uncomfortable. In general, we manage the patient's anxiety with the oral administration of a short-acting benzodiazepine and rarely resort to an intravenous sedative such as propofol (Diprivan, Zeneca Pharmaceuticals, Wilmington, DE, U.S.A.). Local anesthetic is used around the puncture site and in most cases this is all that is required for uneventful angiography. An intravenous dose of a short-acting narcotic such as fentanyl may be necessary in patients who experience pain or in whom balloon angioplasty or stenting is suspected. In rare instances such as children, a more intense sedation or general anesthesia may be necessary.

C.   The most common puncture site is **transfemoral** using the Seldinger technique (Fig. 6.1). If a synthetic graft is punctured, prophylactic antibiotics are important to reduce the risks of graft contamination and infection. Several reports, however, have doc-umented a low complication rate following prosthetic graft punc-tures for angiography. Although the morbidity from direct graft puncture is usually higher than that associated with puncture of a native vessel, alternative approaches such as transbrachial or transaxillary are also associated with higher complication rates.

The Seldinger technique allows:

1.   Placement of a catheter that can be moved to various positions in the arterial tree.

2.   Measurement of pressures across an arterial stenoses (e.g., iliac arteries) to determine hemodynamic significance.

3.   Safe movement of the patient into oblique positions to evaluate the origin of various vessels (e.g., the profunda femoris artery).

D.   Transaxillary or transbrachial angiography also pro-vides access to the arterial system. The risks of this approach include nerve injury, axillary hematoma, and emboli to the cere-bral circulation. However, the transaxillary (transbrachial) route provides excellent access in situations where transfemoral punc-ture is not feasible. Using the transaxillary (transbrachial) ap-proach, the cervical and intracranial circulations as well as the aorta can be studied.

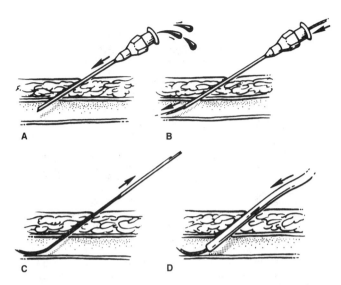

Figure 6.1. Seldinger technique for percutaneous catheter angiography. A: Introductory needle is passed into femoral or axillary artery. B: Smaller flexible guidewire is passed through the introductory needle into the artery. C: Introductory needle is withdrawn over the guidewire, which is left in the artery. D: Larger flexible angiographic catheter, passed over the smaller guidewire, then is manipulated through the arterial system until the desired level of study is reached. Angiographic dye is injected through this catheter.

    E. One final alternative is **translumbar aortography,** which is an exam of last resort and is rarely necessary in current practice. This technique has become even more rare with the current use of MR arteriography in patients with difficult arterial access.
    F. Regardless of the approach selected, angiographic studies should maximize anatomic information and minimize discomfort, contrast load, and procedure time. To attain these goals, the physician ordering the arteriogram should discuss them with the angiographer before the study.
    IV. Angiographic series. The following imaging techniques are suggested for the evaluation of cerebrovascular, peripheral occlusive, visceral occlusive, and aneurysmal disease.
    A. Symptomatic cerebrovascular disease (transient ischemic attacks [TIAs]). Angiographic study of symptomatic cerebrovascular disease begins with an aortic arch injection, with both oblique views, to identify the arch and the origins of the innominate, both common carotid, vertebral, and subclavian arteries. In addition, selective images of both carotid arteries with intracerebral views are done showing the anterior–posterior (AP) and lateral projections. The carotid bifurcation usually is visualized better on the lateral view. The AP view of the intracranial vasculature demonstrates cross-circulation to the opposite hemisphere. In the symptomatic patient, the intracranial

images are essential to identify any central pathology such as an aneurysm, an arteriovenous malformation, a mass (e.g., tumor), or a small-vessel occlusion. In recent years, all of this anatomic information could be gained by gadolinium-enhanced, time-gated magnetic resonance angiography (MRA). MRA is rapidly replacing standard contrast angiography for most patients.

B. Asymptomatic carotid disease. Patients with asymptomatic carotid disease usually have asymptomatic neck bruits and noninvasive carotid studies that suggest a hemodynamically significant stenosis. An increasing number of surgeons are using only duplex ultrasound to define extracranial carotid lesions before endarterectomy. This approach may be safe when the ultrasound study is performed by a laboratory with a proven record of accuracy. Otherwise, standard contrast or MRA should be performed to confirm the duplex imaging.

C. Aortoiliac disease. When occlusive disease appears to be limited to the terminal aorta and iliac arteries, we request an abdominal aortogram with lower-extremity runoff. Specifically, this includes anterior–posterior and lateral views of the abdominal aorta to identify the origins of the visceral (celiac, superior, and inferior mesenteric) and renal arteries. In addition, oblique views of the pelvis, and profunda femoris artery are performed to show the sometimes hidden origins of these vessels. Lastly, anterior–posterior and lateral views of the feet are performed to identify the pedal vessels.

D. Multilevel occlusive disease. In addition to a biplanar aortogram with runoff, patients with multilevel occlusive disease may benefit from oblique views of the femoral artery to better delineate profunda stenoses, which may be hard to see on the AP projection.

A difficult problem with multilevel occlusive disease is determining whether the patient needs aortoiliac or femoropopliteal reconstruction or both. Measurement of a **femoral artery pressure (FAP) gradient** helps make this determination. A transfemoral angiographic catheter measures the distal aortic pressure and is then pulled back across the iliac system into the femoral artery where the femoral pressure is recorded. An iliac stenosis is significant when the resting pressure gradient across the segment is greater than 10 mm Hg or falls more than 15% after provocative maneuvers (reactive hyperemia or injection of a vasodilator).

E. Femoropopliteal and tibial disease. Patients with femoropopliteal and tibial disease often present with an ischemic foot and multiple medical problems including renal insufficiency. **Therefore, the amount of contrast material should be limited** to prevent further renal damage. One approach to such patients is a transfemoral arteriogram of the ischemic leg with measurement of a FAP gradient to detect significant iliac disease. If a pressure gradient is present, extra contrast is injected to image the distal aorta and iliac system. In some patients, a focal iliac stenosis can be dilated by a balloon catheter, and the femoral artery disease treated later with femoropopliteal bypass. Some of these patients also have severe tibial occlusive disease and require arteriography of the leg and foot arteries. Such views can be obtained by proper timing of x-ray exposure, intraarterial injection of vasodilators (e.g., papaverine), or balloon-occlusion arteriography. In most cases, proper exposure times are sufficient to show the runoff. When conventional runoff views are inadequate, magnetic resonance angiography provides definition of distal tibial and foot arteries.

F.   Renal artery occlusive disease. The angiographic views needed for treatment of renal artery occlusive disease depend on the surgical or endovascular procedure that is planned. An aortogram will show both proximal and distal renal arteries and the infrarenal aorta which is commonly used for aortorenal bypass. **A lateral view of the aorta, identifying the origins of the mesenteric arteries, should always be included in case a splenorenal or hepatorenal bypass is necessary.** Selective renal artery injections in oblique views may be needed to further define renal artery anatomy.

Inferior vena cava and renal vein renins may be useful to confirm the presence of a unilateral pressor kidney. These samples are taken 30 to 60 minutes after the patient has been given captopril, 25 to 50 mg orally, to enhance renin ratios. If renal function is poor (creatinine > 2 mg/100 mL or creatinine clearance < 30 mL/min), less than 125 mL of contrast should be used as larger volumes may worsen renal function. Gadolinium-enhanced magnetic resonance imaging allows definition of renal artery anatomy in most cases and avoids exposure to potentially harmful contrast loads.

G.   Intestinal angina. The angiographic evaluation for intestinal angina should include a lateral view of the aorta demonstrating the origins of the mesenteric arteries. Selective catheterizations may help if the aortogram does not define the distal anatomy and venous return of the mesenteric vessels.

H.   Aneurysms

1.   Most patients can undergo open surgical repair of **abdominal aortic aneurysms** based on ultrasound or computed tomography. A preoperative arteriogram is generally reserved for: (a) patients with symptoms consistent with acute or chronic intestinal ischemia, (b) patients with poorly controlled hypertension or worsening renal function, (c) patients with diminished femoral pulses or lower extremity claudication, (d) patients with abnormal anatomy demonstrated on CT scan (e.g., horseshoe kidney), (e) patients with large internal iliac artery aneurysms, and (f) patients in whom stent-graft therapy is considered. **Currently, intraoperative aortography is used for most aortic stent graft deployments.**

Gadolinium-enhanced magnetic resonance aortography has evolved to the point where it is replacing standard contrast aortography in many patients, especially those with renal insufficiency.

2.   Femoral aneurysms. Since patients with femoral aneurysms often have diffuse aneurysmal disease, an abdominal aortogram with runoff is appropriate.

3.   Popliteal aneurysms. These patients often have diffuse aneurysmal disease. If the physical examination and ultrasonography or CT have ruled out proximal femoral or aortic aneurysms, a transfemoral arteriogram with runoff is adequate to define local anatomy before popliteal aneurysm repair is undertaken.

V.   Postangiogram care. Any patient who has undergone angiography should be monitored hourly for at least 4 to 6 hours. Most early complications become evident during this time. Nursing personnel can perform these routine checks, but a physician or physician assistant/nurse practitioner also should examine the patient sometime during this recuperative period. After hospital discharge for outpatient angiography, these individuals are generally on-call for any emergent complications arising outside the hospital. Consequently, their baseline post-procedure exam is helpful if problems occur later. The routine examination should include (a) evaluation of the patient's general appearance and mental status (especially after cerebral studies), (b) heart rate, (c) blood pressure, (d) inspection of puncture sites, (e) palpation of extremity pulses, and (f) hematocrit if any signs of hemorrhage exist.

In addition, adequate hydration must be maintained for 12 to 24 hours, since the angiographic contrast causes a diuresis and can lead to dehydration. The combination of diuresis and the nephrotoxicity of the contrast material can cause renal deterioration. Patients with diabetes mellitus or chronic renal insufficiency are most susceptible to this complication. We maintain an intravenous infusion for 4 to 6 hours after the angiogram, because it is during this period that diuresis and other early complications are most likely to occur. Oral fluids are encouraged for 24 hours after the procedure to maintain hydration in all patients.

VI.   Complications

A.   Neurologic deficits. Aortic arch and selective cervical artery injections can result in transient or permanent neurologic deficits which may be delayed, occurring minutes to hours after the angiogram. Neurologic deficits that happen during the study probably are embolic from dislodged atheroma or catheter thrombus. Delayed neurologic deficits may be secondary to hypoperfusion or thrombosis associated with contrast-induced diuresis and dehydration. Emergent carotid endarterectomy should be considered in the event of an immediate neurologic deficit on the side of a tight carotid stenosis, especially if a post-procedure duplex scan confirms that the internal carotid artery has occluded suddenly.

Sometimes the neurologic change is subtle, such as confusion, mild facial paresis, dysarthria, or dysphagia. If the neurologic deficit is not recognized for several hours (>4 hours) and is not resolving, the patient probably has suffered a stroke. Emergency endarterectomy may not be advised in such cases, since it may worsen neurologic deficits by changing an ischemic infarct to a hemorrhagic infarct. A CT or MRI scan should be done in 12 to 24 hours to define infarct areas, intracranial hemorrhage, and edema.

If a cerebrovascular accident has occurred, several measures can help minimize cerebral edema and stroke progression. Intravenous fluids should be limited to maintenance levels (1 mL/kg/h) so that cerebral edema is not worsened by excessive hydration. Steroids also may be useful during the period of maximum cerebral edema (3 to 7 days). Systemic anticoagulation to prevent distal internal carotid clot propagation should be considered if there are no signs of intracerebral hemorrhage.

B. Hemorrhage. Small hematomas and ecchymosis at the puncture site are not uncommon however expanding hematomas indicate continued bleeding into the perivascular spaces. This complication can be prevented by application of direct pressure over the puncture site for 15 to 30 minutes after the arterial catheter is removed and bed rest of the extremity for 6 hours. Sandbags and ice packs provide a false sense of adequate hemostasis and are of dubious value as they provide diffuse rather than point pressure. Although some physicians use femoral artery pressure clamps, these devices may not compress adequately puncture sites and can cause pressure necrosis of friable skin if applied too tightly and left in place too long. If used, they require close supervision. A variety of percutaneous closure devices are also available to seal arterial puncture sites and are particularly helpful in cases where thrombolytic drugs or other anticoagulants are in effect when the catheter sheath is removed. They have a 2% to 3% complication or failure rate (arterial thrombosis, pseudoaneurysm or local infection/abscess).

Expanding or pulsatile hematomas should be evaluated immediately by ultrasound. Often, an active pseudoaneurysm can be closed by ultrasound-guided compression or ultrasound-guided thrombin injection. In some patients an acute arteriovenous fistula may also resolve with ultrasound-guided compression. **After axillary puncture, any hematoma that compresses the brachial plexus, causing pain or other neurologic change, should be decompressed in the operating room.**

Significant retroperitoneal hemorrhage can occur after translumbar aortography. Early indications of such bleeding may be persistent back pain, tachycardia, hypotension, and anemia. Flank ecchymosis is a delayed finding. Abdominal CT scan will demonstrate a periaortic or psoas muscle hematoma.

C. Diminished pulses. Diminished or absent pulses (compared to baseline) following the angiogram suggest partial or complete arterial occlusion. Although arterial spasm may occur, it is rarely the cause of diminished pulses that persist beyond 30 to 60 minutes. **The most common causes of compromised extremity blood flow after angiography are (a) arterial injury (intimal flap), (b) a clot stripped off the catheter, (c) arterial occlusion associated with a misplaced percutaneous arterial closure device, and (d) compression by a hematoma in the arterial wall or extrinsic to it.**

The acutely ischemic extremity that is painful, pallid, and pulseless requires emergent revascularization. In contrast, an intimal flap may diminish but not obstruct arterial flow. The extremity will be asymptomatic, but pulses and Doppler pressures (ankle–brachial index) will be diminished compared to those prior to the angiogram. Such asymptomatic cases with mild pressure reduction (10 to 20 mm Hg) can initially be managed nonoperatively. Small intimal flaps usually will adhere to the arterial wall and heal in several days to a few weeks. Systemic heparinization for 24 to 48 hours followed by antiplatelet drugs for 4 to 6 weeks has been a successful regimen in our experience. Ankle-brachial indices at rest and after exercise can be followed to document improvement or deterioration. However, we emphasize that the presence of any ischemic symptoms and the absence of previously palpable pulses require emergent intervention to restore normal extremity circulation.

D.   A **pulsatile mass** at the angiogram puncture site is a hematoma or a false aneurysm. This is a difficult distinction to make and an ultrasound is diagnostic.

Any postarteriogram hematoma that suddenly causes pain and local subcutaneous hemorrhage is a ruptured pseudoaneurysm and usually requires urgent surgical evacuation and repair of the artery. Pseudoaneurysm rupture is most likely to occur within 7 to 10 days of the initial angiogram. For this reason, we suggest that all patients with local hematomas remain close to a surgical facility during this time. In some situations, small (<3 to 4 cm) acute hematomas can be eliminated by ultrasound-guided compression. Although this process may take more than an hour, the success rate is over 90%. Pseudoaneurysms that are initially missed and then noted at a later examination should be repaired about 6 to 8 weeks after the arteriogram. By this time, local inflammation generally has resolved and dissection and repair may be easier. Chronic pseudoaneurysms have a developed capsule that is not likely to resolve with ultrasound-guided compression.

E.   Infection. Local infection at arteriogram puncture sites is unusual with meticulous sterile technique. Such technique should include (a) cleansing the site with a surgical scrub soap before the study, (b) standard surgical operative preparation at the time of the study, and (c) standard surgical attire for members of the angiogram team.

Local superficial pustules at the skin puncture site should be incised, drained, and cultured. If cellulitis extends around this site, oral or parenteral antibiotics should be started. Most local infections will be secondary to hospital-acquired *Staphylococcus aureus* or Streptococcus. Abscesses should be incised and drained in the operating room, since hemorrhage from an infected artery may occur and require repair or ligation. **Any elective synthetic bypass, especially aortofemoral grafting, should be postponed until local groin infections are resolved completely.**

VENOGRAPHY

I.   Indications. The use of contrast venography to diagnose deep venous thrombosis (DVT) of the lower extremity has decreased in the past decade. Duplex ultrasound has assumed the primary role in DVT diagnosis at and above the knee. Nonetheless, venography remains useful in defining lower-extremity venous anatomy in patients undergoing deep venous valve reconstruction or venous bypass. With increasing use of chronic subclavian vein catheters for parenteral nutrition and chemotherapy, venography also has been the most accurate method of defining subclavian vein thrombosis.

II.   Patient preparation. Minimal preparation is required prior to venography. Past allergy to contrast material must be ascertained. The extremity must also be examined for a suitable puncture site.

III.   Risks. About 3% of venographic studies will be complicated by minor allergic reactions, contrast-induced thrombophlebitis, or contrast extravasation at the puncture site. Major allergic reactions of hypotension and bronchospasm occur in less than 1% of cases.

IV.   Methods. The quality and safety of contrast leg venography can be optimized by paying attention to several aspects of the technique.

A.   The patient should be positioned at 30 to 45 degrees on a tilt table, with no weightbearing on the affected limb. Weightbearing causes the gastrocnemius and soleus muscles to contract, preventing adequate filling of some deep veins.

B.   Generally, a vein on the dorsum of the foot is punctured with a 21-gauge needle. Rarely, a cutdown exposure of the greater saphenous vein at the ankle is necessary.

C.   Dilute contrast material, ionic or nonionic, is suitable. The usual volume is 60 to 90 mL per extremity.

D.   Views of the superficial and deep veins can be obtained **without** a tourniquet unless leg swelling is severe and causes increased compartmental pressures. In this situation an ankle tourniquet is used to promote better filling of the deep veins.

E.   Exposures of the leg are made with external and internal foot rotation and the same views are obtained over the knee and thigh. Finally, the pelvic film is exposed after the table is returned horizontal and the leg elevated.

F.   The venous system of the lower limb is flushed with 60 mL of normal saline.

V.   Interpretation

A.   The normal venogram will opacify the deep and superficial veins except for the profunda femoris vein, which is rarely filled with contrast material. Deep venous trunks in the calf are paired and have smooth, straight walls except at valve sites, which have a beadlike appearance. The anterior tibial veins are the smallest. Deep muscle venous plexuses are large and fusiform in young people but appear smaller with advancing age. The femoral vein usually is single but may be paired for a variable length. Normally, contrast material should flow quickly up the deep system after leg elevation.

B.   Acute deep venous thrombosis is confirmed by filling defects in the deep veins on more than one view. The contrast column will end abruptly when the thrombosis completely obstructs the vein. Deep veins also may be nonopacified because of external compression from muscle swelling in the fascial compartments. Mixing defects can be seen at major junction sites such as the femoral triangle and iliac bifurcation.

VI.   Postvenographic care. Complete drainage of the leg is performed immediately after filming by the examiner. The filming should proceed rapidly to minimize the contact time between the contrast material and the venous endothelium. This technique will reduce the risk of postvenographic phlebitis to near zero. Patients with positive studies should remain at bed rest with the leg elevated, and systemic heparinization should be continued.

ULTRASOUND AND COMPUTED TOMOGRAPHY

The search continues for noninvasive methods of imaging the vascular system. Currently, ultrasonography and CT scanning have the longest proven value in defining arterial aneurysms and also in detecting various graft complications. In the past, these methods were considered inferior to arteriography for clear identification of stenotic lesions and ulcerated plaques. This limitation has been overcome for the most part by newer duplex scanners with high-resolution imaging capabilities. The entire field of noninvasive vascular diagnosis is also being changed by magnetic resonance imaging (MRI). For example, MRI has proved to be excellent in depicting the anatomic relationships of hemangiomas, arteriovenous malformations, and aortic arch anomalies. Despite the rapid emergence of MR technology, ultrasonography and CT scanning remain safe, cost-effective methods of vascular imaging for most common vascular problems.

I.   Risks. Current ultrasound techniques have very few if any harmful effects. CT scanning may involve the risk of contrast administration and the risk from a small radiation exposure. Likewise, MRI does not appear to have an identifiable risk at present field strengths, provided no metallic substances (pacemakers, artificial joints, etc.) are in the field.

II.   Indications

A.   Abdominal aortic aneurysm diameter can be accurately measured by gray-scale ultrasound to within 3 to 5 mm (Fig. 6.2). In addition to size measurement, ultrasound can identify intraluminal thrombus and reveal a periaortic hematoma from aneurysm leakage. The most common problem in obtaining an accurate abdominal aortic sonogram is interference by overlying bowel gas which compromises the image. In the past, sonography was limited by its inability to define aneurysm position in

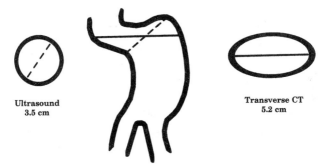

Ultrasound
3.5 cm

Transverse CT
5.2 cm

Figure 6.2.   Variations in the measurement of abdominal aortic aneurysm diameter from ultrasound versus computed tomography (CT). Anterior–posterior measurements on ultrasound are accurate to within 3 to 5 mm of actual size measured at operation. CT measurements are also accurate but may overestimate size if they are made at an oblique angle. This problem arises since CT scans make measurements perpendicular to the body axis while aneurysms are often tortuous.

relation to the renal arteries and to detect iliac aneurysms. **Current ultrasound can image the mesenteric, renal, and iliac arteries in most patients. If ultrasound cannot define the aneurysm position in relation to the renal arteries, a CT scan may be performed.** CT is also useful in defining other abdominal pathology in patients with unexplained symptoms (e.g., retroperitoneal fibrosis, tumors). In the acute setting, CT can evaluate hemodynamically stable patients with a high suspicion of a leaking aneurysms. Many emergency departments currently use on-site ultrasound to quickly ascertain the presence or absence of an abdominal aortic aneurysm in patients with hypotension and acute abdominal/back pain.

B.   Peripheral aneurysms of the common femoral and popliteal arteries can be accurately defined by ultrasound.

C.   Graft complications such as abscesses, a perigraft hematoma, graft dilation, and pseudoaneurysms can be delineated by ultrasound or CT. Ultrasound is especially useful in the groin and lower limb, while CT is preferable in the abdomen or chest. Nonetheless, high-resolution ultrasound can provide excellent images of most abdominal grafts, including the common iliac areas. Arteriography is necessary to define arterial anatomy before most arterial reconstructions for graft complications. Also, indium[111]-labeled leukocyte scans can help document and localize prosthetic vascular graft infections.

DIGITAL SUBTRACTION ANGIOGRAPHY

Digital subtraction angiography (DSA) refers to a technique where contrast is injected into the circulation and multiple, timed fluoroscopic images of arteries are taken at short intervals. A computer subtracts the early images from late images so that bone and other soft tissues are eliminated. Therefore, the only images recorded are those of contrast-filled arteries. The images can be enhanced, displayed on a video monitor, and stored. Two main methods of DSA have been developed:

I.   Intraarterial DSA involves direct injection of the contrast into the arterial bed of interest. This technique provides the best images of arteries and has become a standard part on nearly all contrast angiograms.

II.   Intravenous DSA involves injection of the contrast material into the venous system and waiting for the bolus to circulate to the arterial system before images are taken. We rarely use this technique which provides images with less density of contrast opacified because of time delay for contrast to circulate to the arterial system. The time delay introduces artefacts from movement and breathing. In addition, intravenous DSA opacifies all of the vessels in a given area of interest, precluding selective views. This technique does avoid the need for arterial access and may still be useful in patients who do not have suitable arterial access sites for catheterization.

MAGNETIC RESONANCE IMAGING

MRI relies on the principle that hydrogen nuclei (protons), when subjected to a magnetic field, align themselves in the direction of the field's poles. However, bursts of radio waves of appropriate frequency will alter this alignment (excitation). Following each radio frequency burst, the protons realign themselves with the magnetic field. This realignment (relaxation) is associated with the emission of a faint radio signal of their own. A computer translates these signals into an image of the scanned area which reveals varying densities of protons that correlate with different tissues (e.g., soft tissue and bone).

The physics of MRI are well suited for imaging vascular disease. In rapidly moving blood, the hydrogen nuclei do not line up in the applied magnetic field and thus produce little or no signal when stimulated by a radio frequency burst. The result is a natural contrast between the blood and the vessel wall.

MRI can study several nuclei of biologic significance, including hydrogen, sodium, phosphorus, calcium, oxygen, carbon, chlorine, and potassium. Hydrogen is ideally suited for MRI because it has the greatest sensitivity of the stable nuclei and is the most abundant atomic nucleus in the body. **Phosphorus MR spectroscopy (P^{31}-MR)** analyzes the tissue content of adenosine triphosphate (ATP), and adenosine diphosphate (ADP) making P^{31}-MR useful in studying the effects of ischemia on the depletion of high-energy phosphates. Techniques for blood flow measurement by MRI are also in various developmental stages.

The role of MRI/MRA in vascular imaging has evolved rapidly and it is used commonly in many vascular centers. Visualization of the aorta is the area where MRI has shown its greatest promise. Mesenteric and renal arteries can also be readily seen in patients with occlusive disease. **The development of the low-nephrotoxic contrast agent gadolinium (Gd)** has added significantly to the clarity of MR arterial images and has broadened the clinical usefulness and confidence in MRA. Early attempts to image extra- or intracranial vessel achieved limited success because of the complex three-dimensional anatomy of these systems. However, recent computer software advances (i.e., time-gated, gadolinium-enhanced) have brought brachiocephalic MR imaging to a level comparable to standard contrast arteriography. In addition, MRI is superior to CT scanning in evaluating cerebral edema and has the potential to accurately stage strokes and to determine the optimal time for any cerebrovascular operation in such patients.

Obviously, MRI offers several advantages in evaluating cardiovascular disease: (a) noninvasive imaging, (b) blood flow velocity estimation, (c) avoidance of any nephrotoxic contrast medium, and (d) multidimensional images (transverse, sagittal, and coronal planes). Despite these advantages, several important limitations currently exist. The major limitation remains cost ($800,000 to $2,000,000). In addition patients dependent on metallic life-support systems (e.g., pacemakers) are excluded, since the magnet creates problems with their operation. Intracranial magnetic arterial aneurysm clips also preclude MRI scanning. Patients with joint prostheses or intraabdominal clips have been evaluated by MRI without problems. Finally, some patients become claustrophobic. Some authors also caution that less expensive but effective methods of vascular imaging must not be abandoned during the current rapid proliferation of this new diagnostic modality.

BALLOON ANGIOPLASTY AND STENTING

One of the most active topics in the treatment of vascular disease remains nonoperative dilatation and stenting of arterial stenoses by inflatable balloon-tip catheters. This procedure has most commonly been called **percutaneous transluminal angioplasty (PTA)** and usually is performed by vascular radiologists. In recent years, an increasing number of surgeons and cardiologists have also applied the technique in the peripheral vascular system. PTA generally uses polyethylene catheters that have an inflatable balloon near the tip. The balloon angioplasty represents a variation of the transluminal arterial dilatation described originally by Dotter and Judkins. The older Dotter technique used a relatively large no. 12 French Teflon catheter introduced over an inner no. 8 French catheter and passed through the stenosis to dilate it. No balloon was involved. Gruntzig popularized balloon catheters in the late 1970s, and their use has become common practice. Larger balloon catheters usually are only no. 5 to 7 French, but the balloon tip inflates to a predetermined diameter (4 to 25 mm) at 3 to 20 atm pressure. Even smaller catheters (no. 4 French) are available for small tibial lesions. The smaller catheter size obviously reduces local complications at the arterial puncture site, and the rigidity and pressure characteristics of the balloon allow for greater force to be exerted in dilating the stenosis.

I. **Mechanisms of balloon angioplasty** (Fig. 6.3). The mechanisms by which percutaneous balloon angioplasty dilate a stenotic artery are complex. First, balloon dilatation disrupts the plaque and the artery wall, with partial separation of the plaque from the media, rupture of the plaque and possibly the media, and stretching of the adventitia to increase the lumen cross-sectional area. Second, the intimal plaque protrudes into the lumen, accounting for the angiographic appearance of local flaps and dissection channels. Third, remodeling occurs by adherence of the intimal flaps with little change in plaque volume. Thus, long-term patency depends on sufficient stretching of the vessel and an adequately remodeled lumen. Restenosis may occur because of insufficient dilatation (compliance), from extension of dissection channels into nondilated segments, and from intimal hyperplasia. **A variety of metallic stents (Table 6.1) are available to improve the initial dilation, treat local dissections, and possibly improve patency. Stents are categorized broadly according to their means of expansion (balloon expanding versus self-expanding).**

II. **Indications.** Since its revival in the late 1970s, PTA has been used successfully to dilate or recanalize arteries or grafts in every anatomic region. PTA is generally safer than surgery and less expensive since hospitalization is shorter. However, PTA is generally less durable than operative revascularization (Fig. 6.4). Restenosis rates after angioplasty vary with anatomic location but range between 15% and 50% within 2 to 3 years. Regardless of one's opinion, PTA is a reasonable therapeutic option for selected patients. Based on our reported experience and other studies, we suggest that the following indications are justified based on long-term follow-up. We agree with others that success must be documented by significant improvement of both clinical symptoms **and** hemodynamic measurements (ankle/brachial indices, Doppler wave forms, pulse volume recordings, exercise distance, or transcutaneous oxygen measurements).

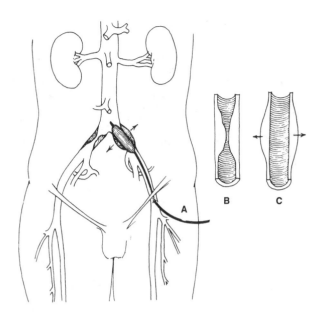

Figure 6.3.   Percutaneous transluminal angioplasty (PTA). A: By the Seldinger technique, a catheter with an internal flexible guidewire is passed to and gently insinuated through the area of arterial stenosis. B,C: The balloon is inflated to several atmospheres of pressure. When the PTA is complete, the arterial lumen is larger and the local artery is stretched.

A.   Iliac stenosis. A focal common iliac artery stenosis (1 to 3 cm in length) is considered an ideal lesion for dilation, especially in a patient with unilateral claudication and good femoropopliteal runoff. The best results are achieved when PTA is limited to lesions that appear hemodynamically significant by either a 10-mm gradient at rest or a 15% pressure drop after either intraarterial injection of a vasodilator agent or after reactive hyperemia following tourniquet occlusion for 5 minutes. Hemodynamic improvement is achieved in 80% to 90%, but long-term functional success falls to 60% at 4 to 5 years. These results can be enhanced in select patients with balloon **angioplasty plus metallic stenting** of the lesion (e.g., Palmaz stent; Johnson and Johnson, Warren, NJ, U.S.A.). Generally, patients with diffuse bilateral aortoiliac disease or common iliac artery occlusion require fewer reinterventions with arterial bypass grafting than with angioplasty.

B.   Femoral, popliteal, and tibial lesions. Balloon angioplasty of infrainguinal arterial lesions is less successful than PTA for iliac artery stenosis. Success is more likely if the lesions are more proximal in the leg, are focal, are less than 3 cm in length, and associated with good distal runoff. Initial clinical

Table 6.1. Stents used in the treatment of occlusive vascular disease

Method of expansion	Examples	Material
Balloon expandible	Palmaz (Johnson and Johnson)	Stainless steel
	Intrastent (Schneider, Boston Scientific, Natick, MA)	Stainless steel
Self-expanding	Wallstent (Intratherapeutics, St. Paul, MN)	Cobalt-based alloy jacket (tantalum or platinum core)
	Gianturco (z-stent) (Cook, Inc., Bloomington, IN)	Stainless steel
	Memothermflex (Bard Access Systems, Plymouth, MN)	Nitinol (nickel, titanium alloy)

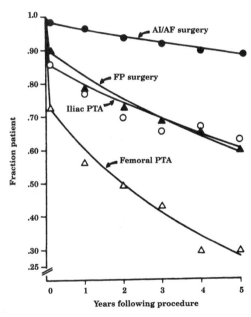

Figure 6.4. Limb patency rate among survivors of surgical procedures or percutaneous transluminal angioplasty (*PTA*) during a 5-year period. *AI/AF*, aorto-iliac or aortofemoral; *FP*, femoropopliteal. These primary results of PTA and surgery have not changed significantly since this graph was compiled in 1984. (Adapted from Doubliet P, Abrams HL. The cost of underutilization: percutaneous transluminal angioplasty for peripheral vascular disease. *N Engl J Med* 1984;310:95–102.)

and hemodynamic improvement ranges from 50% to 75% but diminishes to as low as 30% at 5 years. Smokers and diabetics have particularly poor results.

Despite these disappointing results, PTA represents a reasonable option for younger claudicants with focal superficial femoral stenosis or high-risk patients whose rest pain may be relieved more safely by PTA of one or more sequential short femoropopliteal stenoses. Angioplasty of distal popliteal and tibial vessels using smaller balloon catheters has the same limited effectiveness as PTA of superficial femoral arteries. Recanalization of noncalcified superficial femoral occlusions less than 10 cm long has been possible, but recurrent stenosis or occlusion is common. Thus, saphenous vein femoropopliteal bypass remains the most durable treatment for most superficial femoral, poplitial, and tibial artery occlusions.

C.   Combined disease. In a high-risk patient with a focal iliac stenosis and a superficial femoral artery occlusion, we usually dilate the iliac stenosis to improve inflow and then performed a distal femoropopliteal/tibial bypass to achieve limb salvage. This approach avoids an abdominal or retroperitoneal procedure such as aortofemoral or ileofemoral bypass, which is often difficult for an elderly, debilitated patient. In other cases of combined femoropopliteal and tibial disease, a standard femoropopliteal bypass can be performed and a tibial stenosis can be dilated in the operating room through the popliteal arteriotomy under fluoroscopic control.

D.   Renal artery disease. For years, balloon angioplasty of the renal arteries was more effective when performed for **fibromuscular dysplasia** than for atherosclerotic occlusive lesions. Currently however, PTA plus stenting appears to improve the initial results for proximal renal artery atherosclerotic lesions as well.

PTA is probably the treatment of choice for renovascular hypertension due to fibromuscular dysplasia (FMD). The mechanism of dilation in dysplastic stenosis is presumably stretching, shearing, and rupture of the fibrous septa. PTA is particularly attractive when the FMD extends into intrarenal branches that are difficult to repair surgically. Since FMD tends to be a disease of younger women, PTA usually delays the need for surgical revascularization until the patient is older. Initial technical success is possible in 80% to 90% of lesions, and blood pressure becomes normal or improves in slightly more than 90% of patients. In short-term follow-up (3 years) of patient with FMD, success with PTA is comparable to surgical bypass and in some patients, PTA can be successfully repeated.

Focal unilateral atherosclerotic stenosis beyond the renal aortic orifice can be dilated **without stenting** in 50% to 60% of patients, but PTA alone of bilateral atheromatous stenoses, especially ostial lesions, succeeds in less than 50% of patients. Ostial lesions are extensions of severe aortic disease that cannot be effectively dilated by a balloon. Currently, renal balloon angioplasty plus stenting appears to achieve better early results. The durability of renal artery stenting, however, has not been proven. In general, 10% to 40% of atherosclerotic lesions treated by PTA and stenting restenose within two years. Nonetheless, blood pressure is improved in 80% to 85% of atherosclerotic patients who have good renal dilation with significant improvement in the pressure gradient across the lesion. Although some have successfully improved renal function by dilating high-grade stenoses in solitary renal arteries, we have generally avoided PTA in solitary kidneys and have not found PTA to be a durable method of preserving renal function in patients with atherosclerosis.

Since the complications of renal PTA include perforation or dissection of the artery or thrombosis a vascular surgeon should be available to handle such problems when they occur. In addition, close monitoring of blood pressure is essential for at least 6 to 12 hours since significant hypotension can occur after successful PTA of high-grade renin-stimulating stenoses.

    E. Other applications. Additional uses for PTA are evolving. Success has been achieved in relieving atherosclerotic stenoses of the axillary, subclavian, and mesenteric arteries. **The dilatation of atherosclerotic carotid bifurcation lesions has been performed with increasing frequency and is currently being compared to carotid endarterectomy in a multicenter, randomized trial (CREST: Carotid Revascularization Endarterectomy versus Stent Trial).** Cerebral microembolism presents a small but real danger, and long-term results (5 to 10 years) of carotid PTA remain unknown. In contrast, high intimal-carotid fibromuscular lesions may be more suitable for either percutaneous or intraoperative balloon dilatation. In addition, the following types of anastomotic stenoses may be relieved by balloon dilatation: splenorenal or mesocaval shunts, saphenous vein grafts, renal transplants, renal dialysis angio-access, and synthetic grafts. Again, the durability of such angioplasties is often limited, but even temporary success may be important in very ill patients.

    III. Complications. The complications of PTA occur in 3% to 5% of patients. Thrombosis and local arterial dissection are the main problems associated with PTA. Dissection can frequently be treated with the immediate placement of a stent, but thrombosis requires urgent surgical intervention. Any angioplasty should be planned so that a vascular surgeon is available to manage any significant complications.

    IV. Use of antiplatelets and anticoagulants. There is no consensus regarding the administration of antiplatelet and anticoagulant agents around the time of angioplasty. A regimen that is followed by many angiographers is as follows:

    A. Antiplatelet therapy is begun 24 to 48 hours before angioplasty. Aspirin, 81 or 325 mg (i.e., one children's aspirin or one adult aspirin) daily are common doses and are generally continued for 2 to 3 months after the procedure.

    B. Systemic heparin (2,500 to 5,000 units) is administered intraarterially during the procedure.

    C. Warfarin sodium (Coumadin) therapy has been used for 1 to 3 months for angioplasties at low-flow sites such as the popliteal and tibial arteries, as well as a variety of venous sites. However, such therapy places the patient at increased risk for bleeding complications, and no prospective, randomized data to date support its long-term use after angioplasty.

THROMBOLYTIC THERAPY

Despite widespread interest in thrombolytic drugs, their role in peripheral arterial and venous disease remains relatively selective in many practices. Enthusiastic reports of the early 1980s have been balanced by more critical analyses from clinical trials. Although we have used thrombolytic agents in a variety of clinical settings, we tend to use them for indications that have been supported by these randomized trials. Their use became more limited when urokinase was removed from the marketplace in 1998 by the U.S. Food and Drug Administration. Newer agents are already filling the vacuum left when urokinase was discontinued.

Currently, alternatives to urokinase include recombinant tissue plasminogen activator (rt-PA), streptokinase, anisoylated plasminogen–streptokinase complex (APSAC), pro-urokinase, and t-PA mutants (e.g., reteplase). Since withdrawal of urokinase, rt-PA has become the primary peripheral thrombolytic agent. The use of any of these agents must be undertaken with careful consideration of their pharmacokinetics, indications, and possible complications. They are an adjunct, and not a substitute, for standard medical or surgical therapy.

I. Pharmacokinetics. These drugs are plasminogen activators that lead to clot lysis by enhancing the fibrinolytic system via conversion of plasminogen to its active form, plasmin. These fibrinolytic agents not only act on plasminogen within a clot but also on plasminogen throughout the circulation. A systemic fibrinolysis may result. **rt-PA** acts primarily on plasminogen bound to fibrin clot. Although systemic fibrinogenolysis occurs with t-PA, it happens to a less degree than that observed with streptokinase. This advantage reduces bleeding complications. **Reteplase,** a third-generation t-PA mutant, has improved clot penetration, longer half life and faster initiation of thrombolysis compared to rt-PA. **Pro-urokinase** converts Lys-plasminogen to plasmin. High concentrations of Lys-plasminogen are present in thrombus; and thus, pro-urokinase focuses its actions on fibrin complexes. **Streptokinase and APSAC,** which are seldom used anymore, must first form an activated complex with plasminogen which completes the conversion of excess plasminogen to plasmin.

These agents can be administered intravenously or intra-arterially in full systemic doses or lower regional infusions. For peripheral arterial occlusions, regional catheter delivery of the drugs into the thrombus is preferable. Rt-PA can be effective at relatively low doses (0.05 mg/kg/h for 12 hours). This dose is lower than that tried initially in the STILE trial (0.1 mg/kg/h) where higher doses were associated with more bleeding from puncture sites. Efficacy is also reasonable at even lower doses: 2 mg the first hour, followed by 1 mg/h, which further minimizes bleeding complications. For reteplase, a clot-lacing dose of 5 units is recommended and followed by 0.5 to 2.0 units/h. **(Note that rt-PA doses are mg, and reteplase doses are units.)**

Pro-urokinase is a good replacement for urokinase. Generally, 4 mg of pro-urokinase is similar to the previous single ampule urokinase dose of 240,000 units. Lacing the thrombus with 4 mg of pro-urokinase is reasonable followed by 2 to 8 mg/h. At a dose of 4 mg/h, the thrombolysis and complication rates for pro-urokinase are similar to those of urokinase at 4,000 IU/h.

Two common laboratory tests to document a lytic state are measurement of thrombin time and fibrinogen level. When clot lysis occurs, fibrin split products generally rise, also. However, changes in the constituents of the fibrinolytic system do not correlate with bleeding complications. Hemorrhagic problems usually occur at the arterial puncture site and are related to catheter size and manipulation.

The half-life for most thrombolytic drugs is short: streptokinase, 10 to 12 min; urokinase, 11 to 16 minutes; t-PA, 4 to 6 minutes; and reteplase, 15 minutes. Consequently, the effects of the drugs dissipate rapidly, although depleted fibrinogen levels may take at least 24 hours to normalize. This is especially true for pro-urokinase which has a prolonged half life in some instances, lasting for days. In our experience, the need to use (**ε-aminocaproic acid (Amacar**; Quad Pharmaceuticals, Inc., Indianapolis, IN, U.S.A.) or fibrinogen concentrates to reverse the thrombolysis rarely occurs.

Whether the thrombolytic drug should be administered concomitantly with heparin is debatable. Those who favor concomitant heparin state that it prevents clot accumulation around the infusion catheters. On the contrary, heparin may increase the risk of hemorrhage at the catheter infusion site. We generally start heparin (1,000 units/h i.v. without a loading dose) at the onset of regional lytic therapy to avoid **pericatheter thrombus formation.** For reteplase, it is recommended that heparin be avoided or administered at very low doses (e.g., 200 to 500 units/h).

II.   Contraindications. Since thrombolytic drugs can lyse recent clots anywhere in the body and result in serious bleeding, they generally should not be used in the presence of **(a) an active bleeding site, (b) a recent stroke, (c) operation or organ biopsy within the past 10 days, (d) a coagulopathy, and (e) a cerebral tumor.** Patients with acute ischemia and neuromotor impairment should undergo emergency surgical revascularization as thrombolytic therapy takes several hours and may delay reperfusion.

III.   Indications. Definite indications for lytic therapy are difficult to define. Prospective, randomized studies have confirmed benefit in selected patients with acute DVT and with pulmonary embolus (see Chap. 21). Thrombolytic infusions can alleviate acute subclavian vein thrombosis associated with central venous catheters, effort thrombosis, or thoracic outlet syndrome. Thrombolytic agents are also used commonly to clear fresh thrombus in central venous lines.

The benefits of thrombolytic therapy for arterial thrombosis are controversial. **The STILE (Surgery versus *Thrombolysis for Ischemia* of the *Lower Extremity*) trial** suggested that patients with **acute ischemia** (0 to 14 days) who were treated with thrombolysis had improved amputation-free survival and shorter hospital stays. Surgical revascularization was more effective and safer than thrombolysis for patients with **chronic ischemia** (>14 days). There was no difference in efficacy or safety between urokinase and rt-PA. However, this study was stopped early because of an increased incidence of adverse effects in patients assigned to thrombolysis. Also of importance, failure of catheter placement occurred in 28% of patients who were randomized to lysis in the STILE trial.

Another multicenter clinical trial (**TOPAS: Thrombolysis Or Peripheral Arterial Surgery**) examined patients with acute arterial occlusions of less than 14 days' duration. Although amputation-free survival between thrombolysis and surgery was not significantly different, two secondary outcomes were interesting. First, patients undergoing thrombolysis had a decreased need for open surgical procedures, a benefit that extended into the follow-up period. Second, thrombolytic results appear superior in patients with bypass graft occlusions compared to those with native artery thrombosis.

Other uses of thrombolytics for acute arterial occlusion are situations for which surgery has traditionally poor results, or for which high operative mortality makes a nonoperative approach attractive. Acutely thrombosed popliteal aneurysms with tibial artery thrombosis, thrombosis of autogenous vein grafts, and lower-extremity arterial embolism associated with myocardial infarction are examples; although our experience with thrombolysis in these situations has not been uniformly successful.

IV.   Complications. Regional thrombolytic therapy is complicated by bleeding, thrombosis, or embolism in 10% to 15% of patients. In our experience, bleeding at the angiographic catheter site has been the most common problem. Distal emboli are often small and sometimes can be resolved with continued thrombolytic administration. Nonetheless, about 5% to 10% of patients will require surgical intervention to manage these complications. Unfortunately, regional low-dose infusions have not eliminated these problems.

SELECTED READING

Ahn SS, Obrand DI, Moore WS. Transluminal balloon angioplasty, stents, and atherectomy. *Semin Vasc Surg* 1997;10:286–296.

Bettmann MA. Principles of angiography. In: Loscalzo J, Creager MA, Dzau VJ, eds. *Vascular medicine,* 2nd ed. Boston: Little, Brown, 1996:483–508.

Cambria RP, Kaufman JA, L'Italien GJ, et al. Magnetic resonance angiography in the management of lower extremity arterial occlusive disease: a prospective study. *J Vasc Surg* 1997;25:380–389.

Karch LA, Mattos MA, Henretta JP, et al. Clinical failure after percutaneous transluminal angioplasty of the superficial femoral and popliteal arteries. *J Vasc Surg* 2000;31:880–887.

Ouriel K, Veith FJ, Sasahara AA. A comparison of recombinant urokinase with vascular surgery as initial treatment for acute arterial occlusion of the legs. *N Engl J Med* 1998;338:1105–1111.

Ouriel K, Veith FJ, Sasahara AA. Thrombolysis or peripheral arterial surgery: phase I results. *J Vasc Surg* 1996;23:64–75.

Pentecost MJ, Criqui MH, Dorros G, et al. Guidelines for peripheral percutaneous transluminal angioplasty of the abdominal aorta and lower extremity vessels. *Circulation* 1994;89:511–531.

Porter JM. Thrombolysis for acute arterial occlusion of the legs. *N Engl J Med* 1998;338:1148–1150.

Strandness DE Jr, van Breda A, eds. *Vascular diseases: surgical and interventional therapy.* New York: Churchill Livingstone, 1994.

The STILE Investigators. Results of a prospective randomized trial evaluating surgery versus thrombolysis for ischemia of the lower extremity: the STILE trial. *Ann Surg* 1994;220:251.

Treiman GS, Schneider PA, Lawrence PF, et al. Does stent placement improve the results of ineffective or complicated iliac artery angioplasty? *J Vasc Surg* 1998;28:104–114.

Tumeh SS, Seltzer SE, Wang A. Computed tomography in vascular disorders. In: Loscalzo J, Creager MA, Dzau VJ, eds. *Vascular medicine*, 2nd ed. Boston: Little, Brown, 1996:509–552.

Van Jaarsveld BC, Krijnen P, Pieterman H, et al. The effect of balloon angioplasty on hypertension in atherosclerotic renal-artery stenosis. *N Engl J Med* 2000;342:1007–1114.

Preoperative Preparation

Many patients who undergo vascular surgery have multiple medical problems that increase operative risk. Preoperative preparation must include accurate assessment of anesthetic risk and optimization of specific medical problems. This chapter focuses on assessing perioperative anesthetic and cardiac risk, managing medications, optimizing pulmonary function, and controlling diabetes mellitus.

I. Perioperative risk. A key factor in achieving excellent results from elective vascular surgery, open or endovascular, is accurate assessment of anesthetic risk. Although clinical sense and experience contribute a great deal to an initial impression of anesthetic risk, more objective data also assist with assessment of operative risk.

A traditional approach to correlating a patient's preoperative physical status with anesthetic morbidity and mortality is the American Society of Anesthesiologists (ASA) classification (Table 7.1). The ASA grading system refers only to a patient's **general physical condition** and does not consider the type of anesthesia, extent of operation, or experience of the surgeon. In 1977, Goldman developed an index to evaluate perioperative cardiac risk by reviewing 1,000 patients having undergone noncardiac, general surgical procedures (Table 7.2A). When this scoring system was applied prospectively to 99 patients undergoing elective aortic surgery, the **rates of cardiac complications were higher across all classes of patients having aortic surgery than patients in Goldman's original study** (Table 7.2B). This finding reflected the incidence of significant coronary artery disease (CAD) in patients undergoing aortic reconstruction.

A. Cardiac problems are the leading cause of death after vascular surgery and occur in 3% to 6% of elective cases. Hertzer and colleagues at the Cleveland Clinic defined the prevalence of CAD in vascular surgery patients. They **showed that severe but correctable CAD was present in 25% of patients presenting for surgical management of peripheral vascular disease** (abdominal aortic aneurysm, 31%; cerebrovascular disease, 26%; arteriosclerosis obliterans of the lower limbs, 21%). Severe, correctable CAD was present in about 50% of patients with angina pectoris and 30% of patients with a previous myocardial infarction (MI).

1. Eagle and associates identified key clinical markers of increased cardiac risk in patients undergoing vascular operations: (a) angina pectoris, (b) prior MI, (c) congestive heart failure, (d) diabetes mellitus, and (e) age greater than 70 years. The risk for a perioperative cardiac event increases with the number of Eagle Criteria present (Table 7.3). With three or more criteria, the risk of a perioperative cardiac event is 30% with 77% of these patients having severe CAD on coronary angiography.

Table 7.1. Dripps–American Society of Anesthesiologists Classification

Class	Clinical description	48-h mortality(%)
1	Normal healthy	0.08
2	Mild systemic disease	0.3
3	Severe systemic disease with limited activity but not incapacitated	1.8
4	Incapacitating, constantly life-threatening systemic disease	7.8
5	Moribund, not expected to survive 24 h with or without operation	9.4
E	Denotes emergency case	—

Adapted from Vacanti CJ, Van Houton RJ, Hill RC. A statistical analysis of the relationship of physical status to postoperative mortality in 68,388 cases. *Anesth Analg* 1970;49:564–566.

Table 7.2A. Multifactorial cardiac risk index

Criteria	Points
History	
Age > 70 years	5
Myocardial infarction in past 6 months	10
Physical exam	
S_3 gallop or jugular venous distention	11
Aortic valve stenosis	3
Electrocardiogram	
Rhythm other than sinus	7
5 or more premature ventricular contraction/min	7
General status	
P_aO_2 < 60 mm Hg or P_aCO_2 > 50; K^+ < 3meq/liter or HCO_3 < 20 meq/liter; BUN > 50 or creatinine > 3 mg/dl; Chronic liver disease; Bedridden or malnourished	3
Operation	
Intraperitoneal, intrathoracic, or aortic surgery	3
Emergency operation	4
Total possible	53

BUN, blood urea nitrogen; K^+, potassium; HCO_3^-, bicarbonate; P_aO_2, partial pressure of oxygen; P_aCO_2, partial pressure of carbon dioxide.
Adapted from Goldman L, Caldera DL, Nassbaum SR, et al. Multifactorial index of cardiac risk in noncardiac surgical procedures. *N Engl J Med* 1977;297: 845–850.

Table 7.2B.   Cardiac risk index: categories of increasing risk

Class	Points	Abdominal aortic surgery		General surgical procedures		
		Patients	Cardiac complications	Patients	Cardiac complications	P value
1	0–5	56	4 (7%)	537	5 (1%)	0.01
2	6–12	35	4 (11%)	316	21 (7%)	NS
3	13–25	8	3 (38%)	130	18 (14%)	NS
4	>26	0	—	18	14 (78%)	—
Total		99	11 (12%)	1,001	44 (4%)	0.01

NS, not significant.
Adapted from Jeffrey CC, Kunsman J, Cullen DJ, Brewster DC. A prospective evaluation of cardiac risk index. *Anesthesiology* 1983;58:462–464.

Table 7.3.   Eagle criteria

Clinical criteria	Number of criteria present– % risk for cardiac event
Angina pectoris Prior myocardial infarction Congestive heart failure Diabetes mellitus Age > 70 years	0 criteria–2% risk 1 or 2–10% risk 3 or more–30% risk

From Eagle KA, Coley CM, Newell JB, et al. Combing clinical and thallium data optimizes preoperative assessment of cardiac risk before major vascular surgery. *Ann Int Med* 1989;110:859–866, with permission.

2. In 1996, the American College of Cardiology and the American Heart Association recognized the need to develop guidelines for preoperative cardiac evaluation. **They developed three classes of clinical predictors of increased perioperative cardiac risk: major, intermediate, and minor** (Table 7.4). These predictors stratify patients most likely to benefit from preoperative coronary assessment and treatment. Using these predictors, it is recommended that preoperative cardiac assessment be selective and based on the presence or absence of clinical markers.

3. Estimation of the patient's **functional capacity** is not so important in patients with major clinical predictors because all of these patients should undergo preoperative cardiac testing. However, functional capacity becomes important in sorting out which patients with intermediate or minor predictors will benefit from a cardiac assessment. Functional capacity is expressed in metabolic equivalent levels (METs). One MET is equivalent to a middle-aged person in a sitting and a resting state (Table 7.5). Cardiac risk is increased in persons who are unable to meet a 4-MET demand such as performing work around the house during daily activities. The following are examples of how clinical predictors (Table 7.4) are combined with functional capacity assessment (Table 7.5) to determine the need for preoperative cardiac testing:

    a. **Patients with major clinical predictors should see a cardiologist before the operation for definite preoperative cardiac testing (e.g., consideration of a cardiac catheterization) regardless of functional capacity.**

    b. Patients with intermediate clinical predictors and good functional capacity (>4 METs) can generally undergo **intermediate risk operation** (carotid endarterectomy) with little likelihood of perioperative MI.

    c. If these same patients with intermediate predictors and good functional capacity (>4 METs) are having a **high-risk operation** (aortic or lower extremity peripheral vascular), they should undergo noninvasive cardiac testing.

Table 7.4.   Clinical predictors of increased perioperative cardiac risk

Major
  Unstable coronary syndromes (myocardial infarction within
    30 days, unstable or severe angina)
  Decompensated congestive heart failure
  Significant arrhythmias (high-grade atrioventricular block, symp-
    tomatic ventricular arrhythmias, supraventricular arrhythmias
    with uncotrolled ventricular rate)
  Severe valvular disease

Intermediate
  Mild angina pectoris
  Prior myocardial infarction based on history or Q-waves on ECG
  Compensated or prior congestive heart failure
  Diabetes mellitus

Minor
  Advanced age
  Abnormal ECG (left ventricular hypertophy, left bundle branch
    block, ST-T abnormalities)
  Rhythm other than sinus (atrial fibrillation with controlled
    ventricular rate)
  History of stroke
  Uncontrolled systemic hypertension

ECG, electrocardiogram.
Adapted from The American College of Cardiology and the American Heart
Association. Guidelines for perioperative cardiovascular evaluation for non-
cardiac surgery. *Circulation* 1996;93:1278–1317.

Table 7.5.   Estimated energy requirements for various activities

1 MET
  Sitting at rest
  Eat, dress, or use the toilet
  Walk indoors around the house

4 METs
  Light work around the house
  Walk a block or two on level ground
  Climb flight of stairs or walk on slight incline
  Brisk walk on level ground
  Heavy work around the house
  Moderate recreational activities (golf, bowling, dancing)

10 METs
  Strenuous sports (swimming, tennis, jogging)

MET, metabolic equivalent.
Adapted from Hlatky MA, Boineau RE, Higginbotham MB, et al. A brief self-
administered questionnaire to determine functional capacity. *Am J Cardiol*
1989;64:651–654, and Fletcher GF, Balady G, Froelicher VF, et al. Exercise standards: a statement for healthcare professionals from the American Heart Association. *Circulation* 1995;91:580–615.

d. Patients with intermediate predictors and poor functional capacity (<4 METs) should undergo noninvasive cardiac testing regardless of the vascular procedure planned.

e. If the patient has no major or intermediate predictors (Table 7.4) and can meet more than 4 METs, surgery is generally safe and the patient does not need preoperative cardiac testing.

f. If the patient has no major or intermediate predictors but has poor functional capacity (<4 METs), cardiac testing should be strongly considered if an aortic or peripheral vascular procedure is planned.

4. Previous coronary evaluation or revascularization. If the patient has undergone previous cardiac evaluation within the past 2 years and the findings were favorable, then repeat testing is not needed unless the patient has experienced a change or has new cardiac symptoms. If the patient has undergone coronary revascularization within the past 5 years and has no recurrent symptoms or sign of cardiac ischemia, then further cardiac testing is generally not necessary.

5. Selective noninvasive cardiac testing can be used to determine further preoperative management, including intensified medical management, cardiac catheterization or postponement of elective surgery. Hopefully, the findings result in a recommendation to proceed with the operation. Of course, the risk of underlying pathology to the patients must also be considered. The risk of dying from a large aortic aneurysm is different than from occlusive disease of the legs causing claudication. Current methods used for preoperative noninvasive cardiac testing include:

a. Two-dimensional echocardiography (2-D echo) is an excellent technique for evaluating resting left ventricular function and valve abnormalities. Studies have shown that a left ventricular ejection fraction of less than 35% increases the risk of noncardiac surgery. Patients with severe diastolic dysfunction are also at risk. **The use of dobutamine stress testing with 2-D echo has become an important tool in patients who cannot walk or exercise.** This technique provides an opportunity to assess left ventricular motion and function under stress conditions. Of course, valvular dysfunction can be assessed at the same time.

b. Exercise stress testing with the use of a bicycle or treadmill provides significant information about a patient's functional capacity and risk of perioperative MI. Poor functional capacity associated with observed myocardial ischemia suggest a patient at very high risk for a perioperative cardiac event. Myocardial ischemia can be assessed during exercise stress testing using a 12-lead ECG looking for ST-segment changes or nuclear imaging (e.g., thallium or sestamibi). During nuclear myocardial imaging the radioisotope is given intravenously preceding the exercise test. Normally perfused myocardium absorbs the radioisotope promptly and is visualized on an initial scan following the stress test. Ischemic myocardium, beyond a fixed stenosis takes up the isotope more slowly ("cold spot") but does visualize on a delayed scan done hours later (redistribution). Previously infarcted myocardium fails to absorb the isotope on either the initial or late scan.

c. **Pharmacologic stress tests such as the dipyridamole or adenosine thallium** are performed in patients who are unable to exercise. During these tests, the pharmacologic agent (dipyridamole or adenosine) is administered intravenously, followed by an intravenous bolus of radioisotope. These drugs cause coronary vasodilatation but without increasing myocardial oxygen consumption. The rationale for these tests is that atherosclerotic vessels have fixed stenoses and cannot dilate. Thus, normally perfused myocardium is visualized on the initial scan, while ischemic myocardium takes up the isotope more slowly ("cold spot") but does visualize on a delayed scan (redistribution). Previously infarcted myocardium does not absorb the isotope on either the initial or late scan. Pharmacologic stress testing has a sensitivity of 85% to 90% and a specificity of 65% to 80% in detecting important coronary stenosis confirmed with coronary arteriography. Patients on theophylline should have this medication withdrawn for 72 hours before dipyridamole testing, since dipyridamole will not increase coronary blood flow effectively in the presence of theophylline.

d. **Ambulatory ECG monitoring.** Detection of ischemia with preoperative ECG monitoring (24 or 48 hours) has been shown to correlate with increased risk of perioperative cardiac events. In patients who have baseline ECG abnormalities, this method is not useful. In addition, this technique has not been shown to add significantly to the previously described preoperative tests.

In general, patients should be considered for coronary angiography when they have clinical predictors (Table 7.4) of severe CAD and poor functional status assessments (Table 7.5) and have evidence of ischemia during noninvasive cardiac testing.

4. **Preoperative coronary revascularization.** Following this selective approach, about 5% to 8% of patients with peripheral vascular disease will need preoperative coronary angiography and some type of revascularization. In a Mayo Clinic series of 2,452 elective abdominal aortic aneurysm repairs, just over 4% of patients underwent preoperative coronary revascularization. In most cases, the revascularization required coronary artery bypass grafting (CABG), but in 15% of cases coronary angioplasty was sufficient. This entire group underwent aneurysm repair without any major cardiac events. The average time between coronary revascularization and aortic surgery was 10 weeks for those having CABG and 10 days for those undergoing coronary angioplasty.

In our experience this with selective approach, operative mortality for abdominal aortic aneurysm repair has been about 1% to 2% for patients with a negative history of CAD and 3% to 5% for those with a positive history of CAD.

5. Conduction abnormalities must be defined before operation. First-degree atrioventricular block, right bundle branch block, left bundle branch block, and bifascicular or trifascicular block are usually chronic conditions and seldom progress to complete heart block. Thus, temporary pacing is usually not required for these conduction disturbances. In contrast, patients with second-degree, Mobitz type II or, third-degree atrioventricular block should have perioperative pacing support. Whether such pacing is temporary or permanent largely depends upon the discretion of the cardiology and anesthesia consultants. Permanent pacemakers are usually required for complete heart block or intermittent complete heart block.

Placement of central venous catheters or monitoring devices (e.g., Swan–Ganz catheter) places a patient with left bundle branch block at risk for induced right bundle branch block and can precipitate complete heart block. This unusual possibility should be recognized and pacing capability made available prior to placement of such catheter in patients with left bundle branch block.

Patients with **implanted permanent cardiac pacemakers** may present a problem during the operation as electrocautery may adversely affect the pulse generator. To prevent this possibility the rate of the pacemaker can be converted to a fixed-rate prior to the operation. Complexities involving the operation of pacemakers mandate that the surgeon and anesthesiologist consult preoperatively with the patient's cardiologist to establish a safe perioperative management plan.

B. Carotid occlusive disease is present in 10% to 20% of patients presenting with aortic or femoropopliteal atherosclerosis and abdominal aortic aneurysms. Often the carotid disease is asymptomatic and detected initially by cervical bruits. Controversy continues over whether asymptomatic carotid disease should be ignored or whether carotid bruits should be evaluated by noninvasive testing and selective arteriography to ascertain the exact nature of the lesions. Most studies suggest that there is no significant increase in risk of perioperative stroke in patients with asymptomatic bruits. These studies, however, do not define the anatomy of the carotid lesions and leave doubt about whether high-grade (greater than 80%) bilateral carotid lesions may increase stroke risk.

Our approach to asymptomatic cervical bruits in patients facing elective aortic or coronary reconstruction is noninvasive classification of the degree of stenosis by ocular pneumoplethysmography (OPG) or duplex scanning. High-grade lesions (greater than 80% and bilateral) with poorly compensated distal cerebral pressures (positive OPG result) are generally considered for carotid endarterectomy before elective aortic or coronary surgery. Obviously, patients with large or symptomatic aneurysms, unstable angina pectoris, or threatening leg ischemia must have these more pressing problems operated urgently, accepting the risk of stroke. After the more critical operation, elective repair of asymptomatic hemodynamically significant carotid disease can be considered.

C. Pulmonary complications (Table 7.6) are a leading cause of postoperative morbidity and mortality. Studies have

Table 7.6. Pulmonary risk reduction strategies

Preoperative
Smoking cessation for at least 8 weeks
Treat airflow obstruction in patients with COPD or asthma
(Beta-agonist inhalers)
Antibiotic and delay elective surgery if respiratory infection is
present
Patient education regarding lung expansion

Intraoperative
Limit duration of surgery to <3 h
Use of epidural anesthesia
Substitute less invasive procedures when possible

Postoperative
Deep-breathing exercises or incentive spirometry
Continuous positive airway pressure if mechanically ventilated
Epidural anesthesia

COPD, chronic obstructive pulmonary disease.
Adapted from Smetana GW. Preoperative pulmonary evaluation. *N Engl J Med*
1999;340:937–944.

shown that pulmonary complications are at least as common as
or more common than cardiac complications. Most patients
undergoing vascular operation have a degree of chronic lung
disease from smoking.

1. The initial **history and physical examination** will
identify the patients at highest risk of pulmonary problems.
They often are dyspneic at rest or report dyspnea with minimal exertion or exhibit chronic cough and sputum production.
Other typical findings include a hyperinflated chest with dis-
tant breath sounds and use of accessory neck and abdominal
muscles to assist with breathing. Patients with reactive airway disease may have wheezing. A simple bedside assessment
of the degree of airway obstructive disease can be made by
having the patient take a deep inspiration and then expire as
quickly as possible while the examiner listens with a stethoscope. Normal complete expiratory time is less than 3 seconds.
For patients with obstructive lung disease, this time is often
4 to 8 seconds. This simple bedside test also can be used to
monitor clinical improvement during bronchodilator therapy.

2. A **chest x-ray** may reveal important anatomic information such as an occult lung cancer, cardiomegaly, interstitial
fibrosis, or giant lung blebs.

3. Pulmonary function testing and measurement of
arterial blood gases need not be routine but are indicated
for patients with chronic lung disease. One of the most reliable predictors of high pulmonary risk is the forced expiratory volume at 1 second (FEV_1). Significant postoperative
pulmonary complications can be expected in patients with an
FEV_1 of less than 15 mL/kg or less than 1 L. If the FEV_1 is less
than 70% of that predicted, the spirometry should be repeated
after administration of an inhaled bronchodilator. An increase
of at least 15% in FEV_1 indicates that preoperative bron-

chodilator therapy may enhance pulmonary function. This improvement may be significant for the patient who has marginal lung function and requires elective surgery. Although measurement of arterial blood gases need not be routine, baseline values may help in patients with severe chronic obstructive pulmonary disease (COPD). For example, an elevated P_aCO_2 (>45 mm Hg) is associated with increased perioperative pulmonary risk.

D. Renal function should be checked routinely by serum creatinine level. Many vascular patients take diuretics, which cause intravascular volume depletion. This chronic dehydration places them at increased risk for acute renal failure after angiography or operation. Consequently, rehydration appears to be the single most important factor in reducing postoperative renal failure.

E. Diabetes mellitus, a common metabolic disease of many vascular patients, often becomes difficult to control when patients are hospitalized for diagnostic tests, treatment, and surgery. When diabetics enter the hospital, their activity level decreases and diet usually changes. Consequently, the insulin administered should be adjusted. Wide swings in blood sugar levels may result, especially when patients receive insulin but miss meals because of diagnostic tests or other preoperative preparations.

F. Poor nutritional status has been correlated with increased postoperative complications, sepsis, and mortality. Few physicians think of vascular patients as being poorly nourished. Nonetheless, certain vascular patients tend to be malnourished and need repletion of nutritional deficits.

1. Chronic intestinal angina from mesenteric ischemia leads to fear of eating and subsequent weight loss. This weight loss usually occurs over several months and may amount to 20 to 50 lb in some patients.

2. Severe lung disease requires extra expenditure of energy because accessory neck and abdominal muscles are used to assist with breathing. Pulmonary cachexia often is obvious on examination. Because the weight loss usually is insidious, the severe degree of malnutrition may not be appreciated.

3. Multiple complicated vascular procedures or serious postoperative infections also place increased caloric demands on the body. Again, the weight loss may be gradual and the severity of the malnutrition may be missed.

4. Chronic alcoholism and associated liver disease may result not only in poor nutrition but also in altered clotting function. If hypersplenism is present, the platelet count may be low. Liver-dependent clotting factor deficiency and thrombocytopenia can be life-threatening problems in patients who require extensive thoracic or abdominal aortic surgery. Patients with chronic liver disease also become more hypoalbuminemic in the postoperative period and may develop peripheral edema, ascites, or anasarca.

5. Patients in the clinical categories above must be nutritionally assessed and may need parenteral or enteral supplemental feedings before or after surgery. A clinical "eyeball" evaluation of nutritional status is unreliable in assessing high-versus low-risk patients. Several objective **criteria for supplemental nutrition** are:

    a. **Weight loss** of 10% in the past 30 days.

    b. **Failure to reestablish** adequate nutrition (35 calories/kg/day) within 5 to 10 days after surgery.

    c. **Compromised immune response** indicated by anergy to common skin tests or total lymphocyte count of less than 800.

    d. Preoperative **serum albumin** of less than 3 mg/100 mL.

II.   Cardiovascular medications. Nearly all patients requiring vascular care are on various combinations of cardiovascular medications. In general, these medications are continued until the day of the operation and remain unchanged following treatment. There are, however, a few points worth mentioning.

    A.   Antihypertensives should be continued until the time of operation, although bed rest, smoking cessation and hospital diet often permit a reduction in the dosage.

    B.   Chronic diuretic therapy depletes both intravascular volume and total body potassium stores. Diuretics generally should be reduced or discontinued 24 to 48 hours preoperatively and potassium replacement should be initiated.

    C.   Beta blockers being administered for hypertension or heart disease should not be abruptly discontinued. Acute withdrawal has been associated with exacerbation of coronary events such as angina, ventricular tachycardia, and fatal MI.

    D.   Antiarrhythmic drugs should be continued until the operation. Their suppressing effect on the myocardium may require alteration in doses of other drugs given during anesthesia.

III.   Optimizing pulmonary function. In patients with chronic lung disease, optimizing pulmonary function before the operation can decrease the incidence of postoperative respiratory complications at least twofold. Preoperative preparation may require that the patient stop smoking, that antibiotics for bronchitis and bronchodilators be administered, and that the patient be instructed in deep breathing.

    A. Ideally, **smoking** should be stopped eight weeks before surgery so that cilia regeneration can occur and any bronchorrhea can be resolved. However, this goal is difficult to attain in many patients who are anxious before hospitalization. Although some patients are too anxious to stop completely, most can be convinced to reduce cigarette consumption before operation. A reasonable request is to reduce smoking to half a pack (ten cigarettes) per day with a commitment to stop when admitted to the hospital. Subsequently, we enforce nonsmoking on admission, treat any anxiety with sedatives, and begin intensive pulmonary care before surgery in patients with severe lung disease.

    B.   Respiratory infections in patients with COPD are caused by *Streptococcal* or *Haemophilus* species and ampicillin, or amoxicillin, (500 mg p.o. t.i.d.-q.i.d.) are effective in treating. Importantly, any respiratory infection must be adequately treated before elective surgery even if this means a delay.

C. **Bronchodilators** remain the cornerstone of drug treatment for patients with COPD. However, we often find that COPD patients are not on optimum doses of inhaled bronchodilators when they enter the hospital for elective surgery. Initial bronchodilator therapy is usually an inhaled beta-agonist delivered by a metered-dose inhaler or nebulization three or four times daily. If bronchospasm is severe, oral or intravenous aminophylline can be considered. Theophylline may also improve the strength of the diaphragm and suppress fatigue in patients with fixed airway obstruction.

D. **Deep breathing maneuvers after surgery decrease the incidence of pulmonary complications.** Preoperative instruction has been shown to be more effective than waiting to teach the proper method until the early postoperative period, when the patient is having incisional pain. Different types of incentive spirometers are popular methods of achieving deep breathing, but the key to deep inspiration is patient motivation, nursing instruction, and adequate pain control after the operation.

IV. **Diabetes mellitus** can be difficult to manage in the perioperative period, when glucose intake is varied and physiologic stress high. In general, stress results in a state of insulin resistance due to increased levels of glucagon, epinephrine, cortisol, and growth hormone. To avoid hypo- or hyperglycemia, the clinician should attempt to maintain the patient's blood glucose level in the range of 150 to 250 mg/100 mL.

A. The **best method to monitor** insulin therapy remains measurement of blood glucose levels. Testing urine glucose without correlation with blood sugars is an inaccurate means of determining insulin requirements, as the incidence of falsely high and falsely low tests is so great.

B. The **perioperative drug management** of the diabetic depends on whether the patient's usual therapy has been insulin or oral hypoglycemics.

1. **Patients who are insulin-dependent** and scheduled for surgery early in the morning (before 9 a.m.) should not take their insulin the morning of surgery. They may be asked to bring their insulin with them if they are a morning admission. The blood sugar level is checked on arrival at the operating room. If the blood sugar is more than 100 mg/dL, the patient should receive one-half the usual intermediate-acting insulin. If the blood sugar is less than 100 mg/dL, the patient should receive a dextrose containing solution once an intravenous line is established.

In general, blood glucose levels are managed with intermittent doses of intravenous regular insulin and frequent checks during the operation.

2. **Insulin-taking patients who are NPO** ("nothing by mouth") after breakfast and scheduled for a procedure later in the day should be asked to take one-half the usual dose of intermediate-acting insulin instead of the full dose **(no regular insulin)** at breakfast.

3. Patients taking oral hypoglycemic agents should be advised **not** to take the oral agents on the morning of surgery.

4. The so-called **brittle diabetic** can have wide variations in blood sugars despite frequent glucose monitoring and little change in insulin dose. In this setting blood glucose is optimally controlled with a continuous intravenous insulin drip. An infusion of 1 to 4 units of regular insulin per hour generally results in good control. In the acute postoperative period, various sliding scales exist that allow the infusion of insulin to change according to blood glucose levels. **Prolonged, severe hypoglycemia can cause severe neurologic damage and must be avoided if one is to use continuous intravenous insulin.** To avoid an accidental rapid insulin infusion, we recommend mixing only 10 units of regular insulin in 250 mL of D5W or D5NS and infusing at a rate of 25 to 100 mL/h (1 to 4 units), with control by an infusion pump. One should also infuse a dextrose containing solution when using an insulin drip.

V.   Preoperative weight reduction. Obesity makes operative dissection more difficult than usual, especially in the abdomen and retroperitoneum. In our experience, it also increases wound complications in the groin. Consequently, we insist that obese candidates for **elective** vascular surgery lose excess weight. Obviously, obese patients who require urgent treatment for symptomatic aneurysms or limb salvage cannot wait to lose excess weight before an operation. However, moderately obese patients who require elective operation for claudication or asymptomatic aneurysms generally may be followed until excess weight is lost.

Patients who are 15 to 40 lb above their ideal weight are considered moderately obese. Morbidly obese patients (100 lb overweight) seldom can be expected to lose substantial weight before elective surgery. Therefore, the benefits of elective abdominal or extremity vascular reconstruction in excessively obese patients must be weighed carefully against the increased risks of perioperative complications.

Occasionally, some physicians remark that weight reduction in preoperative patients is extremely difficult to achieve and may be unsafe. They are concerned that insistence on weight loss may discourage the patient from returning to them for further treatment. The added cost of dietary consultation often is mentioned. Finally, the danger of excess weight loss and protein catabolism before major surgery also is raised as an objection to preoperative weight reduction.

In our experience, safe preoperative weight reduction can be accomplished in approximately eight of ten moderately obese patients who require an elective operation. Ideally, we strive to bring the patient's weight to within 10% of ideal weight. The following guidelines for preoperative weight reduction are effective:

A. The **importance of preoperative weight reduction** as a means to facilitate operative dissection and to decrease postoperative complications must be explained to the patient. We emphasize that elective surgery can be safely postponed until excess weight is lost.

B. A **definite time period** for the diet is proposed and a tentative surgery date is selected. Most moderately obese patients will need to lose 10 to 30 lb. To ensure safe, gradual weight reduction, we recommend a weight loss of 1 to 2 lb/week. Thus, elective surgery is postponed for 6 to 8 weeks for most patients. Obviously, some patients will need 3 to 6 months of dieting. We also have found it important to recheck patients every 6 to 8 weeks to ensure that they are losing weight and not having any problems with the diet.

C. The diet should be low-calorie (800 to 1,200 calories/day) but **balanced.** We use a relatively low-fat, low-cholesterol **1,000-calorie diet.** Strict starvation or diets that do not have a balance of carbohydrates, protein, and fat are not safe for older patients with vascular disease. Adherence to such diets may result in severe catabolism and deficiencies in vitamins, minerals, and trace elements.

D. Although consultation with a dietician may be helpful in selected cases, a simple **explanation of the diet** by the physician and office nurse generally will suffice and saves the patient the extra time and cost of a dietary consultation. In our experience, patients seem to respond best to the firm insistence on and explanation of a diet by the primary surgeon.

E. **A specified amount of weight** to lose is marked on the front page of the diet. Patients are instructed to take a baseline reading of their weight on a home scale and then to lose the specified weight.

F. **Alcoholic beverages** are commonly an overlooked source of calories. This fact should be emphasized to patients who drink regularly, as they usually must reduce alcohol intake to lose weight.

G. It is extremely difficult to lose weight and stop **smoking** at the same time. Consequently, we allow chronic smokers to continue some smoking while they diet. We make an agreement with the patient that smoking will stop when the patient is hospitalized for elective surgery. Some physicians criticize this relatively late discontinuance of smoking; however, this approach usually results in successful weight reduction and has not led to increased pulmonary morbidity in our experience.

SELECTED READING

Eagle KA, Brundage BH, Chaitman BR, et al. Guidelines for perioperative cardiovascular evaluation for noncardiac surgery: an abridged version of the report of the American College of Cardiology/ American Heart Association Task Force on Practice Guidelines. *Mayo Clin Proc* 1997;72:524–531.

Eagle KA, Brundage BH, Chaitman BR, et al. Guidelines for perioperative cardiovascular evaluation for noncardiac surgery. Report of the American College of Cardiology/American Heart Association Task Force on Practice Guidelines. *Circulation* 1996;93: 1278–1317.

Eagle KA, Froehlich JB. Reducing cardiovascular risk in patients undergoing noncardiac surgery. *N Engl J Med* 1996;335:1761–1763.

Elmore JR, Hallett JW Jr, Gibbons RJ, et al. Myocardial revascularization before abdominal aortic aneurysmorrhaphy: Effect of coronary angioplasty. *Mayo Clin Proc* 1993;68:637–641.

Hertzer NR, Beven EG, Young JR, et al. Coronary artery disease in peripheral vascular patients: a classification of 1000 coronary angiograms and results of surgical management. *Ann Surg* 1984;199: 223–233.

Hoeg JM. Evaluating coronary heart disease risk. Tiles in the mosaic. *JAMA* 1997;277:1387–1390.

Inzquierdo-Porrera AM, Gardner AW, Powell CC, et al. Effects of exercise rehabilitation on cardiovascular risk factors in older patients with peripheral arterial occlusive disease. *J Vasc Surg* 2000;31:670–677.

L'Italien GJ, Paul SD, Hendel RC, et al. Development and validation of a Bayesian model for perioperative cardiac risk assessment in a cohort of 1,081 vascular surgical candidates. *JACC* 1996;27:779–786.

Mangano DT, Goldman L. Preoperative assessment of patients with known or suspected coronary disease. *N Engl J Med* 1995;333:1750–1756.

Samain E, Farah E, Leseche G, et al. Guidelines for perioperative cardiac evaluation from the American College of Cardiology/American Heart Association task force are effective for stratifying cardiac risk before aortic surgery. *J Vasc Surg* 2000;31:971–979.

Smetana GW. Preoperative pulmonary evaluation. *N Engl J Med* 1999;340:937–944.

Perioperative Management

After the initial patient evaluation and preoperative preparation, the next phase of management may involve an operation. Perioperative management encompasses not only anesthesia but also vascular monitoring and early postoperative care. A carefully administered anesthetic is just as important as an appropriate and technically successful operation. The vascular surgery team should understand at least the basic concepts of anesthesia for vascular patients. To avoid early postoperative failures and reoperation, those caring for the vascular surgery patient must understand techniques of vascular monitoring that will detect perioperative problems. Finally, the vascular surgery team must have an understanding of postoperative cardiorespiratory support and common multiorgan dysfunctions that may threaten patient survival.

This section emphasizes the principles of perioperative management that we have found useful. This section should be especially valuable to surgical house staff and nurses, who often are the first to recognize and treat perioperative problems.

Anesthesia

Improved anesthetic management has been a key factor in the reduction of operative morbidity and mortality in vascular surgery. The preoperative assessment of the patient and his or her comorbidities form the basis for selecting a successful anesthetic. The anesthesia team must be aware of the aspects of the operation that are most stressful to cardiac, cerebral, and renal function in order to manage the patient effectively. Communication between the surgery and the anesthesia teams must be maintained for the smooth conduct of any major vascular operation.

This chapter focuses on carotid and aortic operations, since these arterial reconstructions represent the most difficult challenges in anesthetic management. Appropriate anesthesia for other arterial and venous operations is discussed briefly.

I. Perioperative physiologic monitoring. Perioperative physiologic monitoring provides objective data critical to assessment and maintenance of multiorgan function. The magnitude of the operation and the patient's medical condition determine the extent of such monitoring. It should be recognized that information gathered from invasive monitoring may be misleading or imprecise and may not influence the ultimate outcome of the patient. It is important to understand the limitations of such monitoring.

A. All patients should have at least one large-caliber (14- or 16-gauge) intravenous line and electrocardiographic (leads II and V5), temperature, and blood pressure monitoring. A urinary catheter and collection system to measure hourly urine output is needed for operations that last longer than 2 to 3 hours.

B. Major vascular cases usually require the addition of an indwelling radial artery line and a central venous catheter. The arterial line allows easier blood sampling for measurements of arterial blood gases, hematocrit, sodium, potassium, and glucose, as well as continuous observation of the systemic blood pressure. The central venous line allows measurements of central venous pressure and central infusion of medications.

C. Pulmonary capillary wedge pressure measured with a **Swan–Ganz pulmonary artery catheter (PAC)** is a reliable guide to left-sided (left atrium and left ventricle) filling pressures and left ventricular function. The PAC also allows the measurement of cardiac output and some provide mixed venous oxygen saturations (SvO_2) as an indicator of oxygen delivery and end-organ extraction. Furthermore, some PACs allow rapid initiation of ventricular pacing if necessary. **Consequently, patients with ventricular dysfunction, unstable angina, or recent myocardial infarction generally require a Swan–Ganz pulmonary artery catheter.** Some anesthesiologists prefer a PAC in all major aortic reconstructions where an aortic cross-clamp is necessary and blood loss may be significant. If there is question about the need for a PAC, the surgeon

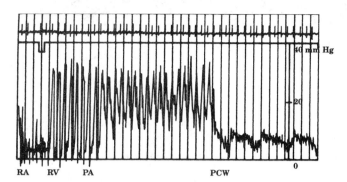

Figure 8.1.   Swan–Ganz pulmonary catheter tracings as the catheter is advanced from the right atrium (*RA*) through the right ventricle (*RV*) and pulmonary artery (*PA*) to a wedged position in a pulmonary artery (*PCW*). The pressures shown are within normal limits. Abnormal values are discussed in the text.

and anesthesiologist should discuss the indications for such monitoring and the surgeon's operative plan. When it is unclear whether a Swan–Ganz catheter will be needed, an introducer can be placed in a central vein at the start of the operation allowing for a PAC to be placed if necessary. Figure 8.1 illustrates the pressure tracings as the Swan–Ganz catheter is floated through the right heart to a wedge position in a pulmonary artery. The use of pulmonary artery pressures in managing cardiac function is discussed further in Chapter 10. Although there are complications related to the use of a PAC, most of the risks are incurred with the process of obtaining central venous access. Therefore, once the decision to place a central venous catheter has been made, the decision to use a PAC is less difficult.

Oximetric pulmonary artery catheters allow continuous monitoring and display of Svo$_2$. This measurement is an early indicator of change in the patient's physiologic course and it may be used to follow the effectiveness of specific interventions. A decrease in Svo$_2$ indicates worsening oxygen delivery (e.g., myocardial infarction) or increased end-organ extraction (e.g., sepsis). Svo$_2$ of less than 60% mandates a reassessment of the patient looking for a source or explanation of this critical level. Svo$_2$ can then be followed as an early measure of treatment success (e.g., the initiation of an inotropic agent). Oximetric pulmonary artery catheters are significantly more expensive than the standard catheters. Therefore, they should be placed in cases where such physiologic detail will be put to appropriate and effective use to improve patient care and not just to record another number in the chart.

Despite all the physiologic information that this technology provides, the value of the Swan–Ganz pulmonary artery catheter is debatable as some prospective studies have shown its routine use not to improve mortality.

D. Pulse oximeters, which attach to a finger or toe, are also used to continuously determine arterial oxygen saturation of hemoglobin. Pulse oximetry functions by positioning any pulsating arterial vascular bed between a two-wavelength light source and a detector. A familiar plethysmograph wave form results. Because the detected pulsatile waveform is produced from arterial blood, the amplitude of each wavelength related to reduced versus oxyhemoglobin allows continuous beat-to-beat calculation of arterial hemoglobin oxygen saturation. The instrument's ability to accurately calculate saturation can be impaired by (a) hypothermia, (b) hypotension (mean blood pressure, <50 mm Hg), and (c) vasoconstriction by drugs. The placement of an additional pulse oximeter probe on another site is recommended (alternate extremity or more central location such as ear or nose).

E. Transesophageal echocardiography (TEE) is another option for monitoring cardiac function in the operating room. It is the most sensitive method to detect myocardial ischemia manifest by the development of myocardial wall motion abnormalities. TEE is also able to more accurately assess ventricular filling. This method requires additional expertise and training to gain a working understanding of the technique and the information provided.

F. Core temperature monitoring is critical for all major aortic or vascular cases that last for more than 2 to 3 hours. Hypothermia (<35°C) is associated with risk for cardiac events including ventricular tachycardia. The mechanism for this is related to an elevated level of circulating catecholamines. In addition, hypothermia leads to a systemic coagulopathy by adversely effecting the enzymes which participate in the clotting cascade. Esophageal, intravenous or bladder thermistor monitoring are all generally accurate. Warming the operating-room to 75°F before the patient enters and using warm-air plastic drapes (Bair Hugger; Augustine Medical, Inc., Eden Prairie, MN, U.S.A.) are helpful in maintaining core temperature.

II. Patient positioning. Positioning of the patient on the operating table is critical if pressure-related injuries of the skin are to be avoided. The most common pressure-related problems in our experience have been heel ulcers. These pressure sores generally occur on the lateral heel. They usually affect patients with impaired lower-extremity arterial perfusion or with a prolonged ischemic time during the operation. Pressure-related heel ulcers can be prevented by elevating the legs on soft towels so that they do not rest on the operating table, or by placing a soft pad under the heels.

Another potential problem occurs when the upper extremities are tucked along the side of the patient, and pressure from the edge of the operating table causes an ulnar neuropathy. This bothersome problem can be prevented by gently wrapping the elbow region with a soft pad to keep pressure off of the ulnar nerve.

Positioning of the head, eyes, ears, and neck should also be performed with care. Patients with carotid disease or musculoskeletal conditions such as arthritis may be particularly susceptible to injury secondary to poor positioning. Gentle positioning of the neck in the neutral position is best when possible and the eyes should always be taped to avoid abrasions.

Any limitations of range of motion involving the neck or extremities should be known before positioning the patient. Positioning after induction of anesthesia should not involve any motion that goes beyond what the patient can achieve while conscious. The risk of injury to the skin should be minimized by carefully accounting for the electrocardiogram (ECG) leads, catheter connectors, and jewelery that may be in contact with the skin of the patient. **The patient's skin should not be directly exposed to metal.**

III.   Aortic surgery. The determinants of safe anesthesia for aortic surgery include careful control of the patient's blood pressure, intravascular volume, and myocardial performance within context of the patient's baseline. As these patients commonly have coronary artery disease, hypotension or hypertension can result in myocardial ischemia. Therefore, the anesthesiologist must be aware of the stages of the operation and their hemodynamic consequences. **From the surgeon's standpoint, he or she must be aware of specific organ system performance and response during the operation as this often provides insight into the response of these systems in the postoperative period.** Some of the most useful information regarding the patient's physiologic responses can be obtained during the operation (e.g., during transesophageal echocardiography). Furthermore, the surgeon must understand how the anesthesia team manages the patient during critical parts of the operation and be willing to contribute information that he or she deems important.

Anesthesia may consist of a regional technique, a mixed regional and general technique, or a general anesthetic technique. Some centers have satisfactorily used continuous epidural anesthesia with a mixture of local anesthetics (e.g., bupivacaine) and narcotics supplemented with general anesthesia and endotracheal intubation. Epidural catheters appear to be safe in vascular patients who will be heparinized after the catheter insertion for their vascular operation. Epidural or subdural hematomas are a very rare complication, provided an atraumatic puncture is made. We have also found that a continuous epidural narcotic (e.g., fentanyl) infusion is a safe and highly effective method of controlling early postoperative pain for 48 to 72 hours after abdominal or lower-extremity operations. General endotracheal anesthesia may offer the greatest control of the hemodynamics and respiratory system for patients with significant pulmonary and cardiac disease. Although balanced general anesthesia with nitrous oxide, narcotics, relaxants, and barbiturates provides excellent operative conditions, a small amount of an inhalation agent or an intravenous vasodilator frequently is required to manage hypertension. An epidural anesthesia may influence fluid requirements and adversely effect blood pressure.

A.   Causes of hypotension. Unexplained hypotension during the operation must be met with a calm but rapid assessment of the patient for possible causes. During this period the surgeon should stop what he or she is doing.

1.   Palpation of the aorta should be performed to confirm what the anesthesia monitors indicate. If there is a strong aortic pulse and the monitors do not confirm this, attention should be focused on the monitoring systems (e.g., compression or occlusion of the arterial line).

2. Myocardial infarction or arrhythmia should be indicated by findings on ECG or TEE.

3. Tension pneumothorax from preoperative line placement will be accompanied by distended neck veins and high airway pressures.

4. Cardiac tamponade from right atrial injury during preoperative line placement will also be accompanied by distended neck veins but more normal airway pressures initially.

5. Malignant hyperthermia is a rare but devastating complication accompanied by increases end-tidal CO_2 and in the patient's core temperature.

6. Manipulation or withdrawal of the intestines from the abdomen may also cause hypotension which usually can be corrected with a fluid bolus or a one-time dose of ephedrine or a phenylephrine.

7. Blood pressure may decrease when the inferior vena cava is compressed or retracted for exposure of the lumbar sympathetic chain during a lumbar sympathectomy. Compression of the inferior vena cava results in decreased venous return to the heart and the surgeon should inform the anesthesia team prior to performing this maneuver.

B. One of the most stressful steps of the operation for the myocardium is the **aortic cross-clamp,** which acutely increases afterload. Blood pressure and pulmonary capillary wedge pressures increase and the ECG often shows ST-segment changes or ventricular irritability. The healthy heart can tolerate these changes fairly well, however, the impaired heart is at a high risk. In the case of a severely impaired heart, the blood pressure and cardiac output may actually decrease. Therefore, immediately after aortic cross-clamp, afterload must be reduced by titration of peripheral vasodilators such as sodium nitroprusside or nitroglycerin. Inotropic support should be added if necessary to stabilize the hemodynamics.

With aortic cross-clamp, renal cortical blood flow and urine output may decrease in spite of an infrarenal clamp placement. This effect can usually be prevented by establishing a diuresis before the cross-clamp with hydration and mannitol (12.5 to 25.0 g intravenously). The preoperative pulmonary wedge pressure and left ventricular function must be considered when determining whether the patient is adequately volume-loaded. If this treatment is not effective, 10 to 20 mg of furosemide (Lasix, Hoechst Marion Roussel, Kansas City, MO, U.S.A.) is given. During any diuresis, potassium must be carefully monitored and supplemented to prevent serious arrhythmias that result from hypokalemia. Hypokalemia during the cross-clamp must be cautiously treated as decreased renal function after restoration of flow may impair potassium excretion. Once again, the surgeon should inform the anesthesia team before placing or releasing the aortic cross-clamp.

C. Blood loss

1. Significant blood loss may occur when the aneurysm sac is opened after aortic clamping. Back-bleeding from lumbar arteries and the inferior mesenteric artery can be brisk. While these vessels are being oversewn,, additional fluid resuscitation may be necessary and should be mentioned to the anesthesia team if bleeding is excessive.

2. Blood loss is usually substantial enough in aortic cases to require transfusion. The alternative to bank blood transfusions is **autotransfusion.** When more than 2,500 mL is autotransfused, clotting factors and platelets must be checked and administered as necessary. The use of the thromboelastogram (TEG) can also provide a qualitative analysis of the ability of the blood to clot, which can be used to guide platelet and factor replacement. Empirical transfusion of blood products may be necessary but should be carefully considered. Fresh plasma and platelets may be especially important initially when the graft is opened. Failure to replenish these factors may result in problematic anastomotic, graft, or retroperitoneal hemorrhage. The hemoglobin used to initiate transfusion of red blood cells should be determined on an individual basis for each patient based on the severity of underlying diseases, age, and surgery. **The surgeon and anesthesiologist should communicate openly about the transfusion of blood and blood products.**

D. Fluid replacement. Throughout the procedure, adequate amounts of fluid must be given continuously. Fluid replacement should be guided by indices of ventricular filling and maintenance of a good cardiac index. The large incision, prolonged exposure of the abdominal contents, and the usual blood loss create large fluid shifts. Lactated Ringer's solution is administered at 750 to 1,000 mL/h, in addition to blood and colloid as needed. Patients can become hypothermic (<34°C) during long operations; therefore, blood and fluids should be warmed. In addition, we prevent hypothermia by using an upper-body heating tent (Bair Hugger) during the operation. (This special heating blanket can also be used in the early postoperative period to rewarm the trunk and lower extremities.)

E. One of the most critical times of the entire operation is at aortic unclamping. Profound hypotension can occur. The surgeon should warn the anesthesia team several minutes before unclamping. Hypotension can be minimized by intravascular volume loading, avoidance of myocardial depressants and vasodilators as well as inhalation agents prior to release of the cross-clamp. Opening the graft slowly also may minimize sudden changes in blood pressure. Occasionally, small amounts of sodium bicarbonate will be necessary, but acid metabolites from ischemic limbs are not the primary cause of "declamping shock." Generally, we also give intravenous calcium chloride, which rapidly increases myocardial contractility, cardiac output, and blood pressure. **If one reverses heparin with protamine at the end of the operation, it must be administered slowly (e.g., use an initial test dose) as it can cause hypotension or bradycardia. In rare cases, protamine may lead to severe bronchospasm and hemodynamic instability.**

IV. Carotid artery surgery. Anesthesia for carotid artery surgery must be administered skillfully to avoid dangerous swings in blood pressure and cerebral perfusion. The surgeon must understand basic control mechanisms for cerebral blood flow, methods of monitoring cerebral perfusion, and the effects of different anesthetic agents on cerebral metabolism. The surgeon must keep the anesthesia team informed of operative steps that affect blood pressure or interrupt carotid blood flow.

   A. Cerebral blood flow. The major determinants of cerebral blood flow in the normal brain are:

1. **Local metabolic factors.** Accumulation of local metabolic products causes vasodilation of adjacent blood vessels and increased local flow.
2. **Arterial oxygen tension (P_aO_2).** Within wide limits, P_aO_2 does not significantly influence cerebral blood flow.
3. **Arterial carbon dioxide tension (P_aCO_2)** affects cerebral blood flow throughout its physiologic range. As P_aCO_2 is decreased, cerebral blood flow also decreases, and vice versa.
4. **Cerebral perfusion pressure** (mean arterial pressure minus intracranial pressure or venous pressure). Within wide ranges of perfusion pressure, cerebral blood flow is maintained in a steady state by autoregulation.

   In diseased states, these control mechanisms are altered. Autoregulation is altered so that the acceptable mean arterial pressure is different and the point at which autoregulation becomes lost is also altered. Blood vessels in ischemic brain are maximally vasodilated, and therefore blood flow becomes a direct function of perfusion pressure. During carotid clamping, normotension to slight hypertension should optimize cerebral perfusion. In addition, normocarbia to slight hypocarbia seems preferable. Raising the P_aCO_2 may dilate normal brain arterioles and increase intracranial pressure so that flow is diverted from ischemic to normal areas (intracranial steal).

   B. Monitoring. In our experience, the best method to assess adequate cerebral perfusion during carotid cross-clamping has been a continuous electroencephalogram (EEG). Carotid artery stump pressures may not correlate with the EEG changes. Chapter 11 describes indications for use of an intraluminal shunt.

   C. Anesthetic agents. The goals of anesthesia for carotid surgery include (a) consistent blood pressure control, (b) regulation of P_aCO_2 to maximize blood flow to ischemic areas, and (c) rapid emergence from anesthesia for a postoperative neurologic examination in the operating room.

   We routinely use general anesthesia because blood pressure, arterial blood gases, and the patient's airway are easily controlled by this technique. We also prefer general anesthesia in a teaching setting where instructional comments may bother patients. One of the most common anesthetic techniques for carotid surgery is **balanced anesthesia** of barbiturates, nitrous oxide, narcotics, and muscle relaxants. Volatile agents and barbiturates may offer some protection against ischemia because cerebral oxygen demand is reduced. Beyond the level of an isoelectric EEG, which reflects an absence of functioning neurons, barbiturates have no cerebral metabolic effect or protection.

   In contrast, some surgeons prefer local or regional anesthesia as a safe technique that allows immediate detection of neurologic change when the carotid artery is clamped. Regardless of whether one prefers general or regional anesthesia, either technique can achieve safe results. In our opinion, the choice lies with the experience and judgment of the surgeon and the anesthesia team.

All volatile anesthetics are considered cerebral vasodilators, with halothane being the most potent and isoflurane the least. Most of the intravenous agents for anesthesia are cerebral vasoconstrictors. The effects these agents have on the abnormal cerebral vasculature is variable. As a result, the impact of one anesthetic choice versus another may be less important as long as the hemodynamics are kept adequate. The ability of either volatile or intravenous agents to suppress metabolism and provide cerebral protection occurs only at anesthetic depths that could impair hemodynamic stability. Halothane can cause hypotension and myocardial depression. Deep anesthesia with a volatile agent such as halothane may also increase intracranial pressure and promote intracerebral blood flow steal from ischemic areas. Prevention of ischemia may be more beneficial than any attempt with anesthetics to prolong the brain's tolerance to ischemia. Light levels of anesthesia with any combination of volatile or intravenous agents with EEG monitoring can be successful. Postoperative neurologic evaluation usually is delayed because the patient is slower to awaken when deeper anesthetic techniques are used or longer-acting intravenous agents are administered.

V. Lower-extremity arterial reconstructions. Lower-extremity arterial reconstructions can be performed under a general or regional anesthetic. In our experience, continuous catheter epidural anesthesia is an excellent method for femoropopliteal bypass grafting. In the early postoperative period, the epidural catheter may be left in place for additional pain relief or for reoperation if early graft thrombosis occurs.

The indication and appropriateness of a regional technique should ultimately be decided by the anesthesiology team. The surgeon should give appropriate input on the choice of a regional anesthetic and any potential ramifications. Patient acceptance of a regional anesthetic as well as its safety must be considered. Many factors may reduce the advisability of a regional technique, such as dementia, risk of pulmonary aspiration, or previous neurologic injury. Prolonged sedation is often required in many of these lower-extremity arterial reconstructions. In addition, some patients may have cardiovascular conditions that may disqualify them for regional anesthesia because of venous and arterial dilation (hypertrophic cardiomyopathy or severe aortic stenosis).

The use of regional anesthesia in patients undergoing intraoperative anticoagulation is still controversial. Most studies reveal a low complication rate. The risk for patients taking aspirin or mini-dose heparin also appears very small. However, current use of Coumadin or clopidogrel (Plavix, Sanofi Pharmaceuticals, Inc. New York, NY, U.S.A.) is a relative contraindication to an epidural catheter insertion due to a potential risk of serious bleeding into the epidural space with attendant neurologic damage. The use of a preoperative bleeding time or activated partial thromboplastin time (aPTT) has been advocated by some in these circumstances.

VI. Arterial embolism. Arterial embolism often occurs in critically ill patients who are poor risks for general anesthesia. In such cases, femoral thromboembolectomy may be accomplished under local anesthesia. However, general anesthesia is preferred for most thromboembolectomies, especially when operative arteriograms or an associated arterial bypass or patch angioplasty is planned.

VII. Lower-extremity venous procedures. Lower-extremity venous procedures require general or regional anesthesia. A spinal or epidural anesthetic is adequate for most varicose vein operations, which generally last 1 to 2 hours.

SELECTED READING

Brewster DC, O'Hara PJ, Darling RC, et al. Relationship of intraoperative EEG monitoring and stump pressure measurements during carotid endarterectomy. *Circulation* 1980;62(Suppl 1):I4–I7.

Bush HL Jr, Hydo LJ, Fischer E, et al. Hypothermia during elective abdominal aortic aneurysm repair: the high price of avoidable morbidity. *J Vasc Surg* 1995;21:392–402.

Clagett GP, Valentine RJ, Jackson MR, et al. A randomized trial of intraoperative autotransfusion during aortic surgery. *J Vasc Surg* 1999;29:22–31.

Cullen ML, Staren ML, el-Ganzouri A, et al. Continuous epidural infusion for analgesia after major abdominal operations: a randomized, prospective, double blind study. *Surgery* 1985;98:718–728.

Ereth MH, Oliver WC Jr, Santrach PJ. Perioperative interventions to decrease transfusion of allogeneic blood products. *Mayo Clin Proc* 1994;69:575–586.

Frank SM, Fleisher LA, Breslow MJ, et al. Perioperative maintenance of normothermia reduces the incidence of morbid cardiac events. A randomized clinical trial. *JAMA* 1997;277:1127–1134.

Mangano DT, Layug EL, Wallace A, et al. Effect of Atenolol on mortality and cardiovascular morbidity after noncardiac surgery. *N Engl J Med* 1996;335:1713–1720.

Mannucci PM. Hemostatic drugs. *N Engl J Med* 1998;339:245–253.

Valentine RJ, Duke ML, Inman MH, et al. Effectiveness of pulmonary artery catheters in aortic surgery: a randomized trial. *J Vasc Surg* 1998;27:203–212.

Wiklund RA, Rosenbaum SH. Anesthesiology. First of two parts. *N Engl J Med* 1997;337:1132–1141.

Wiklund RA, Rosenbaum SH. Anesthesiology. Second of two parts. *N Engl J Med* 1997;337:1215–1219.

Youngberg JA, Lake CL, Roizen MF, et al., eds. *Cardiac, vascular and thoracic anesthesia.* Philadelphia: Churchill Livingstone, 2000.

Vascular Monitoring

The success or failure of a vascular operation often can be recognized by simple examination of the patient in the operating or recovery room. Numerous techniques are available for intraoperative and postoperative vascular monitoring, and this chapter describes the methods we currently use. Although the ideal methods of vascular monitoring can be debated, few surgeons would argue against some type of objective assessment of immediate technical results. **The best time to detect and correct a technical problem is in the operating room, before the patient departs for the recovery area.**

INSTRUMENTATION

Our vascular monitoring is accomplished by the following techniques.

I. Pulse volume recorder (PVR) or other air plethysmograph. The PVR is a segmental plethysmograph that provides a pulse volume tracing that correlates directly with arterial pressure (Fig. 9.1). The tracing can be made by application of a blood pressure cuff to the distal extremity at the calf or ankle level. A baseline tracing is made before the operation begins (Fig. 9.1). For aortic reconstructions (e.g., aortic aneurysms), the calf cuffs can be left in place if the lower limbs are only prepped to the thighs. Sterilized cuffs can be used in the operative field following femoropopliteal bypass grafting. Tracings are recorded when the arterial reconstruction is completed.

Interpretation of PVR tracings is fairly simple. If normal PVR tracings existed before operation, they should show no worsening after the procedure. A flat or diminished pulse contour (<5 mm) suggests significant obstruction. This obstruction may be the result of an anastomotic stenosis, a distal intimal flap, or distal thromboemboli. Corrective measures should be undertaken and the PVR tracing should be repeated when the obstruction has been relieved (Fig. 9.1).

II. Continuous-wave Doppler and duplex scanning. The continuous-wave Doppler system represents one of the simplest methods to evaluate arterial perfusion before and after arterial reconstruction. The Doppler unit allows evaluation of the quality of the arterial signal and measurement of arterial pressures in the limb. It is particularly useful when pulses are not palpable. Also, it is a good method to assess arterial flow signal quality after carotid endarterectomy and renal reconstruction.

A. A triphasic or biphasic signal with a crisp upstroke is normal. Significant arterial obstruction is associated with a monophasic, dampened signal. These Doppler patterns are illustrated in Figure 5.1.

B. Ankle blood pressures can be obtained by application of a blood pressure cuff at the ankle and auscultation of the dorsalis pedis or posterior tibial arteries with the Doppler unit.

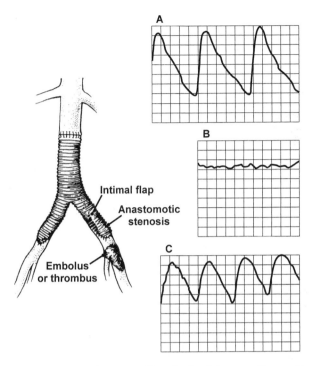

Figure 9.1. Pulse volume recordings during intraoperative monitoring of arterial reconstructions. A: Baseline tracings at the calf document normal preoperative pulse volume recording. B: When arterial reconstruction is completed, a flat or severely attenuated pulse volume recording (<5 mm) indicates an obstructive problem. Usual intraoperative problems are intimal flap, anastomotic stenosis, twisted or kinked graft, or distal thromboembolus. C: After the problem is corrected, pulse volume recording should return to a more normal-appearing tracing.

C. The **primary advantages** of the Doppler system are its ability to provide an audible arterial signal and accurate distal limb blood pressures. In addition, most Doppler units are small, easily transported by one person, and relatively inexpensive. With limited training, most paramedical personnel can detect arterial signals and measure pressures with a Doppler unit. Doppler probes may be sterilized and used in the operative field to examine abdominal or extremity vessels when necessary.

D. Several **disadvantages** of the Doppler system for perioperative vascular monitoring must also be mentioned. Unless the Doppler unit is attached to some type of strip recorder, no permanent paper copy of the signal is recorded. Also, some experience is necessary for interpretation of the biphasic, triphasic, and monophasic quality of Doppler arterial signals. This experience is critical in examination of severely ischemic limbs in which monophasic arterial signals may be confused with low-intensity venous sounds. Finally, Doppler signals and ankle pressures may be depressed in the immediate operative and postoperative period, when the patient is often cold and vasoconstricted.

   E.   The combination of B-mode ultrasound imaging and continuous-wave or pulsed Doppler flow velocity analysis (**duplex scanning**) can be used for intraoperative assessment of carotid endarterectomy, infrainguinal bypass grafts, and renal and visceral artery reconstructions. Our experience with intraoperative duplex ultrasound after carotid endarterectomy and renal revascularizations has enhanced detection and correction of technical problems. These technical defects can generally be corrected immediately and thus the risk of early postoperative arterial thrombosis at the operative site can be reduced. We have detected significant defects after 5% of carotid endarterectomies and after 10% of renal reconstructions. **When major defects (>50% luminal compromise on gray-scale image and more than three times normal peak systolic velocity) were corrected following carotid endarterectomy, the postoperative outcome was uncomplicated. Failure to correct major defects resulted in a 50% occlusion rate at the operative site in the early postoperative period.** For lower extremity bypass grafts, duplex scanning can quickly detect anastomotic problems, incompletely cut valves (nonreversed grafts), and overall low graft velocities.

III.   Electroencephalogram (EEG). The EEG represents one of the most sensitive detectors of cerebral ischemia during carotid artery clamping for endarterectomy. Excellent correlation has been established between ischemic EEG changes and reduction of regional cerebral blood flow (rCBF) to a critical level of 17 to 18 mL/100 g/min. In patients under general anesthesia, severe EEG ischemic changes have been associated with postoperative neurologic deficit.

   Despite evidence of its reliability for cerebrovascular monitoring, the continuous EEG has not gained widespread use during carotid endarterectomy, and some authors have recently questioned its benefit. It probably is not necessary if routine intraluminal shunting is used, although it can detect shunt malfunction. For surgeons who shunt selectively, internal carotid stump pressures have been a common technique to assess adequate cerebral collateral flow during carotid clamping (stump pressure, >50 mm Hg). In our experience, internal carotid stump pressures may not correlate with ischemic EEG changes. Consequently, we prefer EEG monitoring if selective shunting is used.

IV.   Ocular pneumoplethysmography (OPG). The ocular pneumoplethysmograph is abnormal when a hemodynamically significant carotid stenosis or occlusion is present. After successful carotid endarterectomy, the OPG should revert to normal. Thus, the OPG may be used to ascertain carotid patency after endarterectomy. However, neither OPG nor continuous-wave Doppler will detect intimal flaps or thromboemboli that may be related to postoperative neurologic deficits. These lesions may not cause significant stenosis or occlusion of internal carotid flow and may be missed by an OPG. **In most practices, duplex ultrasound has**

become the preferred method to check the endarterectomy site in the operating room or recovery area. For patients with profound, early neurologic deficit contralateral to the operated side, we return to the operating room for an examination of the endarterectomy site, ultrasound or arteriography, and any indicated surgical correction.

V. Arteriography. Intraoperative arteriography remains the primary method to check the distal anastomosis of a newly placed graft and visualize distal runoff. A PVR, continuous-wave Doppler unit, or duplex ultrasound machine also can assess graft function. **An arteriogram is essential when the noninvasive tests suggest inadequate distal flow or any disturbance in flow along the graft or at the distal anastomosis.** For example, an operative arteriogram may be necessary to better define lower leg and foot runoff when a distal femorotibial bypass is undertaken and preoperative arteriograms have not clearly shown the distal anatomy. Likewise, a retrograde arteriogram may be useful to ensure that thrombectomy of an occluded aortofemoral limb is complete.

If operative arteriography is anticipated, the following guidelines may ensure an adequate study.

A. An x-ray technician should be notified well before the need for the arteriogram.

B. Any electric coil heating pads or blankets, metal instruments, retractors, or sponges with radiopaque markers should be removed from the arteriogram field as they will obstruct the detail of the angiogram.

C. The graft **proximal to the angiogram injection** site should be clamped temporarily while the contrast material is being injected. This clamping prevents the inflow of blood that may dilute the contrast material and diminish the quality of the arteriogram.

D. Usually 20 to 50 mL of full-strength contrast is administered: one-half of the volume over 5 seconds and one-half of the volume over the next 10 seconds, with x-ray exposure as the final milliliter is injected.

E. The needle or catheter that was used for contrast injection should then be flushed with heparinized saline and the proximal occluding clamp removed.

F. During each exposure, a surgeon standing 1 ft from the x-ray tube receives an absorbed dose equivalent to 0.24 to 1.40 mrem, which is about one-half an operative cholangiogram. With a maximum yearly permissible dose of 5,000 mrem, one could safely perform 3,500 operative arteriograms per year! Fluoroscopy, however, increases radiation exposure more than four times that of nonfluoroscopic x-rays.

VI. Electromagnetic and ultrasonic transit flowmeters. Blood flow through arteries and grafts can be measured by an electromagnetic flow probe. Various sizes are available to fit different diameters of vessels and grafts. Common sources of error include inaccuracies due to distortion of the velocity profile by vessel bifurcations or angulations, poor probe fit, interference from adjacent metal instruments, and lack of calibration. Ultrasonic transit time flowmeters may even be more reliable and easy to use than electromagnetic flowmeters.

SELECTION OF MONITORING

Table 9.1 outlines the purpose, data, and techniques of appropriate vascular monitoring in the preoperative, intraoperative, and early postoperative periods.

I.   Carotid endarterectomy. The preoperative assessment of the patient who undergoes carotid surgery must begin with a complete baseline neurologic examination. All patients have a baseline preoperative carotid duplex ultrasound and/or OPG. During operation, continuous EEG monitoring is used. If carotid clamping causes severe focal ischemic EEG changes, an intraluminal shunt is inserted immediately. When the carotid endarterectomy is completed and blood flow is restored, a continuous-wave or pulsed Doppler with or without an ultrasound image can be used to assess flow velocity and any residual obstructing lesions. Although we do not routinely perform operative arteriograms, other surgeons advocate them. About 5% of endarterectomy sites need immediate revision for stenosis, occlusion, or intimal flap. However, neither duplex imaging nor angiography detect all abnormalities. The best method to ensure a good result remains a careful endarterectomy with adequate direct visualization of the internal carotid artery endpoint of the plaque.

In the early postoperative period, the neurologic examination remains the best single indicator of success. **If a focal neurologic deficit complicates the operation, immediate duplex ultrasound or intraoperative arteriography are the best methods to ensure that a technical mishap has not occurred.** If the postoperative neurologic deficit is not focal and one wants to ascertain whether the endarterectomy site is patent and not severely narrowed, a duplex scan is the best emergent test to detect carotid occlusion.

II.   Aortic grafting. Preoperative baseline data should include complete pulse examination. Doppler signal analysis and ankle pressures **(ankle-brachial indices)** or PVRs are also useful, especially when pulses are already decreased or absent. These data should be rechecked in the operating room before beginning the procedure. When the aortic graft is open, pulses, PVR tracings, or Doppler signals should be rechecked. We also use an electromagnetic flowmeter to measure graft flow, which normally ranges from 500 mL/min to over 1,000 mL/min. Flows of less than 250 mL/min combined with diminished calf PVRs (<5 mm) and monophasic or absent ankle Doppler signals usually suggest a problem with the reconstruction, uncorrected distal disease, or a distal thromboembolus. If easily palpable pedal pulses are present, their palpation is adequate for continued postoperative monitoring. If pedal pulses are not palpable because of uncorrected femoropopliteal disease, ankle or calf PVRs or Doppler ankle pressures will be necessary to ensure adequate arterial perfusion.

III.   Lower- and upper-extremity revascularization. Revascularization of upper and lower extremities includes bypass grafting and thromboembolectomies. In general, distal pulses are not palpable before operation. Therefore, ankle PVRs or Doppler signal analysis and distal extremity pressures (ankle-brachial indices) are needed as baseline measurements. Figure 9.2 demonstrates the intraoperative value of the PVR in construction of

Table 9.1. Techniques of perioperative vascular monitoring

Time	Purpose	Data	Techniques
Preoperative	Establish baseline	1. Appearance of patient 2. Pulse examination 3. Quality of arterial signal 4. Limb pressure (ABIs) 5. PVR tracings 6. Degree of carotid stenosis	(1, 2) Physical exam (3, 4) Continuous wave Doppler (5) Plethysmography (PVR) (6) OPG and or duplex scan
Intraoperative	Ensure successful reconstruction	1. Appearance of extremity 2. Pulse examination 3. Quality of arterial signal 4. PVR tracings 5. Adequate cerebral perfusion 6. Anatomy 7. Flow	(1, 2) Physical exam (3) Continuous wave Doppler (4) Plethysmography (PVR) (5) EEG (6) Arteriogram (6, 7) Duplex scanning (7) Electromagnetic flowmeter
Postoperative	Recognize/define early failures	1. Appearance 2. Pulse examination 3. Quality of arterial signal 4. Limb pressure (ABIs) 5. PVR tracings 6. Carotid patency	(1, 2) Physical exam (3, 4) Continuous wave Doppler (5) Plethysmography (PVR) (6) Duplex scanning

PVR, pulse volume recorder; EEG, electroencephalogram; ABI, ankle–brachial index; OPG, ocular pneumoplethysmography.

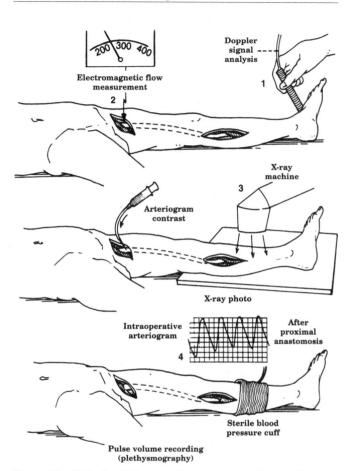

Figure 9.2. Methods of intraoperative assessment of femorodistal bypass. Continuous wave Doppler signal analysis or duplex ultrasonography (*1*) with a sterile probe is the simplest method to assess graft patency and ensure distal flow. Electromagnetic flow measurement (*2*) is useful for vein grafts but cannot be done over polytetrafluoroethylene (PTFE) synthetic conduits. An operative arteriogram (*3*) is the "gold standard" method to check the anatomy of the distal anastomosis and runoff. Finally, we use a sterile blood pressure cuff to check a distal pulse volume recording (*4*).

femoropopliteal bypasses. During operation, the success of revascularization may be judged by return of palpable pulses, an improved PVR tracing, or a better Doppler signal. Doppler pressures are generally 20 to 30 mm lower than they will be once the patient rewarms and vasoconstriction resolves. With *in situ* saphenous vein bypass grafts of the lower limb, we generally measure flow rates proximally and distally with an electromagnetic flowmeter. A high proximal flow rate (200 to 300 mL/min) with a lower distal vein flow rate (e.g., 80 mL/min) suggests an intervening arteriovenous fistula via a side branch that needs ligation. Generally, femoropopliteal grafts have a flow rate of at least 100 to 150 mL/min, whereas femorodistal grafts may remain patent with flow rates of less than 100 mL/min. **Because polytetrafluoroethylene (PTFE) is an electrical insulator, flow rates cannot be measured over PTFE grafts by an electromagnetic flowmeter. Duplex ultrasound is another alternative monitoring method for femoropopliteal and tibial bypasses.**

IV. Renal and visceral reconstructions. Adequate flow through renal and visceral revascularization can be assessed by continuous-wave Doppler, an electromagnetic flowmeter, or duplex scanner. A sterile continuous-wave Doppler probe is a simple and accurate method to ascertain the presence of flow and quality of the arterial signal. In addition, we generally measure flow, which is usually 150 to 350 mL/min for renal arteries and 350 to 1,000 mL/min for visceral vessels such as the celiac or superior mesenteric arteries. Duplex ultrasound has also become an accurate method to assess renal and visceral reconstructions.

SELECTED READING

Brewster DC, O'Hara PJ, Darling RC, et al. Relationship of intraoperative EEG monitoring and stump pressure measurements during carotid endarterectomy. *Circulation* 1980;62:I1–I7.

Donaldson MC, Ivarsson BL, Mannick JA, et al. Impact of completion angiography on operative conduct and results of carotid endarterectomy. *Ann Surg* 1993;217:682–687.

Dougherty MJ, Hallett JW Jr, Naessens JM, et al. Optimizing technical success of renal revascularization: the impact of intraoperative color-flow duplex ultrasonography. *J Vasc Surg* 1993;17:849–856.

Hallett JW Jr, Berger MW, Lewis BD. Intraoperative color-flow duplex ultrasonography following carotid endarterectomy. *Neurosurg Clin North Am* 1996;7:733–740.

Harada RN, Comerota AJ, Good GM, et al. Stump pressure, electroencephalographic changes, and the contralateral carotid artery: another look at selective shunting. *Am J Surg* 1995;170:148–153.

Johnson BL, Bandyk DF, Back MR, et al. Intraoperative duplex monitoring of infrainguinal vein bypass procedures. *J Vasc Surg* 2000; 31:678–690.

Miller A, Marcaccio EJ, Tannenbaum GA, et al. Comparison of angioscopy and angiography for monitoring infrainguinal bypass grafts: results of a prospective randomized trial. *J Vasc Surg* 1993; 17:382–398.

Mills JL, Fujitani RM, Taylor SM. Contribution of routine intraoperative completion angiography to early infrainguinal bypass patency. *Am J Surg* 1992;164:506–511.

O'Hara PJ, Brewster DC, Darling RC, et al. The value of intraoperative monitoring using the pulse volume recorder during peripheral vascular reconstructive operations. *Surg Gynecol Obstet* 1981;152:275–281.

Papanicolaou G, Toms C, Yellin A, et al. Relationship between intraoperative color-flow duplex findings and early restenosis after carotid endarterectomy. *J Vasc Surg* 1996;24:588–596.

Walsh DB. Technical adequacy and graft thrombosis. In: Rutherford RB, ed. *Rutherford's vascular surgery*, 5th ed. Philadelphia: WB Saunders, 2000:708.

Wellman BJ, Loftus CM, Kresowik TF, et al. The differences in electroencephalographic changes in patients undergoing carotid endarterectomies while under local versus general anesthesia. *Neurosurgery* 1998;43:769–775.

Yu A, Gregory D, Morrison L, et al. The role of intra-operative duplex imaging in arterial reconstructions. *Am J Surg* 1996;171:500–501.

Early Postoperative Care

Most life-threatening complications of major vascular surgery occur in the early postoperative period (24 to 48 hours). Fortunately, early recognition and treatment can resolve most of these problems. In this chapter, we focus on methods of recognizing these problems and discuss the principles of treatment that have been most successful in our experience. The management of specific complications of each type of operation is outlined in other chapters.

I. Equipment. The intensive care unit or recovery room should be equipped with ventilators and monitors of cardiac rhythm, mean arterial, central venous, and pulmonary artery pressures. The unit also should have facilities for rapid determination of arterial blood gases, hemoglobin and hematocrit, serum sodium, serum potassium, and blood glucose. An urgent coagulation profile should be available for patients with bleeding problems.

II. Ventilatory support may be necessary in some patients following vascular operations. In patients who are not breathing on their own, controlled mechanical ventilation provides a preset tidal volume at a controlled rate. For the patient with respiratory drive who is not ready for extubation, an assist-control technique allows spontaneous breathing supplemented by pressure-assisted ventilations. A commonly used method of assist-control is intermittent mandatory ventilation (IMV), during which the ventilator delivers a preset tidal volume at selected intervals (breaths per minute). Between mandatory ventilations, the patient breathes spontaneously with the assistance of pressure support.

Most patients require some amount of continuous positive airway pressure (CPAP) or positive end-expiratory pressure (PEEP) in conjunction with assisted ventilation. Although PEEP improves alveolar expansion and arterial oxygenation, high levels (>10 to 15 cm H_2O) may adversely effect cardiac output by decreasing venous return to the heart. Furthermore, high levels of PEEP may cause **barotrauma** to the lung predisposing the patient to acute respiratory distress syndrome (ARDS). Even moderate or high airway pressures may have an adverse effect on the lung after a few hours. Therefore the current trend in patients who require more than a few hours of mechanical ventilation is to use lower tidal volumes (5 to 7 cc/kg) and PEEP (<7 cm H_2O) reducing overall airway pressures and the risk of barotrauma.

Extubation requires consideration of the patient's oxygenation and ventilation status. Oxygenation is assessed by measurement of P_aO_2 in relation to the percent inspired oxygen (FIO_2) administered. In general a patient should not be extubated if they require more than 40% inspired oxygen to maintain a P_aO_2 of 70 to 80 mm Hg. This relationship is quantified as a **P_aO_2/FIO_2 ratio.** A P_aO_2/FIO_2 ratio of less than 200 indicates very poor oxygenation and qualifies as acute lung injury. Ventilation represents the work required to exhale enough CO_2 to prevent respiratory acidosis. One useful measure of ventilation and work of breathing is the **rapid-shallow breathing index.** This index is calculated by dividing the spontaneous, nonassisted respiratory rate (f, breaths per minute) by tidal volume (V_t, liters). In general, an index of greater than 100 suggests that the work of breathing is too great and the patient is not ready to be extubated.

Before extubation one must consider the patient's clinical condition and ability to protect their airway. Specifically, to confirm that the patient (a) is awake/alert enough to protect their airway, (b) does not have secretions too copious to clear, (c) does not have residual airway edema from a traumatic intubation, (d) does not have unexplained acidosis or bleeding, (e) does not have residual effects of muscle relaxants (paralytics), and (f) does not have ongoing signs or symptoms of myocardial ischemia. If there is a question about the patient's readiness for extubation, an experienced member of the surgery, anesthesia, or intensive care unit team should be consulted. Importantly, determining a patient's readiness for extubation must be individualized, with heavy reliance on clinical experience.

Once the patient is extubated, pulmonary complications can be reduced by simple methods. **Adequate pain control (preferably with an epidural catheter), early ambulation, and frequent deep breathing exercises remain the best means to prevent atelectasis.** Incentive spirometers are available to assist the patient with pulmonary toilet. Ideally, patients should be instructed preoperatively as to the use of such devices. Elevating the patient's head and chest 30 to 45 degrees increases functional residual capacity, while inhaled bronchodilators or mucolytic agents may assist patients with chronic obstructive pulmonary disease. Chest percussions and postural drainage are helpful for patients with thick pulmonary secretions but need not be performed in all patients. Occasionally, endotracheal stimulation and suctioning are necessary to help the patient with deep breathing and clearance of secretions. Suctioning should be done after the patient is well-oxygenated, as desaturation and arrhythmias may occur.

III. Cardiac problems. Since the majority of vascular patients also have coronary artery disease or chronic hypertension, postoperative cardiac problems are common.

A. Hypertension is one of the most common early postoperative problems. The causes may be multiple: increased sympathetic tone, incisional pain, or elevated renin-angiotensin activity. The danger of severe hypertension is increased cardiac work or afterload (cardiac work = stroke volume × heart rate × systolic blood pressure). Myocardial ischemia, cardiac failure, or stroke may occur if severe hypertension is not controlled promptly.

For practical purposes, we suggest maintaining the patient's systolic blood pressure at ±15% of its preoperative level. Systolic blood pressure readings from a radial arterial monitor tend to be higher than auscultated values and are subject to positional changes. Before administering antihypertensives, a manual brachial blood pressure measurement should be taken and compared to the arterial line readings.

1. Pain control with a small intravenous dose of a narcotic (e.g., morphine, 2 to 5 mg) may alleviate moderate hypertension. If continuous epidural analgesia is used, the catheter position, patency, and dosage should be checked to ascertain that adequate narcotic is being delivered.

2. Otherwise, intravenous **sodium nitroprusside** (Nipride, Roche Laboratories, Nutley, NJ, U.S.A.), a direct vasodilator, lowers blood pressure immediately and has a short duration of action (1 to 10 minutes). Initially, we begin administration at 0.5 to 1.0 µg/kg/min, increasing to a maximum of 10 µg/kg/min. Table 10.1 shows the doses of selected cardiovascular medications. **Nitroprusside should be administered in an intensive care setting, where blood pressure can be monitored continuously.** In addition, care must be taken not to flush the i.v. line containing nitroprusside, as such a bolus can cause sudden and severe hypotension. If this mishap does occur, the nitroprusside infusion should be stopped, the patient's legs elevated, and intravenous phenylephrine (Neo-Synephrine, Sanofi Pharmaceuticals, Inc., New York, NY, U.S.A.), administered. Since nitroprusside is metabolized to thiocyanate in the liver before renal excretion, it must be used with caution in patients with hepatic or renal insufficiency. **Prolonged infusion (3 to 4 days) or high doses (>10 µg/kg/min) can lead to cyanide intoxication.** We normally begin other antihypertensives if nitroprusside is needed for more than 6 to 12 hours. Other choices for quick control of hypertension are esmolol (Brevibloc, Baxter Pharmaceutical Products, Inc., Liberty Corner, NJ, U.S.A.), a short-acting beta-blocker, or nifedipine (Procardia, Pfizer Inc., New York, NY, U.S.A.), a calcium channel blocker. Hydralazine (Apresoline, CIBA, Summit, NJ, U.S.A.) is a direct vasodilator that may be taken orally but has a relatively quick onset of action (1 to 2 hours). A potential limitation of hydralazine or other direct vasodilators is reflex tachycardia which may require stopping the medication or the careful addition of a beta-blocker.

3. Occasionally, severe hypertension occurs during transport to the recovery room. If a nitroprusside infusion is not immediately available, labetalol can be given intravenously over a 2-minute period in doses of 20 mg (or up to 40 to 80 mg for subsequent injections) and repeated at 10- to 15-minute intervals. Labetalol possesses alpha$_1$-, beta$_1$-, and beta$_2$-receptor blocking activity and should be used cautiously in the setting of congestive heart failure and/or reactive airway disease.

4. A variety of **long-term antihypertensives** are available, and the selection of certain agents in the early postoperative period will depend on the individual patient. If the patient has been on specific antihypertensives, they generally can be resumed orally, even if the patient has not resumed feedings. In patients who are fluid overloaded, a diuretic (e.g., intravenous or oral furosemide) may help decrease blood pressure. A variety of beta-blockers, calcium channel blockers, and angiotensin-converting enzyme inhibitors can also be used as oral intake resumes.

B. **Tachycardia** is a common postoperative problem that increases myocardial oxygen consumption and risk for myocardial infarction. This is especially true if the patient is also

Table 10.1.   Infusion rates of commonly used cardiovascular drugs

	Nitroprusside	Nitroglycerine[a]	Esmolol	Diltiazem	Dobutamine	Dopamine	Lidocaine
Starting dose	0.5–1 μg/kg/min	5.0–50 μg/min	0.5 mg/kg/min over 1 min	0.25 mg/kg, repeat if no effect	2–10 μg/kg/min	1–2 μg/kg/min	50–100 mg i.v. bolus
Maintenance	2–4 μg/kg/min	50–200 μg/min	0.05–0.2 mg/kg/min	5–10 mg/h	5–15 μg/kg/min	3–10 μg/kg/min	1 mg/min
Maximum	10 μg/kg/min	>200 μg/min	>0.2 mg/kg/min	15 mg/h	20 μg/kg/min	20 μg/kg/min	2–4 mg/min

[a] The starting and maximum doses for nitroglycerin are μg/min (not μg/kg/min).
Note: If the patient is on multiple drips, consider normal saline as diluent to prevent free water excess and hyponatremia.

hypertensive. An analgesic may help if the patient is having pain and should be tried initially while more data is being gathered. **In the surgical patient, hypovolemia (or anemia) often is the cause of tachycardia and should be at the top of the list of differential diagnoses.** Low urine output, blood pressure, and central filling pressures are indicators that more fluids are required to treat the tachycardia.

When intravascular volume is adequate, tachycardia may be caused by cardiac failure or increased sympathetic tone. A low cardiac output and an elevated pulmonary capillary wedge pressure (PCWP; >18 mm Hg) suggest left ventricular dysfunction which may be associated with an increased heart rate. In this setting careful balance of fluids and cardiac medications will be necessary to treat the tachycardia. If tachycardia persists in this setting, transesophageal echocardiography (TEE) may give additional useful information about myocardial function and volume status.

If the cardiac output is normal and the PCWP is not elevated, then cardiac dysfunction is less likely and a beta-blocker may control the tachycardia. This may be especially true if the patient was on a beta-blocker preoperatively. Administration of an intravenous beta-blocker [esmolol, 50 to 200 μg/kg/min; metoprolol, 5-mg increments up to 15 mg; propranolol (Inderal, Wyeth–Ayerst Laboratories, Philadelphia, PA, U.S.A.), 1-mg increments every 2 minutes] with continuous ECG and blood pressure monitoring can effectively slow the heart rate. Generally, only a few doses are necessary, and the patient can then be started on an oral beta-blocker. In patients with chronic obstructive airway disease, nonselective beta-blockers may cause bronchospasm. If an oral beta-blocker is needed, metoprolol [Lopressor (Novartis Pharmaceuticals Corporation, East Hanover, NJ, U.S.A.), 50 mg p.o. b.i.d.] may cause less bronchospasm than propranolol because it is a cardioselective beta-adrenergic agent. As beta-blockade may mask the sympathetic signs (e.g., tachycardia) of hypoglycemia, propranolol must be administered carefully in insulin-dependent diabetics.

C. Low cardiac output (CO) with hypotension in the early postoperative period generally results from hypovolemia. Primary myocardial dysfunction is the other cause of low cardiac output and is more common in patients who have a reduced ejection fraction (less than 40%) at baseline or who have sustained perioperative myocardial ischemia. Arrhythmias also may decrease cardiac output. Table 10.2 summarizes low CO states in the early postoperative period.

  1. Recognition and treatment of low perfusion states are facilitated by the application of **basic principles of cardiovascular physiology.** Specifically, the following formulas define arterial (C_aO_2) and venous (C_vO_2), oxygen content as well as oxygen delivery (DO_2) and extraction (OER). The application of these formulas and principles is often necessary in the early postoperative care of vascular patients:

CO = heart rate × stroke volume
Stroke volume = preload × contractility/afterload
Oxygen Content (C_aO_2 or C_vO_2) = Hb × Sat × 1.34
$$+ (PO_2 \times 0.003)$$

**Table 10.2. Low cardiac output
states in the postoperative period**

Etiology	Recognition	Initial treatment
Hypvolemia	Low CVP (0–5) Low PCWP (<10 mmHg) FE_{Na} <1%	Bolus of crystalloid Transfusion of blood
Myocardial dysfunction	High CVP (>15) High PCWP (>18–20 mm Hg) Low Cardiac Index (<2.2 L/m2) FE_{Na} <1%	Afterload reduction Inotropic support
Arrhythmia	12-lead ECG or continuous monitoring	See Table 10.3 (page 116)

CVP, central venous pressure; ECG, electrocardiogram; PCWP, pulmonary capillary wedge pressure.

Oxygen Delivery (DO_2) = CO × C_aO_2 × 10
Oxygen Extraction $C_aO_2 − C_vO_2$
Oxygen Extraction Ratio = $C_aO_2 − C_vO_2/C_aO_2$ × 100

   Preload represents the end-diastolic filling pressures in the left atrium. Because routine measurement of left atrial pressure is not practical, we rely on the best estimation of preload provided by the pulmonary capillary wedge pressure (PCWP). Other measurements such as pulmonary artery diastolic pressure (PAD) and central venous pressure (CVP) are also used to assess preload and volume status but may be less accurate than the wedge pressure. Stroke volume is directly related to preload and is described by the Frank–Starling curve (Fig. 10.1).
   Afterload represents the resistance against which the left ventricle contracts and is inversely related to stroke volume.
   Contractility reflects factors such as baseline ejection fraction, as well as beta-adrenergic agonists and antagonists that modify the force of contraction independent of preload and afterload.
   Systemic blood pressure (BP) depends directly on CO and peripheral vascular resistance (PR):

BP = CO × PR

   Although regulation of CO, blood pressure, and oxygen delivery is a complex physiologic process, clinical recognition and treatment of low-output states can be achieved by application of these simple relationships.
2. Recognition of a low-perfusion state usually is made when blood pressure, urine output, or both decrease. In stressful situations, heart rate may already be elevated and

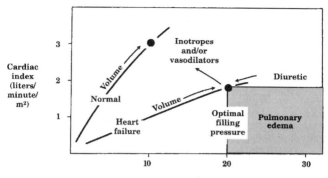

Figure 10.1. Frank–Starling left ventricular function curve relating ventricular filling pressure (pulmonary capillary wedge pressure) to stroke volume (cardiac index). In patients with heart failure and pulmonary edema, cardiac performance can be improved by a combination of inotropes (e.g., dobutamine), vasodilators (e.g., nitroprusside), and diuretics (e.g., furosemide). (Adapted from Marino PL. *The ICU book.* Philadelphia: Lea & Febiger, 1991.)

thus may not change. If fluid resuscitation (5 to 10 mL/kg bolus) does not improve perfusion, more intensive monitoring should be considered if it is not already in place. A low CVP (0 to 5 mm Hg) suggests hypovolemia but is not reliable in assessing left ventricular function or CO. A Swan–Ganz thermistor-tipped pulmonary artery catheter allows measurement of central venous and pulmonary arterial pressures and CO by thermodilation. Afterload of the left ventricle is the peripheral arterial resistance.

3.   Knowledge of the pulmonary capillary wedge pressure and cardiac index allows categorization of patients into subsets that respond to different modes of treatment. Vascular congestion begins when PCWP exceeds 18 to 20 mm Hg. Pulmonary edema occurs when PCWP rises above 30 mm Hg. The normal cardiac output is 3.5 to 8 L/min (the normal cardiac index is 2.7 to 4.3 L/m[25]). However, clinical hypoperfusion becomes evident when the cardiac index drops to the 1.8 to 2.2 L/m^2. Below an index of 1.8 L/m^2, cardiogenic shock becomes a problem.

   a.   Low filling pressures (PCWP, CVP) are the hallmark of hypovolemia. If blood pressure and urine output are low (<90 mm Hg and <0.5 mL/kg/h, respectively), CO usually can be optimized by fluid administration to bring PCWP to the level of 10 to 12 mm Hg. If the patient is symptomatic (tachycardia) and the hemoglobin (Hb) is low (less than 8 to 9 g), blood should be transfused to increase the oxygen-carrying capacity or content of the arterial blood (C_aO_2) and therefore increase oxygen delivery (DO_2).

Otherwise, an intravenous bolus of 5 to 10 mL/kg of a crystalloid solution (Ringer's lactated solution or normal saline) may be given to increase filling pressures. Colloid solutions generally are not necessary unless serum albumin and protein are excessively low. Not uncommonly, patients after aortic surgery are both hypovolemic and hypertensive. As volume is repleted, nitroprusside can be used to control hypertension and vasodilate the patient, who is often cold and vasoconstricted. After hypovolemia is corrected, persistent tachycardia can be treated with a beta-blocker or a calcium channel blocker. It must be remembered that intubated patients on higher levels of PEEP (>5 cm H_2O) may have decreased venous return and ventricular filling. PEEP, which increases intrathoracic pressure, may also falsely elevate central venous and pulmonary artery pressures.

b. Elevated left ventricular filling pressures and low CO suggest impaired contractility. Such patients usually have a PCWP in excess of 18 mm Hg—generally in the range of 25 to 30 mm Hg. Their peripheral vascular resistance is usually high (>1,500 to 1,800 dynes/sec/cm^{-5}). A low mixed venous oxygen saturation (S_vO_2) (<60%) from an oximetric Swan–Ganz is also an indication of low CO and decreased DO_2. Likewise, an oxygen extraction ratio of greater than 30% indicates that tissue DO_2 is inadequate and or tissue extraction is increased. These patients need an adequate hemoglobin and arterial saturation to maximize C_aO_2 as well as afterload reduction and possibly inotropic support to increase DO_2.

(1) Afterload reduction can be accomplished by vasodilation with intravenous infusion of nitroprusside or nitroglycerin. Sodium nitroprusside relaxes vascular smooth muscle in both the arterial and venous systems. When ventricular function is severely impaired, the cardiac response to afterload reduction is an increase in CO. The dose required for a therapeutic response varies from 15 to 400 μg/min (average about 50 μg/min). Nitroglycerin acts primarily on the venous system. The net effect is a sharp fall in heart filling pressures and pulmonary artery pressures. In severe heart failure, CO may be augmented. Afterload reduction can be maintained in the remaining postoperative period with other nonparenteral vasodilators: nitrates, hydralazine, prazosin, minoxidil, and captopril.

(2) Although several **inotropic drugs** are available to increase myocardial contractility, the most useful agents are dobutamine (Dobutrex, Eli Lilly and Company, Indianapolis, IN, U.S.A.), dopamine (Intropin, DuPont Pharmaceuticals, Wilmington, DE, U.S.A.), and amrinone (Inocor, Winthrop Pharmaceuticals, New York, NY, U.S.A.).

Dobutamine, a beta-adrenergic agonist, is the inotropic agent of choice in acute cardiac failure, especially when the etiology is an ischemic injury. Dobutamine acts rapidly, with an inotropic effect similar to that of isoproterenol. However, CO is increased without appreciable change in heart rate, blood pressure, arrhythmias, or infarct size if one already has occurred. In addition to increasing contractility, dobutamine decreases preload and afterload. The starting dose is 2.5 µg/kg/min, which can be increased to 10 to 15 µg/kg/min.

When low CO is complicated by hypotension and oliguria, **dopamine,** another catecholamine, may be preferable to dobutamine. Dopamine not only enhances cardiac contractility but also causes renal and mesenteric vasodilatation at low doses (0.5 to 2.0 µ/kg/min). We have found low-dose dopamine helpful when urine output is low despite apparent adequate intravascular volume. Higher doses (>10 µg/kg/min) elevate peripheral resistance and heart rate.

Amrinone is a phosphodiesterase inhibitor which increases cardiac contractility directly and decreases afterload through vasodilation. Amrinone may be started as a 0.75 mg/kg i.v. bolus over 2 to 3 minutes and maintained at an infusion of 5 to 10 µg/kg/min. Vasodilation and subsequent hypotension may limit the use of amrinone in some patients.

  c. Low CO secondary to bradycardia may require cardiac pacing, since atropine may worsen the risk of arrhythmia.

  d. Arrhythmias are another cardiac problem encountered in the perioperative period. A few general comments about arrhythmias in vascular patients should provide a basis for their initial management (Table 10.3).

  (1) The physiologic consequence of atrial or ventricular arrhythmias is **decreased CO and oxygen delivery** to cerebral, mesenteric, and renal circulations which may be chronically compromised by atherosclerotic disease. More importantly, coronary perfusion is also decreased. Subsequently, uncontrolled arrhythmias may result in severe myocardial ischemia and infarction.

  (2) Every effort must be made to determine the **etiology** of the arrhythmias. Common causes of arrhythmias in the early postoperative setting are hypoxia, hypothermia (<33°C), hypo- or hyperkalemia, acid–base imbalance, and operative cardiac infarction. Each of these etiologies can be explored easily by checking the patient's core temperature, and ordering arterial blood gases, serum electrolytes, and cardiac isoenzymes. In addition, a 12-lead ECG is essential. These tests should be routine on the patient's arrival in the recovery room.

  (3) Table 10.3 outlines general principles of emergency arrhythmia treatment.

  (a) Tachycardia, especially when accompanied by hypertension, requires increased cardiac oxygen consumption, which is poorly tolerated when coronary artery disease is present. Therefore, we strive to keep heart rate below 100 beats/min.

  (b) Bradycardia is not as common as tachyarrhythmias. However, heart rates of less than 50 beats/min will decrease CO and coronary perfusion. If atropine (0.5 to 1.0 mg i.v.) does not speed the rate and if

Table 10.3.   Emergency treatment of common postoperative arrhythmias

Arrhythmia	Treatment of choice	Dose	Alternatives
Ventricular fibrillation	Cardioversion	200–360 J	Plus cardiopulmonary resuscitation or lidocaine
Ventricular tachycardia	Cardioversion	200–360 J	Lidocaine Procainamide Bretylium 5 mg/kg i.v.
Premature ventricular contractions	Lidocaine	50–100 mg bolus; repeat in 10 min; 200 mg total	Procainamide 20–30 mg/min; maximum 17 mg/kg
Supraventricular tachycardia	Carotid massage Adenosine If narrow complex: Verapamil If wide complex: Lidocaine Procainamide	6 mg i.v. bolus; repeat with 12 mg q1–2 min × 2 5–10 mg i.v. over 2–3 min 1.0–1.5 mg/kg i.v. bolus 20–30 mg/min; maximum 17 mg/kg	Digoxin Propranolol Diltiazem
Atrial fibrillation	Diltiazem Digoxin	0.25 mg/kg, 5–10 mg/h 0.5 mg i.v. 0.125–0.250 mg i.v. q4–6h to loading dose of 0.5–1.0 mg	Cardioversion Procainamide Anticoagulants
Digitalis-induced tachyarrhythmia	Dilantin (Parke-Davis, Morris Plains, NJ, U.S.A.)	50 mg i.v. q5min to 250 mg	
	Potassium	10–20 mEq/h via central line to keep serum potassium at >4.0 mEq/L	

hypotension becomes a problem after adequate volume replacement, cardiac pacing may be necessary.

(c) **Premature ventricular contractions (PVCs)** are a fairly common early postoperative arrhythmia, especially if the patient is cold and acidotic. We treat PVCs (lidocaine, 50 to 100 mg i.v.) when they are multifocal, occur at a rate of more than six per minute, or are associated with runs of ventricular tachycardia or bigeminy. Persistent PVCs may require a continuous lidocaine infusion (1 to 4 mg/min) until chronic antiarrhythmias are started.

IV. **Bleeding.** During or after an operation the most common causes of bleeding are (a) technical failure of hemostasis, (b) anticoagulants, (c) dilutional thrombocytopenia, (d) consumptive or disseminated intravascular coagulation, and (e) defects in clotting factors. Table 10.4 lists common laboratory tests to check various steps in the hemostatic scheme. The clinical situation and the results of these tests will identify the cause of bleeding and correction may then be accomplished by directed therapy.

A. **Technical failure of hemostasis** should be recognized before the wounds are closed. Wound hematomas that appear in the first 6 hours after operation usually are the result of unligated blood vessels. We recommend early evacuation of large wound hematomas and control of the bleeding site by sterile operative techniques. Undrained hematomas may increase the risk of infection. After intraabdominal vascular surgery, significant internal hemorrhage should be suspected if more than 2 units of blood have to be given to maintain the hematocrit in the first 6 to 12 hours after operation.

B. **Anticoagulants** such as heparin or warfarin sodium (Coumadin, DuPont Pharmaceuticals Company, Wilmington, DE, U.S.A.) may cause oozing from wound edges. Such bleeding usually is not significant when mechanical hemostasis is adequate. Some surgeons prefer to routinely reverse the effect of intraoperative heparin with **protamine sulfate given in a dose of 0.5 to 1.0 mg of protamine per 1 mg (100 units) of heparin.** A partial thromboplastin time (PTT) or activated clotting time (ACT) may be checked to ensure reversal of the heparin effect. Fresh-frozen plasma (FFP) also may be used to counteract heparin or warfarin. The usual dose of FFP is approximately 10 mL/kg of body weight. Rarely, it is necessary to administer intravenous vitamin K (25 to 50 mg) to help stop frank hemorrhage in a patient on Coumadin.

Oozing from wound edges also may be seen in patients on antiplatelet therapy. The effect of antiplatelet drugs persists for 3 to 7 days after they are discontinued. Although platelet dysfunction may cause more wound ecchymosis, generally it is not necessary to administer fresh platelets. If intraoperative wound oozing is excessive, a dose of DDAVP (vasopressin or desmopressin acetate, 0.3 µg/kg i.v. in a single dose) may counteract the antiplatelet effect of aspirin.

C. **Dilutional thrombocytopenia** may present a problem after administration of more than 10 units of packed red blood cells. Dilutional thrombocytopenia can be associated with
(*text continues on page 120*)

Table 10.4. Evaluation of the clotting and fibrinolytic system

Test	Purpose of test	Normal finding	What abnormal test may indicate
Bleeding time (Ivy method)	Measures time to compaction of platelet plug	8 min (2–8 min)	Platelet count <75,000 Abnormally functioning platelets Defective capillaries von Willebrand's disease
Platelet count	Measures number (not function) of platelets	160,000–350,000/mm^3 (50,000 considered adequate for surgical hemostasis if platelet function is normal)	Dilutional thrombocytopenia Consumption of platelets Defective platelet production Heparin-induced thrombocytopenia
Peripheral blood smear	Evaluates number and appearance of platelets	15–20 platelets/HPF of anticoagulated blood 3–4 platelet clumps/HPF of blood smear	Thrombocytopenia (decreased platelets/HPF) Thrombocytopenia (bizarre giant platelets) DIC (fragmented red blood cells)
Prothrombin time (INR)	Measures extrinsic pathway of clotting (factors VII, X, V, II) Usual test to monitor warfarin therapy Not affected by platelets	10–12 sec INR 1.0–1.3	Defective extrinsic pathway of clotting DIC Anticoagulation (warfarin)

Partial thromboplastin time	Measures intrinsic pathway of clotting (factors XII, XI, IX, VIII)	44 sec	Defective intrinsic pathway of clotting Congenital abnormalities of clotting (e.g., hemophilia disorders, von Willebrand's disease) Dilutional coagulopathy from blood transfusion DIC Anticoagulation (e.g., heparin)
Thrombin time	Evaluates presence of adequate fibrinogen	12 sec	Thrombolytic drugs Low fibrinogen levels Increased fibrin split products Anticoagulation (heparin)
Fibrinogen assay	Directly measures fibrinogen levels	200–400 mg/100 ml	DIC Thrombolytic drugs
Fibrin split products	Measures fibrin split products (degradation of fibrin)	<1:40	DIC Primary fibrinolysis (platelet count falls with DIC but not with primary fibrinolysis)

HPF, high-powered field; DIC, disseminated intravascular coagulation; INR, international normalized ratio.

excessive use of autologous blood prepared in a high-speed centrifuge. These rapid autotransfusion machines return packed red blood cells without their accompanying platelets. Platelets should be available and administered when packed red blood cell transfusion exceeds 10 units. In general, a platelet count of greater than 50,000 will be adequate for hemostasis during operation. An appropriate starting dose usually is 6 units of platelet concentrate. After operation, spontaneous bleeding usually does not occur until the platelet count is less than 20,000.

D. Disseminated intravascular coagulation (DIC) or consumptive coagulopathy occurs in a variety of clinical settings associated with increased formation of tissue thromboplastin. The most common situations are (a) massive blood transfusions, (b) major transfusion reaction, (c) massive soft-tissue trauma or ischemia, and (d) sepsis. Thrombocytopenia and DIC also have been reported as an idiosyncratic reaction that some patients have to systemic heparin. **If heparin-induced thrombocytopenia is suspected (platelet count of <70,000 to 80,000 after heparin), all heparin, including small amounts in arterial lines, must be stopped immediately.**

Basically, DIC involves consumption of platelets and coagulation factors (primarily VIII, V, and fibrinogen), increased fibrin split products that act as anticoagulants, and fibrin plugs that damage red blood cells. The **clinical criteria for DIC** include thrombocytopenia, prolonged prothrombin time, low fibrinogen levels, and microangiopathic blood smear. The main feature that differentiates DIC from primary fibrinolysis is the platelet count, which is decreased in DIC.

Despite past claims that heparin is the drug of choice for DIC, the primary treatment remains correction of the underlying clinical problem. Heparin should be reserved for situations in which efforts to correct the underlying cause or replacement therapy (FFP, platelets) have failed to correct overt hemorrhage.

E. Defects in clotting factors may be familial or acquired from liver disease. These coagulation problems usually are evident by history or by abnormal partial thromboplastin or prothrombin times. Specific blood component therapy generally is effective in managing these deficiencies during the perioperative period.

V. Gastrointestinal stress ulceration and hemorrhage is a rare complication of vascular operations. Risk factors include preexisting peptic ulcer disease, prolonged mechanical ventilation (>48 hours), sepsis, hypotension, renal failure, and coagulopathy or use of anticoagulants. The ulcerations usually involve the stomach but may also affect the colon. About 10% of patients with mucosal ulcerations have clinically recognized bleeding, usually 6 to 7 days after the onset of the stress. The bleeding usually is controllable by nonoperative means and almost always resolves if the risk factor (e.g., sepsis) is eliminated. Mortality for operative intervention to control stress hemorrhage exceeds 50%; clearly, in high-risk patients, the key to managing gastrointestinal stress bleeding is prevention.

In high-risk patients, control of gastric pH with H_2-receptor antagonists such as cimetidine (300 mg i.v. q6h) or ranitidine (50 mg i.v. q8h) is important in stress ulcer prophylaxis. However, some studies have shown that altering gastric pH increases the incidence of hospital acquired pneumonia. Alternatives such as antacids [Maalox (Novartis Consumer Health, Inc., Summitt, NJ, U.S.A.), 30 cc every 6 to 8 hours] and sucralfate [Carafate, Hoechst Marion Roussel, Kansas City, MO, U.S.A.), 1-g slurry every 6 to 8 hours] are as effective as H_2-receptor antagonists and may have a lower risk of hospital acquired pneumonia. **Vascular patients who have a routine perioperative course and have no risk factors for stress ulceration or gastrointestinal bleeding do not require prophylaxis.**

VI. Renal failure was once a main complication following abdominal vascular operations; especially following emergency aneurysm repair. Improved resuscitative techniques and the use of mannitol before aortic clamping have nearly eliminated renal failure following elective aortic surgery. Postoperative renal failure is more likely to occur in dehydrated patients with underlying renal insufficiency or diabetes. In such patients, renal function may deteriorate as a result of contrast arteriography and/or the stress of surgery.

A. Recognition of renal failure is relatively simple. The hallmark is decreasing urine output (<15 mL/h) and rising serum blood urea nitrogen and creatinine (CR). Other signs may suggest early renal insufficiency and allow intervention before serious renal deterioration occurs. In general, patients with adequate intravascular volume and CO make 30 to 60 mL of urine per hour or 0.5 mL/kg/h. The normal kidney can concentrate urine as indicated by a urine-plasma osmolarity ratio of more than 1.3 and a urine-plasma creatinine ratio of more than 100. The normal kidney also retains sodium, as indicated by a urine sodium of only 20 to 40 mEq/L.

Early or imminent renal failure should be suspected when the following occur:

1. Urine output is less than 15 mL/h for longer than 2 hours in a patient with adequate intravascular volume (PCWP; 12 mm Hg) and adequate CO (2.7 to 4.3 L/m^2).

2. Polyuria (>60 mL/h) occurs in an volume-depleted patient (high-output renal failure).

3. Urine-plasma CR ratio is less than 10.

4. Rising urinary loss of sodium (urine-plasma sodium ratio approaching 0.9 [e.g., urine sodium 80 to 110 mEq/L]).

5. Failure to concentrate urine (specific gravity of 1.010 or urine-plasma osmolarity ratio of <1.3 and usually near 1.0).

A quick functional assessment of the kidneys (Table 10.5) may be accomplished by calculating the **fractional excretion of sodium (FE_{Na})** from the patient's urine electrolytes and CR levels.

$$FE_{Na} = (Urine_{Na}/Plasma_{Na})/(Urine_{CR}/Plasma_{CR}) \times 100$$

This measurement has been used to categorize acute renal insufficiency into two broad categories: (a) prerenal azotemia ($FE_{Na} < 1\%$), which is indicative of hypoperfusion or hypovolemia, and (b) Renal azotemia ($FE_{Na} > 3\%$), which

Table 10.5.   Functional assessment of perioperative renal function

Type of renal failure	Urine osmolarity (mosm/kg)	Urine Na[a] (mEq/L)	Urine creatinine/ plasma creatinine	FE_{Na}[b]
Renal hypo-perfusion (prerenal)	>Plasma	<20	≥100	<1
Vasomotor nephropathy (acute tubular necrosis)	Isomotic	>20	≤10	>2
Urinary obstruction (postrenal)	Isomotic	Variable		>2

[a] Urine sodium concentration measurement can be misleading if diuretics have been administered shortly before urine collection for analysis.

[b] FE_{Na} = urinary fraction excretion of sodium

$$FE_{Na} = \frac{\text{urinary sodium concentration}}{\text{plasma sodium concentration}} \div \frac{\text{urinary creatinine concentration}}{\text{plasma creatinine concentration}}$$

From Blachey JD, Henrich WL. The diagnosis and management of acute renal failure. *Semin Nephrol* 1981;1:11, with permission.

suggests renal tubular injury or obstruction. Importantly, calculation of FE_{Na} following the use of diuretics or contrast agents is not reliable because of effects on the urine electrolytes. In situations where acute renal dysfunction is suspected, this quick assessment may allow the appropriate treatment to be rendered promptly before permanent renal damage is sustained.

6.   Prerenal failure ($FE_{Na} < 1\%$) generally implies inadequate intravascular volume or low CO. This assessment is made by assessing mean arterial pressure, PCWP (CVP is less reliable), and CO.

7.   Renal causes ($FE_{Na} > 3\%$) usually include injury to the renal parenchyma from prolonged ischemia or embolization of atheromatous material. Also angiographic dye or medications such as aminoglycosides may cause acute tubular injury.

8.   Postrenal failure is caused by an obstruction of the urinary collecting system, usually the ureters. Rarely, ureteral obstruction may result from extrinsic compression by an accidental ligature or by the limb of a bifurcated graft. Imaging tests such as CT scan, ultrasound or renal scan may reveal an enlarged or obstructed ureter. Precise location and degree of obstruction may require a retrograde cystoureterogram.

B.   As soon as a preliminary diagnosis of impending or acute renal failure is made, **certain principles of therapy should be followed.**

1.   Maintenance of fluid and electrolyte balance is paramount if fluid overload and hyperkalemia are to be avoided.

Potassium should be removed from all intravenous fluids. Daily fluid requirements for oliguric or anuric patients are less than generally appreciated. Insensible water loss from skin and lungs is about 500 mL/day or 10 mL/kg/day. Without supplemental nutrition, the patient should lose approximately 1 lb daily. Other losses, such as gastrointestinal drainage, should be measured for volume and sodium concentration and then should be replaced.

In addition to fluid overload, hyperkalemia leading to cardiac dysrhythmias is an immediate threat to life in the setting of acute renal failure. Hyperkalemia (>5 mEq/L) associated with peaked T waves and a widening QRS complex on the ECG requires immediate treatment. **The treatment of symptomatic hyperkalemia is slow intravenous infusion of 10% calcium chloride (up to 10 mL over 10 minutes) as well as intravenous sodium bicarbonate and insulin plus glucose (10 units of regular insulin plus one ampule of 50% dextrose in water).** These manuevers stabilize the myocardium and cause a rapid intracellular shift of potassium. If this therapy is ineffective or if hyperkalemia is recurrent, hemodialysis may be necessary. Control of chronic hyperkalemia may require oral administration of the exchange resin sodium polystyrene sulfonate (Kayexalate, Sanofi Pharmaceuticals, Inc., New York, NY, U.S.A.), 20 g t.i.d. with 20 mL of 70% sorbitol solution.

2.   Maintaining optimal perfusion and oxygen delivery to the kidneys. One of the best ways to treat acute renal dysfunction is to avoid hypotensive episodes and/or significant anemia (hemoglobin < 8 g/dL). These simple principles avoid a second injury to recovering renal parenchyma and allow the best chance for regaining function.

3.   Prevention of infections and other organ dysfunction. Maintenance of the pulmonary, cardiac, neurologic and gastrointestinal systems may be difficult but is extremely important in preventing a "second hit" to recovering renal function. Infections or additional organ systems that fail in the setting of acute renal dysfunction decrease the likelihood of renal recovery and quickly increase the patient's mortality from multiple organ failure (MOF).

4.   Adjustment of dosages for medications excreted by the kidney is essential. Common examples are digoxin and aminoglycoside antibiotics and ranitidine (Zantac, Glaxo Wellcome Inc., Research Triangle Park, NC, U.S.A.). Some of these drugs can be monitored by determination of blood levels.

5.   Hemodialysis may become necessary if the patient develops (a) uncontrollable electrolyte disorders, (b) fluid overload, (c) acid–base abnormalities, or (d) severe uremic symptoms.

VII.   Psychosis. Postoperative psychosis manifested by agitation, mental confusion, and hallucinations is not uncommon in elderly patients who undergo vascular operations. In many patients, this change in mental status is mild and resolves in a few days without specific treatment.

A.   The etiology frequently is normal sensory and sleep deprivation in the unfamiliar hospital surroundings. **Hypoxia,**

hypoglycemia, sepsis, and alcohol withdrawal must also be considered as causes of altered mental function. In these situations, narcotics or benzodiazepines often worsen the problem.

B.   Treatment depends on the etiology and severity of psychosis. If no metabolic problem is identified, close observation or restraints are the best options. In addition, treatment should focus on reestablishing the normal waking and sleeping pattern. In addition, an antipsychotic medication such as haloperidol [Haldol (Ortho-McNeil Pharmaceutical, Raritan, NJ, U.S.A.), 0.5 to 2.0 mg p.o. or i.m.] may help sedate severely agitated patients whose psychosis endangers themselves or others. In this setting, sedation must be carefully monitored; otherwise, patients may become obtunded, making them susceptible to aspiration and atelectasis. The patient's family should be reassured that postoperative psychosis generally clears completely in several days. The patient, who may be bothered by his or her own confusion, hallucinations, or nightmares, also needs reassurance that he or she will soon be better.

Alcohol withdrawal syndrome (AWS) is also an important cause of postoperative psychosis. The signs and symptoms of AWS develop within hours of reduction or cessation of prolonged heavy alcohol consumption. The occurrence and severity of these symptoms is difficult to predict and depends upon the duration of alcohol consumption, the amount of alcohol consumed, history of prior AWS, and coexisting illness. Uncomplicated AWS is characterized by signs of autonomic hyperactivity such as tremor, diaphoresis, tachycardia, and agitation. Headache and insomnia may also manifest during this period. Patients with these symptoms frequently pull out their intravenous lines, nasogastric tubes, and urinary catheters. Therefore, these should be well secured and the patient should be carefully observed or restrained. A quiet environment with dimmed lights may help as noise and light often worsen agitation in such patients. Other therapeutic measures include adequate hydration and administration of thiamine (100 mg i.m. daily) and multivitamins. Hypomagnesemia and hypoglycemia are common electrolyte problems in alcoholics who should be monitored for such abnormalities.

More serious clinical signs such as seizures and/or hallucinations are less common and occur 24 to 48 hours after cessation of alcohol consumption. **Delirium tremens (DTs)** is a dramatic clinical syndrome characterized by disturbances of consciousness and marked autonomic hyperactivity. DTs are usually seen 3 to 4 days after cessation of alcohol and can be life-threatening if not managed appropriately.

Benzodiazepines are generally the best agents for the prevention and management of AWS. Specifically, chlordiazepoxide [Librium (ICN Pharmaceuticals Inc., Costa Mesa, CA, U.S.A.), 25 mg p.o. two or three times daily] and diazepam [Valium (Roche Pharmaceuticals, Humaco, Puerto Rico), 10 mg p.o. two to three times daily] have longer acting metabolites and may provide a smoother withdrawal course. Lorazepam [Ativan (Wyeth–Ayerst Laboratories, Philadelphia, PA, U.S.A.), 1 mg p.o. three to four times daily] has no active metabolites and an intermediate duration of action and is associated with a lower risk of oversedation. Special consideration should be given to patients in the intensive care unit requiring mechanical ventilation. In this setting, intravenous benzodiazepines may be used or alternatively the ultrashort acting agent propofol (Diprivan, Zeneca Pharmaceuticals, Wilmington, DE, U.S.A.). The dose of the medication needed to control symptoms varies from individual to individual. Although some form of medication should be started prophylactically in high-risk patients, increasing the dose should be triggered by the onset of symptoms. Symptom-triggered therapy is recommended because it emphasises repeated patient evaluations and matching the dose with the level of withdrawal experienced. The goal is to minimize signs and symptoms without oversedation by titration of the dose and schedule. **Standardized assessment scales such as the Clinical Institute Withdrawal Assessment (CIWA) exist that allow objective titration of medication and reduce the possibility of over- or undermedicating a patient.**

VIII.   Sepsis. Perioperative sepsis is an uncommon problem after most vascular reconstructions. Patients at risk for infectious complications are those with preoperative chronic lung disease, cirrhosis, malnutrition, graft infections, and ruptured aneurysms. After operation, prolonged use of intravascular and urinary catheters, extended endotracheal intubation, ischemic colitis, and wound hematomas or tissue necrosis often precede local or systemic sepsis. Early recognition and treatment remain the keys to success when sepsis occurs. Specific types of infection tend to present at certain times after operation, and knowledge of these patterns is important in deciding which tests are most likely to identify the septic source.

   A.   Pulmonary atelectasis is the most common cause of fever in the first 24 to 48 hours after operation. Generally the chest examination and x-ray will document the problem, and deep breathing exercises and endotracheal suction will resolve it. In the presence of fever, rales, and an infiltrate that persist beyond 24 hours, we culture the sputum and consider broad-spectrum antibiotics until the results are available for a more specific antibiotic regimen.

   B.   **The second most common source of sepsis in the first few days after surgery is **central venous catheters. The typical presentation of catheter sepsis is a sudden fever spike, chills, and a drop in blood pressure and systemic vascular resistance. The catheter must be removed, and the catheter tip and blood should be cultured. Since bacteremia may seed a new synthetic graft, we generally use broad-spectrum antibiotics that are effective against gram-positive, gram-negative, and anaerobic organisms. Enterococcus is one organism that requires specific treatment (e.g., ampicillin). Usually fever resolves quickly after catheter removal, and culture-specific antibiotics are continued for 5 to 7 days and until repeat blood cultures are negative.

   C.   **Following aortic surgery, any signs of sepsis associated with diarrhea must raise one's suspicion of **ischemic colitis. Proctosigmoidoscopy should be done to inspect the left colon. Evidence of extensive mucosal ischemia, localized tenderness, and systemic sepsis mandate resection of the involved bowel. Mild mucosal ischemia with no signs of sepsis is usually managed with bowel rest, maintenance of normal CO, and antibiotics.

D.   Peripheral intravenous site thrombophlebitis is another common source of fever, usually occurring in 3 to 5 postoperative days. Removal of the intravenous catheter and application of local heat will be sufficient therapy for most cases. A tender, erythematous venous cord with pus at the intravenous site requires operative excision of the septic vein.

E.   A urinary tract infection (UTI) should be suspected when patients develop a fever after a Foley catheter has been in place or after its removal when urinary retention occurs. The clinical presentation of a UTI is often delayed until postoperative days 7 to 10, when the patient may be out of the hospital.

F.   Wound infections generally do not become apparent until 5 to 7 postoperative days. Because lower-extremity infections may involve underlying grafts, these infections may require drainage and debridement in the operating room.

G.   Intraabdominal sepsis also may not become apparent until 10 to 14 days after laparotomy. Patients with fever at this time and no other explanation should undergo an abdominal CT scan to search for an abscess. If acute acalculous cholecystitis is suspected by up-per abdominal tenderness, hepatobiliary scintigraphy (technetium-iminodiacetic acid scan) or ultrasound may help confirm the diagnosis before operation.

H.   Finally, unexplained fever after 5 to 14 postoperative days may be related to a superficial or deep **venous thrombophlebitis** of the lower limb. Usually, a careful examination of the leg will reveal some tenderness, swelling, or venous cord. A duplex ultrasound can be used to establish the diagnosis. Diagnosis and treatment are presented in more detail elsewhere (see Chaps. 4, 5, and 21).

I.   Some patients succumb to so-called **multiple organ failure** and **sepsis.** They generally manifest simultaneous and progressive failure of the heart, lungs, kidneys, and sometimes liver. Generally, the common denominator in multiple organ failure is a period of shock or a low CO. Cardiogenic shock results in splanchnic vasoconstriction which may manifest as stress ulceration of the stomach, centrilobular liver necrosis, nonocclusive bowel ischemia, ischemic colitis, and perhaps ischemic pancreatitis and acalculos cholecystitis. Obviously, prevention of multiple organ failure depends on maintaining perfusion pressure throughout the perioperative period. In addition, septic focus, such as an abdominal abscess, must be eliminated to reverse the downhill clinical course.

SELECTED READING

Attlee JL. Perioperative cardiac dysrhythmias: diagnosis and management. *Anesthesiology* 1997;86:1397–1424.

Burchell SA, Yu M, Takiguchi SA, et al. Evaluation of a continuous cardiac output and mixed venous oxygen saturation catheter in critically ill surgical patients. *Crit Care Med* 1997;25:388–391.

Cook D, Guyatt G, Marshall J, et al. A comparison of sucralfate and ranitidine for the prevention of upper gastrointestinal bleeding in patients requiring mechanical ventilation. *N Engl J Med* 1998;338:791–797.

Johanningman JA, Davis K Jr, Campbell RS, et al. Use of the rapid/shallow breathing index as an indicator of patient work of breathing during pressure support ventilation. *Surgery* 1997;122: 737–741.

Kress JP, Pohlman AS, O'Connor MF, et al. Daily interruption of sedative infusions in critically ill patients undergoing mechanical ventilation. *N Engl J Med* 2000;342:1471–1477.

Krieger BP, Isber J, Breitenbucher A, et al. Serial measurements of the rapid-shallow breathing index as a predictor of weaning outcome in elderly medical patients. *Chest* 1997;112:1029–1034.

Mayo-Smith MF. Pharmacologic management of alcohol withdrawal: a meta-analysis and evidence-based practice guidelines. *JAMA* 1997;278:144–151.

National Conference on Standards and Guidelines for Cardiopulmonary Resuscitation and Emergency Cardiac Care. Adult advanced cardiac life support. *JAMA* 1992;268:2171–2183.

Niemann JT. Cardiopulmonary resuscitation. *N Engl J Med* 1992; 327:1075–1080.

Ryan TJ, Anderson JL, Antman EM, et al. ACC/AHA Guidelines for the management of patients with acute myocardial infarction: Executive Summary—A report of the American College of Cardiology/American Heart Association Task Force on Practice Guidelines. *Circulation* 1996;94:2341–2350.

The Acute Respiratory Distress Syndrome Network. Ventilation with lower tidal volumes as compared with traditional tidal volumes for acute lung injury and the acute respiratory distress syndrome. *N Engl J Med* 2000;342:1301–1308.

Tobin MJ. Mechanical ventilation. *N Engl J Med* 1994;330:1056–1061.

Ware LB, Matthay MA. Medical progress: the acute respiratory distress syndrome. *N Engl J Med* 2000;342:1334–1349.

Specific Arterial Problems

Cerebrovascular Disease

A surgeon with vascular expertise is a key member of the health care team that treats patients with cerebrovascular disease. This involvement in the care of such patients has been the direct result of the success of carotid, aortic arch branch, and vertebral artery reconstructions for the relief of symptomatic stenotic or ulcerated arterial lesions, aneurysms, and vascular tumors located in the neck. The surgeon may also be consulted to evaluate patients with asymptomatic but high-grade (>70% stenosis) carotid disease. Recently, some surgeons have also become involved in the selection and performance of carotid stent angioplasty.

In this chapter, we discuss the management of common clinical presentations that suggest extracranial carotid or vertebral artery disease. We have also selected certain principles of operative care that facilitate a smooth, safe operation for the patient. Finally, the management of the most common early and late postoperative complications of carotid operations is summarized.

COMMON CLINICAL PRESENTATIONS

I. Transient ischemic attacks. Approximately 75% of patients who suffer a stroke have experienced some type of preceding transient neurologic symptom. For strokes that occur in the carotid artery distribution, these transient ischemic attacks (TIAs) are usually hemiparesis, hemiparesthesias, transient monocular blindness **(amaurosis fugax),** or difficulties with speech. TIAs of the vertebrobasilar artery distribution are characterized by dizziness, bilateral eye symptoms, ataxia, facial numbness, or some bilateral extremity weakness and numbness. Classically, a TIA is defined as acute neurologic symptoms that last less than 24 hours and completely resolve. However, the duration usually is measured in minutes, not hours. The term **reversible ischemic neurologic deficit (RIND)** has been used to describe neurologic symptoms that last longer than 24 hours but then rapidly resolve completely.

A. The **outcome of TIAs** depends on the underlying etiology. TIAs are not specific for carotid artery stenosis or ulcerated plaques. Only about 50% of patients with TIAs will have a tight carotid stenosis (<2 mm), occlusion, or ulcerated plaques. If untreated, TIAs associated with significant carotid disease will result in a stroke for one of three patients in 5 years. **Most of these associated strokes, however, occur within days to weeks, especially when the TIAs are frequent.** The remaining 50% of patients with TIAs have thromboembolism from the heart, aortic arch, intracranial vascular disease, or no evident etiology. TIAs from thromboembolism or hypercoagulability also commonly lead to a stroke. However, patients with no evident etiology for their TIAs and normal carotid arteriograms may follow a more benign course; they seldom suffer a stroke.

Visual symptoms occur in approximately 25% of patients presenting with symptomatic carotid bifurcation atheroma. Amaurosis fugax is the most common ocular symptom. Rarely, the deterioration in visual acuity is due to ischemic neurovascular glaucoma. Unfortunately, permanent visual loss without warning affects one of four patients with ocular manifestations. This tragic outcome emphasizes the importance of identifying severe carotid stenosis or ulceration and correcting it before retinal artery occlusion or ischemic optic neuropathy has caused permanent visual loss.

B.   The natural history of TIAs can be altered by anticoagulation, surgical therapy or carotid stent angioplasty in selected patients. Antiplatelet drugs such as aspirin and clopidogrel retard platelet aggregation and may prevent microemboli that cause TIAs. Aspirin therapy reduces the risk of continuing TIAs, stroke, and death by approximately 20% compared to controls. In a randomized, blinded trial of clopidogrel (Plavix, Sanofi Pharmaceuticals, Inc., New York, NY, U.S.A.) versus aspirin in patients at risk of ischemic events (CAPRIE), clopidogrel (75 mg daily) reduced the relative risk for ischemic stroke, myocardial infarction and vascular death by 24%. Heparin or warfarin sodium (Coumadin, DuPont Pharmaceuticals Company, Wilmington, DE, U.S.A.) can also control TIAs in at least 90% of patients with recent onset. Warfarin also has proved effective in reducing serious cerebral infarct from 45% in untreated patients to 24% in treated individuals over 5 years. Of course, the main disadvantage of long-term Coumadin therapy is compliance and bleeding complications in about 15% of patients.

Surgical therapy also provides excellent long-term relief of TIAs that are the result of carotid stenosis of greater than 70% in diameter reduction. In general, the symptoms of 90% of patients with classic carotid symptoms of contralateral motor or sensory loss, ipsilateral eye symptoms, or dysphasia are relieved by carotid endarterectomy. In contrast, relief of nonspecific symptoms such as dizziness, syncope, and mental confusion is achieved in less than 50% of such patients. However, the chance of relief of such nonhemispheric symptoms is greater in patients whose carotid stenosis is hemodynamically significant by ocular pneumoplethysmography (Gee-OPG) than in those individuals with OPG-negative lesions (70% versus 30%, respectively). The total incidence of perioperative and late stroke is about 5% to 10% in operated patients compared to 25% to 35% in nonoperated patients.

C.   Because untreated TIAs may lead to stroke, we recommend some type of anticoagulation, surgery or stent angioplasty for patients with TIAs. The **choice of therapy** is influenced by answers to the following questions:

1.   Are the symptoms actually transient ischemic episodes or some other neurologic or psychosomatic complaint? This question is not always easy to answer. TIAs in the carotid distribution classically present with unilateral hemiparsis, hemiparesthesias, speech disturbance, or amaurosis fugax. Amaurosis fugax is described as a graying out of vision, sometimes compared to pulling a shade down over the visual field. The symptoms that present confusion in determining whether a true TIA is being experienced are atypical complaints, especially dizziness and unsteady gait. These vertebrobasilar symptoms are rather common in elderly patients who may experience postural hypotension when arising quickly from a lying, sitting, or stooping position. If a psychosomatic problem is suspected, a careful inquiry about family or work situations may disclose emotional stress that initiates the symptoms. If the patient is unsure of the symptoms, a family member who may have observed an attack should be asked. Noninvasive carotid tests may assist in the selection of patients with atypical neurologic symptoms for arteriography. If these tests indicate a hemodynamically significant carotid lesion, we may suggest arteriography. Correction of a carotid stenosis in the presence of vertebral occlusion may alleviate vertebrobasilar symptoms by improving collateral flow to the posterior brain via the circle of Willis (Fig. 11.1).

2. Are the transient neurologic attacks chronic and stable or repetitive and progressive? If the TIAs are chronic and not progressive, elective evaluation is appropriate. Noninvasive tests generally detect hemodynamically significant carotid lesions. Duplex ultrasonography allows visualization of plaques and measurement of the degree of stenosis. In many patients, carotid duplex scanning may provide enough anatomic and functional information to proceed with carotid endarterectomy without arteriography. However, most symptomatic patients will also undergo gadolinium-enhanced magnetic resonance angiography (MRA) to show the aortic arch, cervical and intracranial cerebrovasculature.

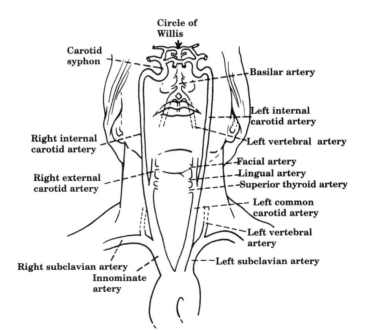

Figure 11.1. Anatomy of the aortic arch and extracranial cervical arteries. The internal carotid artery has no branches in the neck.

Complete elective evaluation for TIAs also may require electrocardiographic monitoring (Holter monitor) to detect arrhythmias or echocardiography to rule out a diseased valve or mural thrombus. Transesophageal echocardiography may also reveal ulcerative atherosclerosis of the aortic arch, which is now recognized as a source of thromboembolic stroke in some patients.

We also have found consultation with a neurologist or ophthalmologist to be helpful in evaluating patients if atypical neurologic or retinal symptoms are present. **Rubeosis iritis, neovascular glaucoma and bright light amaurosis** suggest worsening ocular ischemia and their diagnosis requires a thorough ophthalmologic examination. In patients with atypical neurologic or ocular symptoms, computed tomography (CT) or magnetic resonance imaging (MRI) of the brain is useful to rule out intracranial lesions. Electroencephalography (EEG) is appropriate if a seizure disorder is suspected.

TIAs which continue or progress over 24 to 72 hours are referred to as **crescendo TIAs.** We hospitalize such patients for anticoagulation with heparin (loading dose of 5,000 to 10,000 units, with a continuous hourly infusion of 750 to 1,000 units). If the patient's condition is stable, an urgent MR or standard contrast arteriogram usually is performed within 24 hours after admission. Heparin is withheld for 2 to 4 hours before the study. Operative candidates with severe (>70%) carotid stenosis or shaggy, irregular ulcerative plaques undergo carotid endarterectomy. Carotid stent angioplasty is reserved for patients with excessively high operative risk or anatomic situations where surgical endarterectomy is especially problematic (e.g., severe postradiation skin damage or high recurrent internal carotid stenosis not easily accessible to operative repair). The timing of arteriography, operation or angioplasty must be individualized depending on the patient's medical condition and the availability of an experienced anesthesiologist, operating team and/or interventional radiologist or cardiologist.

Management is more difficult if the neurologic symptoms are progressing without complete resolution. These patients should be considered to have a stroke in evolution. Anticoagulation and emergent carotid surgery for severe carotid lesions may reduce the stroke rate and mortality in this group. However, the differentiation between a **stroke in evolution** or a **completed stroke** is not always clear. Surgery for a completed stroke seldom reverses any established neurologic deficit and may lead to worsening of the stroke and death. A CT scan may help determine whether cerebral infarction has occurred, but CT findings of a stroke may not be positive until 12 to 24 hours after the incident. MRI may be superior to CT scan in the early detection of brain infarction, but CT may be better for identification of hemorrhage.

Although carotid endarterectomy for acute stroke has been discouraged, there has been renewed interest in a more aggressive approach to selected patients with acute stroke. In one series from the Mayo Clinic, carotid revascularization for acute carotid occlusion and profound stroke resulted in a normal neurologic exam (27%) or minimal deficit (12%) in nearly 40% of patients. The surgical mortality of 20% was comparable to the natural history of untreated stroke. Others have also demonstrated good results from early carotid endarterectomy in patients with small, fixed neurologic deficits, even when CT scan has been positive. These more aggressive approaches have been balanced by other studies suggesting that carotid endarterectomy for stroke should be delayed for at least 5 weeks and until the deficit is stable or reaches a plateau in its improvement. Currently, we favor this more delayed approach to carotid surgery for stroke. Long-term follow-up supports the value of carotid endarterectomy in reducing the morbidity and mortality of recurrent stroke. Surgical patients have a recurrent stroke rate of 3% to 5% and a 5-year survival of about 80%, compared to unoperated patients who have a recurrent stroke rate of 25% to 60%.

Treatment of acute ischemic stroke with thrombolytic therapy (tissue-type plasminogen activator) is approved for selected patients when started within 3 hours of onset of symptoms. Unlike positive findings with recombinant tissue-type plasminogen activator (rt-PA) in the treatment of acute ischemic stroke, initial studies with streptokinase have shown no benefit.

3. What is the patient's operative risk? Combined mortality and stroke morbidity for elective carotid endarterectomy should be 2% to 4%. If the patient with chronic TIAs is a poor surgical risk, carotid stent angioplasty, antiplatelet and/or Coumadin therapy are alternatives. Arteriography and surgery should be reconsidered if anticoagulant therapy fails to control the TIAs. For good surgical candidates with classic carotid TIAs, we still recommend elective cerebrovascular arteriography (usually MRA) and elective surgical correction of an ulcerative or stenotic plaque (>70% diameter reduction) that correlates with the exhibited symptoms. **There have now been three randomized clinical trials documenting the superiority of carotid endarterectomy over anticoagulation in preventing neurologic events in symptomatic patients with high-grade (>70%) carotid stenosis** [North American Symptomatic Carotid Endarterectomy Trial (NASCET), European Carotid Surgery Trial, and Veterans Affairs Symptomatic Carotid Endarterectomy Trial]. The NASCET trial demonstrated a 2-year stroke rate of 9% for endarterectomy patients, compared to 26% for the medically treated patients. A more recent report documents a smaller stroke risk reduction for patients with symptomatic 50% to 69% stenosis undergoing carotid endarterectomy. In this update of the NASCET trial, benefit was greatest in men, patients with a recent stroke, and patients with hemispheric symptoms.

II. Asymptomatic cervical bruits. Controversy continues over the natural history and management of asymptomatic cervical bruits.

A.   The **natural history** of a cervical bruit depends on what underlying cardiovascular lesion is causing the noise. A neck bruit may originate from the carotid arteries or be transmitted from the aortic arch or heart (Fig. 11.1). Precise location of the source of the bruit generally requires a duplex ultrasound (see Chap. 5). An echocardiogram (transthoracic or transesophageal) also differentiate carotid bruits from cardiac murmurs.

The degree of narrowing of a carotid stenosis determines whether cerebral blood flow on that side is reduced. Unfortunately, the loudness of a bruit does not correlate with the degree of stenosis. In fact, a tight carotid stenosis with severely diminished flow may have a minimal or inaudible bruit. At present, an accurate noninvasive method to determine the **hemodynamic significance of a carotid bruit** is carotid duplex scanning. Duplex scanning provides a B-mode (brightness-mode, or gray scale) ultrasound image plus a pulsed Doppler analysis of the flow velocity across a lesion. The degree of stenosis can be categorized, and a high-grade (80% to 90%) lesion or occlusion can be identified. These tests are discussed in detail in Chapter 5. Although not used routinely by many vascular labs, ocular pneumoplethysmography (OPG) correlates with internal carotid pressure. In our experience, it provides another confirmatory measurement that the lesion is hemodynamically significant and more prone to causing stroke. Transcranial doppler analysis of collateral flow has also been used to identify poorly collateralized asymptomatic carotid stenosis, but we have not found it essential in patient management.

In a recent analysis of asymptomatic carotid stenosis followed in the NASCET trial patients, the risk of stroke was relatively low. For stenosis less than 60%, the risk was 1.6% annually. For stenosis greater than 60%, it was twice as high (3.2% annually). Annualized stroke risk for asymptomatic internal carotid occlusion was only 1.9%, which was lower than other previously reported series. About one half of strokes were related to the carotid lesion, but the other half were attributed to lacunar stroke or cardioembolic events. The risk factors for large-artery stroke were silent brain infarction, diabetes, and higher degree of stenosis; for cardioembolic stroke, a history of myocardial infarction or angina and hypertension; and for lacunar stroke, age >75 years, hypertension, diabetes, and a higher degree of stenosis. Some patients had more that one stroke of more than one cause, indicating the complexity of predicting the natural history of asymptomatic carotid stenosis.

B.   Our **management of patients with asymptomatic neck bruits** is determined by answers to the following questions:

1.   Is the patient a good operative risk? If so, we recommend noninvasive carotid testing to determine the location and hemodynamic significance of the bruit. If the patient is not, we generally do not pursue further evaluation. The risk of carotid endarterectomy in high-risk patients, especially those with symptomatic cardiac disease, generally exceeds the risk of stroke from an asymptomatic carotid stenosis. Such patients generally should be followed until they become symptomatic with TIAs.

2. Do noninvasive carotid tests suggest a hemo-dynamically significant carotid stenosis? If the answer is yes and the patient is a good surgical candidate, we recommend carotid endarterectomy for carotid stenosis (80% to 99% and OPG-positive). The combination of an asymptomatic systolic carotid bruit and an abnormal OPG on the same side has been correlated with an 3% to 5% incidence of stroke per year. In our experience, the risk of stroke in such cases is considerably higher than the risk of postoperative stroke for elective carotid endarterectomy (1% to 2%). Patients with a normal OPG have a better prognosis, with only a 1% per year incidence of stroke. Patients with asymptomatic carotid bruits in whom noninvasive carotid tests do not suggest a hemodynamically significant stenosis usually are followed. They undergo endarterectomy if symptoms develop or if noninvasive tests demonstrate that the stenosis is progressing into the 80% to 99% stenotic category. The appropriate frequency of such follow-up visits is debatable, but a visit every 6 to 12 months is reasonable.

Although some physicians are hesitant to recommend carotid endarterectomy for patients with asymptomatic carotid bruits, the natural history of this group does not appear to support this nonoperative approach in otherwise healthy adults with good life expectancy. The rationale for prophylactic carotid endarterectomy for high-grade asymptomatic carotid stenosis began with the classic observations of Dr. Jesse Thompson of Dallas. In his nonoperated group, 26.8% eventually had TIAs, 15.2% experienced a nonfatal stroke, and 2.2% had a fatal stroke. On the other hand, 90% of operated patients remained asymptomatic. Only 4.5% of the operated patients developed TIAs and 2.3% experienced a nonfatal stroke.

Subsequently, Strandness and colleagues at the University of Washington used duplex scanning prospectively to study the natural history of carotid arterial disease in asymptomatic patients with carotid bruits. The presence of or progression to a greater than 80% internal carotid stenosis was highly correlated with development of TIA, stroke, and asymptomatic internal carotid occlusion in 46% of patients compared to those lesions of 0% to 79% stenosis (1.5%). The majority of adverse events occur within 6 months of the findings of an 80% to 99% stenosis.

Three randomized trials have addressed the benefit of prophylactic carotid endarterectomy for asymptomatic high-grade carotid stenosis (Carotid Artery Surgery Asymptomatic Narrowing Operation Versus Aspirin [CASANOVA], Veterans Affairs Asymptomatic Carotid Endarterectomy Trial, and Asymptomatic Carotid Atherosclerosis Study [ACAS]). The CASANOVA trial excluded patients with stenosis greater than 90% and those with bilateral high-grade stenoses, two groups most likely to benefit from endarterectomy. A substantial portion (57%) of the medical group crossed over into the surgical arm, but neurologic endpoints leading to this switch were not considered in the final analysis. Thus, the CASANOVA trial did not resolve the dilemma of the critical asymptomatic carotid stenosis. The Veterans trial found a significant reduction in combined TIAs and stroke in the surgical group (8%) versus the medical group (20.6%). However, there was not a statistically significant difference when stroke alone was analyzed (surgical versus medical, 4.7% versus 9.4%). The relatively small sample size was one limitation of this study. Finally, the ACAS trial is the largest of the three studies and has analyzed the outcomes of 1,500 patients with no cerebral symptoms and a greater than 60% diameter reduction of the carotid artery. **Results of the ACAS trial favor carotid endarterectomy over medical therapy.** The 5-year ipsilateral stroke risk was 5% for the surgical group and 11% for the medical group, a relative risk reduction of 53%. The efficacy for women, however, was marginal.

The decision to recommend elective carotid endarterectomy for asymptomatic carotid stenosis also is influenced by the experience of the anesthesiology and the surgical teams. Mortality generally does not exceed 2% to 3% if surgery is performed by an experienced team, and permanent neurologic deficits at the time of operation also should remain in this low range.

3.   Is the patient scheduled for other major surgery? Controversy also continues over whether patients with asymptomatic carotid bruits are at increased risk for perioperative stroke at the time of other major surgery, especially any operation in which prolonged hypotension may occur. The major surgery of most concern has been cardiac and aortic operations. Only 0.5% to 1.0% of patients who undergo major cardiovascular surgery suffer a perioperative stroke. Several studies have shown that cervical bruits are not a good predictor of perioperative stroke. In fact, perioperative strokes often occur in patients who were not suspected of having carotid disease. These strokes also are more commonly diffuse than focal. The conclusion of these studies is that major cardiovascular surgery can be performed on patients with asymptomatic carotid bruits who have not had carotid endarterectomy.

However, we follow a selective approach to such patients. Noninvasive carotid testing is performed to determine the hemodynamic significance of the carotid stenosis. Poorly compensated lesions generally are corrected before elective aortic surgery is attempted. Combined carotid endarterectomy and heart operations, such as coronary artery bypass or valve replacement, are reserved for patients with unstable cardiac disease and severely stenotic or symptomatic carotid disease. Most surgeons agree that patients with symptomatic carotid disease should have carotid endarterectomy before other elective surgery is performed.

III.   Asymptomatic contralateral carotid artery stenosis. Another controversial area in carotid surgery is the management of patients with the asymptomatic contralateral carotid artery stenosis following a carotid endarterectomy. These patients may be at increased risk of TIAs and stroke. The outcome of such lesions again may depend on the hemodynamic significance of the asymptomatic lesion. Conservative management of nonoperated vessels opposite an endarterectomy appears appropriate until symptoms develop or a lesion greater than 80% is detected. We generally repair a hemodynamically significant contralateral carotid stenosis as a staged procedure. The endarterectomies are performed at least 5 to 7 days apart, although most patients require a longer recovery period between operations. If the contralateral stenosis is not hemodynamically significant, if the patient is not a good surgical risk, or if the first endarterectomy was complicated by cranial nerve injury, we follow the patient until symptoms occur or noninvasive studies document progression of the stenosis.

IV.   Asymptomatic ulcerated lesions. The natural history of asymptomatic ulcerated carotid lesions is not easy to define. Carotid ulceration is difficult to detect with duplex ultrasound. This imaging technique can define plaque morphology (homogeneous versus heterogeneous), but these characteristics do not always correlate with surface ulceration. Despite these limitations, some reports suggest that echolucent plaque, detectable by duplex ultrasound, increases the likelihood of future symptoms. Arteriography also is not particularly accurate in defining ulceration which may vary from a slight nonstenotic irregularity to a complicated ulcerated stenosis.

V.   Asymptomatic Hollenhorst plaque. Occasionally a patient is referred for evaluation of an asymptomatic Hollenhorst plaque (cholesterol embolus in a retinal arteriole) noted incidentally on routine retinoscopy, often by an ophthalmologist. Such asymptomatic findings do not appear predictive of future transient or fixed retinal or cerebral symptoms. We generally screen such patients with a carotid duplex scan and do not proceed with further evaluation or treatment unless a high-grade carotid stenosis is detected. Surgically remediable lesions are found in only about 15% of such patients.

VI.   Subclavian steal syndrome. Left subclavian stenosis or occlusion is a common atherosclerotic lesion. Generally, it is asymptomatic and is discovered because the left arm blood pressure is lower than the right. Left arm claudication seldom is a significant problem, since the collateral flow to the left arm usually is well developed. However, for a few patients proximal left subclavian occlusion may cause subclavian steal syndrome. Its clinical features are dizziness, syncope, visual blurring, or ataxia, classically associated with vigorous left-arm exercise. The mechanism of the syndrome appears to be retrograde flow from the left posterior cerebral circulation down the left vertebral artery to the distal subclavian artery and arm. Theoretically, this "stealing" of blood from the brain to the left arm causes intermittent posterior cerebral ischemia.

In our experience, classic subclavian steal syndrome is uncommon. Although many patients with subclavian occlusive disease have retrograde left vertebral flow on arteriography, few have cerebral symptoms with arm claudication. If they do have cerebral ischemic symptoms, we perform a noninvasive evaluation of the carotid system. Subclavian steal syndrome sometimes is relieved simply by correcting a severe left carotid stenosis, which improves collateral flow via the circle of Willis to the posterior brain. **Significant arm claudication may be relieved by carotid–subclavian bypass, subclavian–subclavian bypass,**

subclavian-to-carotid transposition, or transluminal angioplasty.

VII.   Totally occluded internal carotid artery. It is uncertain whether thromboendarterectomy of an occluded internal carotid artery is advisable. Certainly, surgical repair of a thrombosed internal carotid artery in the setting of a completed stroke may be associated with intracranial hemorrhage and a high mortality risk. The natural history of untreated carotid occlusion is still debated. Approximately 25% of patients have subsequent TIAs, and 10% to 15% have a stroke. Many patients, however, remain asymptomatic.

A.   A few reports indicate that **thromboendarterectomy** of a totally occluded internal carotid artery can be achieved with a low morbidity and mortality rate and a 65% to 70% overall patency in severely symptomatic patients. Retrograde filling of the ipsilateral intracranial internal carotid artery to its petrous or cavernous segment appears to be a good sign of operability. Timing of such surgery seems critical. Operation within 4 hours of acute symptoms has been recommended.

B.   An uncommon approach to management of the symptomatic patient with an occluded internal carotid artery is **external carotid artery endarterectomy.** External carotid revascularization may relieve symptoms by increasing both the total and regional cerebral blood flow. The best results of external carotid endarterectomy are achieved when it is performed in the setting of an ipsilateral internal carotid artery occlusion and external carotid artery stenosis. In this setting, this procedure is usually performed to relieve retinal symptoms such as **bright light amaurosis, rubeosis iritis, or neovascular glaucoma.**

C.   Finally, symptomatic patients with total internal carotid occlusion also may be relieved by **extracranial-to-intracranial (EC-IC)** anastomosis of the temporal artery to the middle cerebral artery. EC-IC bypasses generally are performed by a neurosurgeon experienced in microsurgical technique. We continue to see gratifying results in selected patients. However, the international randomized EC-IC bypass study failed to confirm that EC-IC anastomosis is effective in preventing ischemic stroke in patients with atherosclerotic disease in the carotid and middle cerebral arteries. Consequently, EC-IC bypass is rarely performed anymore.

VIII.   Vertebrobasilar insufficiency. Vertebrobasilar insufficiency or nonhemispheric TIAs are characterized by instability of the patient in the upright position, visual changes, and bilateral paresthesias with occasional paresis. They are the result of hypoperfusion of the basilar artery and its branches. Left subclavian stenosis proximal to the left vertebral artery or stenosis of the origin of either vertebral artery may decrease vertebrobasilar flow. Vertebrobasilar insufficiency is especially likely to occur when carotid occlusive disease also is present and collateral flow via the circle of Willis is inadequate. In such cases, we generally repair the carotid lesions in the hope that increased collateral flow will alleviate the vertebrobasilar symptoms. If carotid occlusive disease is not present or the circle of Willis is not intact, direct vertebral artery reconstruction should be considered. Proximal subclavian stenosis is usually corrected by carotid–subclavian bypass, subclavian-subclavian bypass, or subclavian-to-carotid reimplantation. Stenosis at the origin of either vertebral artery may be managed by endarterectomy or reimplantation of the vertebral artery into the side of the common carotid artery. EC-IC anastomosis also may improve the posterior cerebral circulation. Finally, percutaneous balloon angioplasty of focal subclavian stenosis can be successful, but vertebral artery embolization is a potential risk.

   IX.   Pulsatile masses. Pulsatile masses near the carotid artery usually are true aneurysms, carotid body tumors, adjacent lymphadenopathy, or a tortuous carotid artery. Sonography, CT scanning, or MRI can generally differentiate between these etiologies. Carotid aneurysms are rare but dangerous since they may lead to rupture, cerebral embolization, thrombosis, and local pressure symptoms. The best surgical approach is resection and arterial restoration by direct end-to-end anastomosis or an interposition graft. **Carotid body tumors** are uncommon neoplasms of neuroectoderm paraganglion cells of the carotid body and are also referred to as paragangliomas. These tumors arise from the afferent ganglion of the glossopharyngeal nerve and are progressive but rarely malignant neoplasms. Periadventitial excision or carotid artery replacement is recommended for all carotid body tumors. Radiation therapy appears to be of little value in their management and observation is appropriate only for asymptomatic elderly patients who are poor surgical risks.

   X.   Carotid fibromuscular dysplasia (FMD) is a relatively benign, often incidental finding that rarely causes symptoms during when observed. Although carotid FMD may be associated with TIAs, the incidence of subsequent stroke is less than that seen with atherosclerotic carotid occlusive disease. Patients with FMD are more prone to internal carotid dissection. When neurologic or visual symptoms can be attributed to carotid FMD, they generally resolve without operation and recurrence is uncommon. High-grade symptomatic FMD stenoses can be treated by internal carotid balloon angioplasty, and large or symptomatic aneurysms can be resected with vein graft reconstruction.

OPERATIVE MANAGEMENT

   Because carotid endarterectomy is the most common operation for extracranial cerebrovascular disease, we focus on principles of operative care for carotid reconstructions. These same principles also apply to other types of vertebral and subclavian revascularization.

   I.   Preoperative preparation. For elective cases, anticoagulants and antiplatelet medications are usually discontinued at least 48 hours before surgery. The main exception is a patient with multiple recent TIAs or a severe carotid stenosis (<2 mm), who usually remains on heparin or aspirin until operation.

   Although neck infection is rare, several preventive measures are taken. The chin, neck, and anterior chest are shaved on the side of endarterectomy. This area is washed with a surgical scrub solution within 6 to 12 hours of operation. Preoperative parenteral antibiotics are started when the patient goes to the operating room; the antibiotic of choice usually is a cephalosporin or semisynthetic penicillin.

The patient is made NPO ("nothing by mouth") after midnight. Stable or asymptomatic patients are admitted on the morning of operation. Some symptomatic patients will already be hospitalized for heparin anticoagulation. An intravenous infusion of balanced salt solution (e.g., 5% dextrose in Ringer's solution at 100 to 125 mL/h) is begun to maintain hydration. General narcotic premedications that may cause hypotension are avoided.

On the day of surgery, a responsible member of the operating team is present in the operating room from the time the patient enters the room until the patient is transported to the recovery area. An arterial line is generally inserted in the operating room. Selected patients with severe cardiac disease (see Chap. 8) may also receive a Swan–Ganz catheter. A Foley bladder catheter is optional but may assist with blood pressure control since bladder distention may exacerbate hypertension in a labile patient.

II.   Operative principles

A.   General endotracheal anesthesia is our preference, since it both provides the best control of the airway and best facilitates management of cardiorespiratory function. Other experienced surgeons prefer regional cervical block and local anesthesia.

B.   Carotid exposure (Fig. 11.1) must be gentle and meticulous to avoid venous or nerve injury and dislodgement of atheromatous material from a plaque. Figure 11.2 demonstrates the relative positions of the major nerves of the neck that surround the carotid artery.

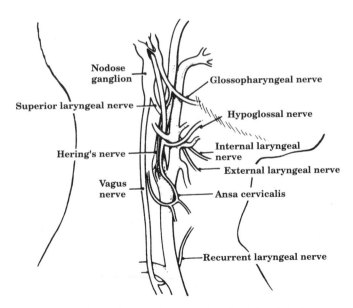

Figure 11.2.   Nerves that may be encountered or injured during carotid endarterectomy. Specific nerve function is discussed in the text.

1. Branches of the **ansa cervicalis** (ansa meaning loop) provides innervation to the strap muscles and may be divided for better exposure, without a resulting neurologic deficit.

2. The **hypoglossal nerve** usually crosses the carotid artery at or near the carotid bifurcation. Most hypoglossal injuries are caused by retraction of the nerve. Clamp injuries may occur if the hypoglossal nerve is not dissected free from the common facial vein before it is divided. Hypoglossal injury results in weakness of the tongue on the operated side, with tongue deviation toward the side of the injury. This deficit may cause biting of the tongue while chewing, and the patient may have some difficulty swallowing or speaking. Bilateral hypoglossal nerve injury may be life threatening, since the tongue may prolapse posteriorly and obstruct the airway when the patient is supine.

3. The **vagus nerve** usually runs in the posterior carotid sheath behind the carotid artery. About 10% of the time it swings anteriorly along the anterolateral surface of the carotid artery (anterior vagus nerve). The nerve must be dissected free from the carotid artery, especially at the proximal and distal extent of carotid dissection, where clamps may accidentally injure it.

  a. Vagal injury is most commonly manifested by hoarseness, as the **recurrent laryngeal nerve** normally originates from the vagus in the chest and runs back to the vocal cord in the tracheoesophageal groove. The recurrent laryngeal nerve loops around the subclavian artery on the right side and the ligamentum arteriosum on the left. Occasionally, the laryngeal nerve is nonrecurrent and originates from the vagus nerve in the neck and passes posteriorly to the carotid artery.

  b. The **external branch of the superior laryngeal nerve** travels behind the carotid bifurcation to the true vocal cord. This nerve innervates the cricothyroid muscle, which maintains the tone of the vocal cord. Injury may be avoided by careful dissection around the external carotid and superior thyroid arteries. Injury results in voice tone fatigue, especially after prolonged speaking or singing.

4. The **greater auricular nerve** is a sensory nerve to the skin overlying the mastoid process, the concha of auricle, and the earlobe. It lies on the anterior surface of the sternocleidomastoid muscle and may be injured when the neck incision is carried toward the mastoid process. Injury results in skin numbness around the lower ear and earlobe.

5. The **mandibular branch** of the facial nerve runs forward from the angle of the mandible and parallel to the mandible. Injury results in weakness of the perioral musculature on the injured side. The patient may drool from the corner of the mouth.

6. With very high internal carotid exposures, the **glossopharyngeal nerve** is at risk for injury. Injury to this nerve is rare but devastating and results in difficulty swallowing which may preclude oral feeding and necessitate placement of a gastrostomy feeding tube. The glossopharyngeal nerve also provides a branch to the carotid sinus called **Hering's nerve,** which usually traverses posterior or deep to the internal carotid artery (Fig. 11.2).

C.   Prevention of thromboemboli obviously is essential if neurologic deficits are to be avoided. We take several measures to avoid thrombus accumulation and embolism.

1.   During gentle carotid dissection, **suction** is used rather than blotting with sponges to keep the operative field dry. Vigorous manipulation of the carotid bifurcation may dislodge loose atheromatous material from an ulcerated plaque.

2.   Before carotid clamping, **heparin** is administered intravenously and allowed to circulate for at least 5 min. Our usual dose is a 5,000-unit bolus.

3.   The inside of the carotid artery is **irrigated** with heparinized saline to wash out any loose atheroma or clot both before a shunt is inserted and before the internal carotid artery is reopened.

4.   Bleeding of the internal and external carotid arteries (back-bleeding) and forward bleeding of the common carotid artery flush out any thrombus or atheroma that may accumulate behind vascular clamps. Carotid blood flow also is reinstituted up the external carotid artery for a few seconds before opening the internal carotid artery. This sequence of reopening the carotid branches should allow any thromboemboli to go out through the external carotid artery and not directly to the brain.

D.   Cerebral protection from clamp ischemia probably is best achieved by two methods: careful blood pressure control and shunting.

1.   In Chapter 8, we emphasized that cerebral perfusion is directly related to **mean arterial blood pressure.** Therefore, during carotid clamping, we remind the anesthesiologist to maintain the blood pressure in a normotensive to mildly hypertensive range. If continuous EEG monitoring is used, a diffuse slowing pattern often can be eliminated by simply raising the patient's mean arterial pressure.

2.   Shunting during carotid endarterectomy remains controversial. Experienced surgeons have demonstrated that with or without shunting, carotid endarterectomy can be performed with a low incidence of permanent postoperative neurologic deficit (1% to 3%). The key question is how to identify the few patients who will not tolerate carotid clamping long enough for the surgeon to complete endarterectomy without a shunt. Under general anesthesia, the two most common methods to assess adequate cerebral perfusion during carotid clamping are carotid stump pressures and EEG monitoring (see Chap. 9). Our experience suggests that carotid stump pressures may not correlate with adequate cerebral perfusion as indicated by EEG monitoring. Consequently, we insert a shunt after carotid clamping if focal EEG changes occur and are not corrected by manipulation of anesthetic agents or blood pressure. If EEG monitoring is not available, a carotid stump pressure below 50 mm Hg may indicate inadequate cerebral collateral flow during carotid clamping. Even without EEG changes, we often insert a shunt to allow for an unhurried endarterectomy and to provide an intraluminal stent which, in our experience, facilitates a better closure of the internal carotid artery. In a teaching situation, we are more likely to use shunting. We also believe that routine shunting is advisable when the contralateral internal carotid artery is occluded. Finally, in patients in whom the internal carotid plaque extends high into the carotid artery, an intraluminal shunt may make endarterectomy excessively difficult. In such cases, the endarterectomy of the distal plaque probably should be performed without a shunt in place. A shunt may subsequently be inserted to complete the operation.

E. The **endarterectomy technique** should achieve the two main goals of carotid artery reconstruction. The first goal is adequate removal of the stenotic or ulcerated plaques. Since atherosclerotic lesions involve the intima and media, we generally remove the plaques down to the external elastic lamina. In our experience, such a deep endarterectomy plane has resulted in the removal of retained media fibers, which may cause recurrent myointimal restenosis, but it has not been associated with late aneurysm formation. The second goal is closure of the arteriotomy so that stenosis or thrombosis does not occur. A primary closure of the arteriotomy is usually adequate for larger (>4.5 mm) internal carotid arteries. Patches are used when primary closure would cause stenosis or in cases of redo endarterectomy. Patch angioplasty may protect against early thrombosis, and we have noted a trend toward more patching by all surgeons in the past ten years. Recent clinical trials indicate that patching is beneficial in the following situations: (a) small internal carotid artery (<3.5 mm), (b) long internal carotid arteriotomy (>3 cm), (c) women who tend to have small arteries, and (d) reoperative endarterectomies. In our opinion, low-power magnifying glasses (magnification of 2 to 4) help us perform a more meticulous endarterectomy and arterial closure. Flow through the internal and external carotid arteries is assessed by a sterile continuous-wave Doppler probe. Absence of flow or an obstructed, monophasic signal indicates thrombosis or stenosis, which requires immediate thrombectomy and a patch. Other methods of intraoperative assessment include arteriography or duplex ultrasound (see Chap. 9).

F. Recognition of postoperative neurologic deficit ideally is made in the operating room if the anesthesiologist can awaken and extubate the patient early. Otherwise, the patient is moved to the recovery area and a neurologic examination of general motor function is made as soon as the patient is responsive. In our experience, the earliest signs of a neurologic deficit may be severe hypertension, difficulty in being awakened from anesthesia, or clumsiness of fine hand movement.

The proper management of an immediate postoperative neurologic deficit must be individualized.

1. First, the patient's general **cardiorespiratory status** must be stabilized expeditiously. This includes stabilization of heart rate, blood pressure, pulmonary ventilation, and blood oxygenation.

2. Treatment then depends on the **location** of the neurologic deficit.

a. If the deficit is a **contralateral hemiparesis,** a technical problem at the endarterectomy site may exist. We generally have returned these patients immediately to the operating room to examine the endarterectomy site. Two tests may help determine whether the arteriotomy should be reopened. First, duplex ultrasound is a sensitive method to ascertain carotid thrombosis or a major filling defect due to thrombus or a technical problem (e.g., residual plaque). Second, an intraoperative carotid arteriogram may also be done if ultrasound is not available or equivocal. If these tests are not satisfactory, reexploration of the artery remains the only way to rule out technical error.

b. If the neurologic deficit is diffuse, the patient may have suffered an **internal capsule stroke,** usually caused by a hypotensive episode. Patency of the carotid arteries should then be assessed with duplex ultrasound. If the operated side is occluded, then reoperation is appropriate. If both carotid arteries appear widely patent, the patient should receive supportive care. A CT brain scan should be performed in approximately 12 to 24 hours to localize the cerebral infarct area and assess the amount of cerebral edema or hemorrhage.

III. Postoperative care

A. Day of surgery. All patients spend the first 12 to 24 hours after cerebrovascular surgery in an intensive recovery area, where vital signs and neurologic status can be continuously monitored. The head of the bed is elevated 30 to 45 degrees to diminish edema and facilitate deep breathing. The patient is kept NPO until the first postoperative morning since reexploration is occasionally necessary. While the patient is NPO, a maintenance intravenous infusion of 5% dextrose in water and one-half normal saline is run at 1 mL/kg/h. Hyponatremia and water intoxication must be avoided in those patients who occasionally develop cerebral edema because of inappropriate secretion of antidiuretic hormone. Patients who have undergone staged bilateral carotid endarterectomies may be insensitive to hypoxia as a result of carotid baroreceptor trauma. Therefore, they must be observed for bradycardia, hypotension, and respiratory distress.

B. Postoperative day 1. If a wound drain has been used, it is removed on the first postoperative day. Patients who are doing satisfactorily resume normal diet, begin ambulation, and restart antiplatelet drugs. The efficacy of long-term antiplatelet therapy after carotid endarterectomy is not known. However, we tend to prescribe a low dose of aspirin (80 to 325 mg daily), especially if the patient has known coronary artery disease, a Dacron patch angioplasty, or contralateral uncorrected carotid disease. If patients have resumed normal activities without complications or hemodynamic instability, they are discharged later the first postoperative day. Older patients with labile blood pressure or other medical comorbidities may stay an additional night.

C. Discharge instructions. Most patients are discharged within 24 to 48 hours after operation. Because the patient's full physical strength may not recover for 2 to 4 weeks, we generally advise patients to convalesce for that period of time before resuming normal working activities. All patients are rechecked as outpatients in 3 to 6 weeks after surgery. They return to their local referring physician for long-term management of any medical problems.

COMPLICATIONS

I. **Early postoperative problems** usually are apparent on the day of surgery and require prompt recognition and treatment.

A. **Immediate postoperative neurologic deficits** are discussed in the section on Operative Management. Occasionally, a patient will do well in the immediate recovery period but develop TIAs between the first postoperative day and the day of discharge. These patients should undergo a head CT scan; if it is negative for intracerebral hemorrhage, they should be anticoagulated with heparin. They should undergo urgent cerebral angiography for detection of any surgically correctable problems. If no anatomic problem is seen, heparin should be continued until symptoms resolve and anticoagulant therapy is established.

B. **Hypertension** is a common postoperative problem occurring in approximately 20% of patients who have carotid endarterectomy. Patients who were hypertensive before operation, especially if poorly controlled, are more likely to have severe postoperative hypertension. The incidence of neurologic deficit and death is significantly higher in these hypertensive patients. Therefore, we strive to maintain postoperative systolic blood pressure in a range from the minimal normal preoperative recording to a maximum of 180 mm Hg. Chapter 10 discusses the use of nitroprusside and other antihypertensives in detail.

C. **Neck hematomas** may compromise breathing and swallowing. Patients with large neck hematomas should be returned to the operating room for evacuation. If a patient's respiratory status and hematoma are stable, no attempt at intubation should be made until the surgical team is ready to operate. In cases where respiration is desperately compromised or bleeding is profuse, nasotracheal intubation and control of bleeding in the recovery room may be necessary to save the patient. Smaller neck hematomas may be left alone and usually resolve in 7 to 14 days. They seldom are complicated by infection. If a pulsatile mass persists after the major portion of the hematoma resolves, a pseudoaneurysm should be suspected and confirmed by ultrasonography.

D. **Local nerve injuries** following carotid operations probably are more common than generally is recognized or reported. Some degree of cranial nerve dysfunction affects 5% to 20% of patients. The mechanism of injury usually is nerve retraction or clamping and not transection. Most injuries involve the hypoglossal or recurrent laryngeal nerves. The injuries often are mild or asymptomatic and will not be detected unless one specifically examines for them. For example, one-third of recurrent laryngeal nerve injuries will go unrecognized unless direct laryngoscopy is performed. **Therefore, all patients who undergo staged, bilateral carotid endarterectomy should be tested by direct laryngoscopy before the second operation.** Fortunately, most cranial nerve injuries resulting from retraction trauma will resolve in 2 to 6 months. Time and reassurance are all the treatment most patients require.

II.   Late complications of carotid artery reconstructions are uncommon or at least seldom cause symptoms.

A.   Recurrent carotid stenosis that is symptomatic is rare, affecting only 1% to 3% of patients after carotid endarterectomy. Asymptomatic restenosis is detectable in 10% to 20% of patients followed by noninvasive carotid testing, and is more common in women and active smokers. The risk of a future stroke in this asymptomatic group appears to be low. Recurrent lesions have a striking predilection for the internal carotid artery near its origin and within the confines of the original endarterectomy site. Early recurrent lesions (<36 months) are predominantly a combination of intimal hyperplasia and surface thrombus. Features of atherosclerosis (abundant collagen, calcium deposits, and foam cells) are more pronounced in late recurrences. An important feature that differentiates primary and recurrent carotid lesions is the presence of surface and intraplaque thrombus in 90% of recurrent stenoses. Recurrent symptoms after carotid endarterectomy generally require repeat angiography. Recurrent stenosis is repaired by repeat endarterectomy and patch angioplasty, or by patch angioplasty alone if an endarterectomy plane is not available. Alternatively, segmental carotid resection and an interposition vein graft may be performed, or even carotid stent angioplasty in select cases.

The need for long-term ultrasound surveillance of carotid endarterectomy sites is debatable. Since early restenosis is often a relatively benign process, asymptomatic restenosis does not mandate reoperation. However, contralateral atherosclerotic asymptomatic 50% to 79% stenoses have a significant risk of becoming symptomatic, especially if they progress. Consequently, we recheck such lesions every 6 to 12 months and caution patients to report any ipsilateral neurologic or ocular symptoms. Since the late results of carotid stent angioplasty are unclear, these patients should be followed regularly (e.g., every 6 months).

B.   Carotid pseudoaneurysm may occur after primary arterial closure or patch angioplasty. In general, such pseudoaneurysms should be repaired since mural thrombus may accumulate and cause cerebral thromboembolism. Large pseudoaneurysms also may cause local pressure symptoms.

SELECTED READING

Albers GW, Bates VE, Clark WM, et al. Intravenous tissue-type plasminogen activator for treatment of acute stroke: the Standard Treatment with Alteplase to Reverse Stroke (STARS) study. *JAMA* 2000;283:1145–1150.

Barnett HJM, Eliasziw M, Meldrum HE. Drugs and surgery in the prevention of ischemic stroke. *N Engl J Med* 1995;332:238–248.

Beebe HG, Kritpracha B. Carotid stenting versus carotid endarterectomy: update on the controversy. *Semin Vasc Surg* 1998;11:46–51.

Bower TC, Merrell SW, Cherry KJ Jr, et al. Advanced carotid disease in patients requiring aortic reconstruction. *Am J Surg* 1993;166: 146–151.

CASANOVA Study Group. Carotid surgery versus medical therapy in asymptomatic carotid stenosis. *Stroke* 1991;22:1229–1235.

Chervu A, Moore WS. Carotid endarterectomy without arteriography (general review). *Ann Vasc Surg* 1994;8:296–302.

European Carotid Surgery Trialists' Collaborative Group. MRC European Carotid Surgery Trial: interim results for symptomatic patients with severe (70–99%) or with mild (0–29%) carotid stenosis. *Lancet* 1991;337:1235–1243.

Evans BA, Sicks JD, Whisnant JP. Factors affecting survival and occurrence of stroke in patients with transient ischemic attacks. *Mayo Clin Proc* 1994;69:416–421.

Executive Committee for the Asymptomatic Carotid Atherosclerosis Study. Endarterectomy for asymptomatic carotid artery stenosis. *JAMA* 1995;273:1421–1428.

Gertler JP, Blankensteijn JD, Brewster DC, et al. Carotid endarterectomy for unstable and compelling neurologic conditions: do results justify an aggressive approach? *J Vasc Surg* 1994;19:32–42.

Hobson RW II, Krupski WC, Weiss DG, et al. Influence of aspirin in the management of asymptomatic carotid artery stenosis. *J Vasc Surg* 1993;17:257–265.

North American Symptomatic Carotid Endarterectomy Trial Collaborators. Beneficial effect of carotid endarterectomy in symptomatic patients with high-grade carotid stenosis. *N Engl J Med* 1991;325:445–453.

North American Symptomatic Carotid Endarterectomy Trial Collaborators. Benefit of carotid endarterectomy in patients with symptomatic moderate or severe stenosis. *N Engl J Med* 1998;339: 1415–1425.

North American Symptomatic Carotid Endarterectomy Trial Collaborators. The causes of stroke in patients with asymptomatic internal carotid artery stenosis. *N Engl J Med* 2000;342:1693–1770.

North American Symptomatic Carotid Endarterectomy Trial. Significance of plaque ulceration in symptomatic patients with high-grade carotid stenosis. *Stroke* 1994;25:304.

Veterans Affairs Cooperative Studies Program 309 Trialist Group. Carotid endarterectomy and prevention of cerebral ischemia in symptomatic carotid stenosis. *JAMA* 1991;266:3289–3294.

Lower-Extremity Claudication

Intermittent claudication of the lower extremities is the most common manifestation of peripheral arterial occlusive disease. The term claudication means "a limp." The patient may limp or claudicate for several reasons. The patient's calf muscles may develop cramping pain with walking. The hip and thigh muscles may cramp or tire. Walking also may be limited because of a feeling of diffuse lower-extremity weakness and numbness.

Although claudication usually is associated with vascular disease, degenerative hip disease or conditions of the spine also may cause a patient to claudicate. Therefore, in the evaluation of lower-extremity claudication, the physician must first question the underlying etiology. Is the claudication caused by arterial occlusive disease or some other problem? The history and physical exam often can answer this question (see Chap. 3). Treadmill walking with measurement of resting and postexercise ankle-brachial indices provides objective data to support or refute the clinical impression (see Chap. 5).

If the initial evaluation suggests arterial occlusive disease as the cause of claudication, the next question concerns how the claudication should be managed. Should therapy be medical, or should a procedure such as percutaneous balloon angioplasty or an operation be recommended? Finally, if an operation is recommended, what operation should be performed?

I. Patterns of disease. Vascular claudication of the lower limb generally is caused by an arterial stenosis or occlusion in one of two main anatomic sites (Fig. 12.1). A common location of stenosis or occlusion is the superficial femoral artery, frequently at the exit of the adductor canal. In diabetics, this infrainguinal disease may also involve the tibial arteries. The other large anatomic category of claudicants has occlusive disease localized primarily to the distal abdominal aorta and iliac arteries with open distal arteries.

Patient history, physical examination, and noninvasive segmental leg pressures and pulse volume recordings usually can identify the primary location of disease (see Chaps. 3 and 5). Since therapeutic decisions are influenced by the location of occlusive lesions, we categorize patients into three patterns of peripheral arterial disease (Fig. 12.2).

A. Aortoiliac disease (type 1). Type 1, the least common pattern (10% to 15%), is limited to the distal abdominal aorta and common iliac arteries. Patients with focal aortoiliac disease are characteristically age 35 to 55, with a low incidence of hypertension and diabetes but a high frequency of heavy cigarette smoking and hyperlipidemia. There has been an alarming increase in premature atherosclerotic aortoiliac disease in younger women (age 35 to 50) who have smoked since adolescence. These patients generally complain of proximal lower-extremity claudication involving the hip and thigh muscles with progres-

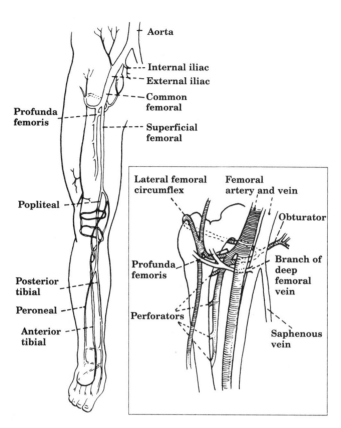

Figure 12.1. Arterial anatomy of the lower extremity. The most common locations of atherosclerotic occlusive disease are the aortoiliac region and the superficial femoral artery. Enlarged drawing of the femoral region demonstrates the major collateral channels of the profunda femoris artery. Branches of the deep femoral vein cross the anterior surface of the profunda femoris artery and must be carefully divided before extensive profundaplasty is attempted.

sion to the calf muscles. In about 15% of such patients, however, the claudication affects only the calves. Diminished femoral pulses and femoral bruits are characteristic physical findings. Weak pedal pulses often are palpable, since the femoropopliteal system is open. Some men have the triad of bilateral hip and buttock claudication, impotence, and absent femoral pulses, which is called **Leriche's syndrome.** Patients with type 2 disease (20%) have aortoiliac atherosclerotic lesions that also involve the external iliac arteries extending to the groins. Final definition of whether the patient has type 1 or 2 aortoiliac disease must be made by arteriography.

Type 1   **Type 2**   **Type 3**

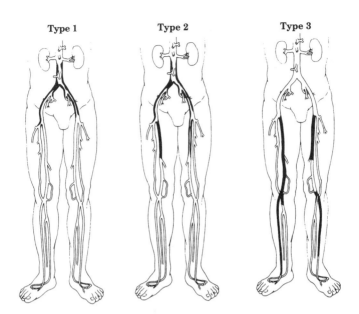

Figure 12.2.   Patterns of aortoiliac and femoropopliteal arterial occlusive disease. Type 1 is limited to the distal abdominal aorta and common iliac arteries. Type 2 is a combination of aortoiliac and femoropopliteal disease. Type 3 involves primarily the superficial femoral, popliteal, and tibial arteries.

B. Combined aortoiliac and femoropopliteal disease (type 2). The majority of patients with lower-extremity claudication (66%) have combined aortoiliac and femoropopliteal disease (type 2), which usually occurs in patients with multiple cardiovascular risk factors: smoking, hypertension, hyperlipidemia, and sometimes adult-onset diabetes mellitus. These patients usually have more incapacitating leg claudication than is seen in aortoiliac or femoropopliteal disease alone and often progress to more severe ischemia problems, such as rest pain, foot ulcers, or gangrene.

C. Isolated femoropopliteal disease (type 3). Patients with isolated femoropopliteal disease generally present with calf claudication that starts after the patient walks and is relieved by stopping for a few minutes. These patients are older (age 50 to 70) and have a higher prevalence of hypertension, adult-onset diabetes mellitus, and associated vascular disease of the coronary and carotid vessels than do those with aortoiliac disease. Like patients with aortoiliac disease, they frequently are cigarette smokers. They generally have good femoral pulses but no palpable popliteal or pedal pulses. Their claudication usually is improved by a supervised walking program and remains stable for long periods of time if significant proximal aortoiliac disease is not present. In fact, the following observations support initial nonoperative management: Patients over 60 years of age with superficial femoral artery occlusive disease (a) have a low likelihood of limb loss (2% to 12% in a 10-year follow-up) if followed closely on conservative treatment, (b) can expect improvement in symptoms (80%) if the initial ankle-to-brachial systolic pressure index (ABI) is greater than 0.6, and (c) should undergo evaluation for angioplasty or reconstructive surgery if the ABI falls below 0.5. Five-year survival is 70% to 80%, and only 20% will require surgical revascularization.

II.   Initial management. The following principles are crucial in determining the best treatment for a patient with intermittent vascular claudication. For most patients, initial treatment is nonoperative. Only 5% to 10% of patients with claudication will require amputation of an extremity due to progression of the disease in 5 years, most of whom continue to smoke or who have diabetes mellitus. **Lower extremity arteriography should be viewed as an invasive intent to treat and is not usually necessary in the majority of patients with recent onset vascular claudication.**

   A.   Determination of initial treatment is based on the duration, disability, and progression of the claudication. Initial management also is influenced by the patient's medical condition.

   1.   Duration. If the leg claudication is of recent onset and is not incapacitating, a trial period of nonoperative therapy is indicated without the need for an angiogram. This approach is recommended particularly for patients who are suspected of having a recent superficial femoral artery occlusion. Although they may experience sudden severe calf claudication when the superficial femoral artery occludes, their claudication usually improves in 6 to 8 weeks if profunda femoris arterial collaterals are well developed. In general, we prefer to follow patients with recent onset of claudication for at least 3 to 6 months to determine whether the claudication will stabilize, improve, or worsen.

   2.   Disability. We generally ask two important questions of the patient about the disability imposed by the leg claudication: Does the leg claudication prevent normal activity, especially the performance of essential daily activities or a job? Does the claudication limit leisure activities that the patient enjoys? In our experience, the answers to these two questions are more helpful in determining patient management than is the distance the patient can walk before he or she is stopped by claudication.

   3.   Progression. It is extremely important to determine whether the claudication is stable or progressing. Patients who have noted rapid progression of claudication over 6 months to 1 year are more likely to need arterial reconstruction than are stable claudicators. Patients with progressive claudication also are more likely to appreciate any relief an operation may provide.

   4.   Assessment of the patient's general medical condition is essential for determining the proper initial management of claudication. Elective operations for intermittent claudication should be reserved for patients who appear to have a low risk of mortality (2% to 3%) and morbidity. This assessment is discussed in detail in Chapter 7. Patients with multiple medical problems and stable leg claudication should be followed until symptoms become incapacitating or the limb is threatened by rest pain, nonhealing ulcers, or gangrene.

B.   Nonoperative management includes a supervised walking program and control or elimination of cardiovascular risk factors.

1.   Regular lower-extremity exercise increases metabolic adaptation to ischemia caused by walking and may enhance collateral blood flow. The result is stabilization or improvement of claudication. A variety of exercise programs can alleviate claudication. A relatively simple program that has helped 80% of our patients emphasizes the following concepts:

a.   Patients are asked to set aside a definite period and frequency of exercise in **addition** to normal daily activities (e.g., 30 minutes, 3 to 5 days per week). Exercise every day may be too much activity for many older patients; consequently, an every-other-day exercise program is ideal.

b.   Patients are instructed to walk at a comfortable (not too fast) pace and stop for a brief rest whenever claudication becomes severe.

c.   This walk–rest routine should be continued for 30 minutes. As the leg muscles adapt to anaerobic metabolism, the frequency and length of rest stops will decrease. After 6 to 8 weeks, most claudicators can double or triple their comfortable walking distance. In bad weather, the patient may use an indoor treadmill, walk inside a shopping mall, or use a stationary exercise bicycle.

2.   Elimination of cigarette smoking improves blood flow to the legs, increases skin temperature, and slows the progression of atherosclerosis. Convincing smokers to quit is not easy; many patients enjoy tobacco smoking too much to be convinced to stop. Although many techniques are available to help patients discontinue smoking, none of them will succeed unless the patient really **wants** to stop. Patients who are convinced that smoking is related to vascular disease and who have good motivation generally will completely stop smoking and not resume tobacco use. Unfortunately, such patients are in the minority. Only 40% of men and 30% of women who stop smoking remain off tobacco use after 1 year. Nicotine skin patches and/or Wellbutrin (Glaxo Wellcome Inc., Research Triangle Park, NC, U.S.A.) or Zyban (bupropion) (Glaxo Wellcome Inc.) may enhance abstinence rates by 10% to 15%. Nicotine dependency programs with inpatient efforts may help inveterate smokers.

3.   Control of hyperlipidemias may slow the progression of peripheral atherosclerosis. In the Scandinavian simvastatin (Zocor, Merck & Co., Inc., West Point, PA, U.S.A.) trial, drug therapy for hypercholesterolemia was associated with a 38% reduction in the development or worsening of claudication. In peripheral vascular disease, the major lipid risk factors are elevated LDL cholesterol and triglyceride levels and low HDL cholesterol levels. Certainly, young adults (age

20 to 45) with severe hyperlipidemias need treatment, as reduction of lipids may slow coronary and peripheral vascular disease.

Normal plasma cholesterol is arbitrarily defined as less than 200 mg/100 mL. However, the risk from serum cholesterol is continuous and increases as the cholesterol level rises. LDL levels greater than 160 mg/dL are considered extraordinarily high and need reduction ideally to less than 100 to 110 mg/dL. Normally, triglycerides should be below 150 mg/100 mL. In general, serum measurements of cholesterol and triglycerides should be determined after a 12-hour fast. A low-fat (35% of calories), low-cholesterol (<300 mg daily) diet remains the cornerstone of treatment. Alcohol may exacerbate hypertriglyceridemia in susceptible persons. Although the past recommendation was at least a 3-month trial of diet management before drugs were added, it is now not uncommon for these drugs to be started earlier.

Details of lipid therapy can be reviewed in other reference sources. However, the HMG-CoA reductase inhibitors or statins (lovastatin, pravastatin, simvastatin, and atorvastatin) currently provide the greatest efficacy in lowering serum lipids with very few side effects (hepatic toxicity and myositis). Cholesterol may also be lowered by the bile acid sequestering resins cholestyramine and colestipol as well as niacin.

4. Control of diabetes mellitus may not retard peripheral atherosclerosis. However, strict control may help the diabetic to more quickly resolve infections and heal minor sores of the lower extremities.

5. Control of hypertension also is important, since stress on the arterial wall is directly related to blood pressure (see Chap. 1). Controlled hypertension also reduces a patient's risk of stroke, heart failure, and renal damage.

6. Pentoxifylline (Trental, Hoechst Marion Roussel, Kansas City, MO, U.S.A.) was the first drug approved by the Food and Drug Administration for the treatment of intermittent claudication. This rheologic agent is a methylxanthine that reduces blood viscosity by improving red blood cell membrane flexibility and inhibits platelet aggregation. Although the benefits of pentoxifylline are still debated, a recent meta-analysis concluded that the drug resulted in an average 29-m increase in initial claudication distance and a 48-m increase in absolute claudication distance compared to placebo.

7. Cilostazol (Pletal, Otsuka Pharmaceuticals, Rockville, MD, U.S.A.) is a more recent medication for intermittent claudication. It is a phosphodiesterase III inhibitor with vasodilator and antiplatelet activity. Three randomized have shown improvements in initial claudication distance and absolute claudication distance in the treated groups compared with placebo.

In our practice, pentoxifylline, 400 mg two or three times daily with meals or cilostazol, 100 mg twice daily, have been combined with a walking program and smoking reduction for selected patients with mild to moderate claudication. If walking is improved after 6 to 8 weeks, the drug is often stopped to ascertain whether exercise and abstinence from tobacco will maintain improvement. If claudication worsens, the drug may be restarted. Common side effects of pentoxifylline are gastrointestinal upset and dizziness. Some patients can tolerate only 400 mg twice daily. For cilostazol, the most common side effects are headache and diarrhea. Cilostazol is contraindicated in patients with class III or IV congestive heart failure.

We emphasize that pentoxifylline or cilostazol cannot prevent the need for surgical revascularization or balloon angioplasty in patients with severe progressive claudication or resting ischemia.

III.   Indications for invasive therapy. Patients must be selected carefully for angioplasty or surgery for lower-extremity claudication. Impairment of occupational performance and significant life-style limitation on a low-risk patient are reasonable indications. In this situation, it is important that a favorable anatomic situation for percutaneous angioplasty or surgical reconstruction be present. The best results are obtained when the occlusive disease is localized to the aorta and iliac arteries with open distal vessels. A focal superficial femoral artery stenosis is also a favorable anatomic lesion for angioplasty.

Occasionally, an active individual with an incapacitating above-the-knee superficial femoral artery occlusion may require an elective femoropopliteal bypass. **In such cases, it must be ascertained that significant proximal aortoiliac disease does not coexist, since inadequate inflow may jeopardize the success of a femoropopliteal graft.** A femoral artery pressure study measuring pressure gradients may detect significant iliac occlusive disease (see Chap. 6).

We generally discourage elective arterial reconstruction for stable claudication if the primary disease is (a) combined diffuse aortoiliac and femoropopliteal arterial disease or (b) severe below-the-knee popliteal and tibial artery disease. An aortoiliac angioplasty/stenting or an aortofemoral bypass without addition of a femoropopliteal bypass generally will not completely relieve claudication when multilevel occlusive disease (type 3) exists. An aortofemoral bypass for claudication in patients with combined aortoiliac and femoropopliteal disease should be recommended only when claudication is rapidly progressive and the aortoiliac disease has advanced to critical stenoses or occlusions. Likewise, below-the-knee femoropopliteal or femorotibial bypasses should be limb salvage procedures, and rarely should they be used to treat claudication alone.

IV.   Preoperative evaluation

A.   The principles of assessing **operative risk** and stabilizing chronic medical problems are discussed in Chapter 7. Mortality for percutaneous angioplasty should be negligible. Operative mortality for elective aortoiliac reconstruction or femoropopliteal bypass for claudication should not exceed 2% to 3%. The primary risk to life during vascular reconstructions is coronary artery disease. Significant coronary artery disease exists in at least 40% of patients with peripheral vascular disease. In general, we recommend that the necessary surgical procedures for significant coronary artery disease be performed before elective aortic surgery is attempted.

B.   The importance of **weight reduction** before elective aortic surgery cannot be overemphasized (see Chap. 7). Truly elective operations (e.g., aortofemoral bypass for life-style-limiting claudication) should be delayed until excess weight is reduced. Weight reduction alone often alleviates some claudication.

C. Before elective surgery, patients should be asked to make a commitment to **stop smoking** before operation and not to resume tobacco use after recovery. They should be informed that the chance of graft failure approaches 30% in patients who continue to smoke regularly.

D. Lower extremity angiography is performed only after the decision has been made to intervene with arterial reconstruction or percutaneous angioplasty. Nonoperative management can be selected and followed with information obtained from the history, physical exam, and noninvasive tests **without** the need for an arteriogram.

V. Selection of proper procedure. The choice of operation or transluminal angioplasty for claudication depends on the general condition of the patient, the extent of the atherosclerotic process, and the experience of the surgeon and or interventional radiologist. The preoperative arteriogram and papaverine femoral artery pressure measurements are the single best determinants of which procedure should be undertaken in a given patient (Table 12.1). A well-trained vascular surgeon should understand the indications and limitations for the following procedures: aortoiliac endarterectomy, aortoiliac or aortofemoral bypass graft, femoropopliteal bypass, lumbar sympathectomy, transluminal angioplasty, and extraanatomic reconstruction such as axillofemoral and femorofemoral bypasses.

A. Aortoiliac endarterectomy. In patients with occlusive disease limited to the distal aorta and common iliac arteries, **aortoiliac endarterectomy** gives excellent long-term results, provided the patient eliminates or controls his or her vascular risk factors. However, such focal aortoiliac disease is treated currently in most patients by percutaneous balloon angioplasty and stenting.

Endarterectomy is contraindicated in the presence of any of (a) aortic or iliac aneurysmal disease, (b) aortic occlusion to the level of the renal vessels, or (c) any occlusive disease in the external iliac or femoral arteries. The 5- and 10-year patency rates are 95% and 85%, respectively.

B. Percutaneous transluminal angioplasty (e.g., balloon dilatation plus stenting) is currently the initial treatment of choice for focal arterial stenoses that cause claudication (see Chap. 6). A focal common iliac stenosis of less than 3 cm in length has been a lesion well suited to treatment by percutaneous transluminal angioplasty. Recanalization of total iliac occlusions and dilatation of distal aortic stenoses also have been reported. Angioplasty results can be enhanced by the addition of stents where plaque resists balloon dilatation or where stenosis is recurrent. In addition, excellent results have been achieved with superficial femoral artery stenoses. **The primary limitation of aortoiliac or distal angioplasty remains restenosis** that affects 20% to 40% of patients within 3 to 5 years. Consequently, current results indicate that it may require repeated angioplasty of focal occlusive lesions to achieve satisfactory, long-term relief of symptoms.

Table 12.1.   Aortofemoral graft for multilevel occlusive disease: Predictors of success and need for distal bypass

Emphasis of evaluation	Predictors of good result with AF bypass alone	Predictors of need for distal bypass
Proximal disease	Absent or severely reduced femoral pulse	"Normal" femoral pulse
	Severe stenosis/ occlusion (arteriogram) (positive femoral artery pressure study)[a]	Mild-moderate inflow disease (arteriogram) (Negative femoral artery pressure study)
Distal disease	Good outflow tract (arteriogram)	Poor outflow tract (arteriogram)
	Index runoff resistance <0.2	Index runoff resistence ≥0.2[b]
Intraoperative	Improved pulse volume recorder amplitude	Unimproved/worse pulse volume recorder amplitude
Clinical	Nonadvanced ischemic symptoms (i.e., claudication, rest pain)	Advanced ischemia (necrosis/sepsis)

AF, aortofemoral.

[a] Femoral artery pressure study. An iliac stenosis is significant when the resting pressure gradient across iliac segment is greater than 5 mm Hg or falls more than 15% after reactive hyperemia or papaverine injection.

[b] $\text{Index runoff resistance} = \dfrac{\text{thigh-ankle pressure difference}}{\text{brachial pressure}}$

Adapted from Brewster DC, Perler BA, Robinson JG, Darling RO. Aortofemoral graft for multilevel occlusive disease: predictors of success and need for distal bypass. *Arch Surg* 1982;117:1593–1600.

C.   The majority of patients with incapacitating claudication will require a **bypass graft of the aortoiliac segments** for durable relief (>5 years). Aortofemoral bypass grafts are preferred to aortoiliac bypass grafts, because, not uncommonly, the external iliac segment eventually is obliterated by progressive arteriosclerosis. Subsequent downstream repair becomes necessary in approximately 25% to 30% of patients who are initially treated by aortoiliac bypass, compared to 10% to 15% of patients who undergo aortofemoral bypass initially. In selected patients with unilateral iliac occlusive disease, unilateral aortoiliac or aortofemoral bypass grafts or endarterectomy may be performed through a retroperitoneal approach. Five-year patency rates of 70% to 80% are encouraging and indicate that iliac-origin arterial grafts are useful in situations where one wants to avoid transabdominal aortofemoral grafting or extra-anatomic femorofemoral or axillofemoral bypasses.

D.   Femoropopliteal bypass for stable claudication is being performed less frequently now than it was in the past. Long-term follow-up of patients with leg claudication from a solitary superficial femoral artery occlusion indicates that nonoperative treatment often stabilizes the problem. In addition, progression of proximal aortoiliac disease may lead to poor inflow to a femoropopliteal bypass and eventual hemodynamic graft failure, often within 5 years. Therefore, patients who undergo femoropopliteal bypass for claudication alone should have a good anatomic situation, which includes normal aortoiliac inflow, a patent popliteal artery above the knee with a two- or three-vessel runoff, and a high likelihood of an available saphenous vein. Autogenous saphenous vein remains superior to all other graft materials for durability of a femoropopliteal bypass.

E. Lumbar sympathectomy alone is not considered adequate treatment of lower-extremity claudication. However, sympathectomy may be beneficial occasionally for ischemic rest pain, microembolic phenomenon, or foot sores when poor runoff and inadequate vein for a bypass are present and the ABI is greater than 0.35.

F. Extra-anatomic axillofemoral or femorofemoral bypasses, in our practice, are useful only in a limited group of patients with claudication. The most suitable candidates are those with the following:

1. Iliac occlusion and a normal iliac artery and normal hemodynamics of the contralateral (donor) leg.

2. Previous postirradiation intestinal obstructions or fistulas that discourage intraabdominal aortofemoral reconstruction.

3. Known extensive postsurgical abdominal adhesions.

Direct aortoiliac arterial reconstruction for claudication is preferable to extraanatomic bypasses. When done by experienced hands, aortoiliac reconstruction is safe and provides a durable result in 85% to 90% of patients at 5 years. In contrast, 5-year patency for femorofemoral bypass and axillofemoral bypass for claudication approaches 50% to 75%.

G. Elective aortoiliac reconstruction for occlusive disease is generally **not combined** with other nonvascular operations. For example, we favor leaving asymptomatic gallstones alone despite the recommendations of others to do a cholecystectomy if there are no mitigating circumstances. Although the morbidity of adding cholecystectomy may be low, additional procedures do increase the risks of complications. Also, postoperative cholecystitis secondary to cholelithiasis is rare in our experience. Most postoperative cholecystitis is acalculous and occurs in patients who have been in shock and have the so-called splanchnic shock syndrome. Occasionally, however, we discover incidentally a gallbladder with cholelithiasis **and** chronic smouldering cholecystitis during operative exploration. If the aortic reconstruction goes well, we may perform cholecystectomy **after** the retroperitoneum and femoral wounds have been closed to cover the prosthetic graft.

VI. Preoperative preparation. In our clinical practice, patients who are scheduled for elective arterial operations for claudications will need the following preparation.

A. Prior to hospital admission. A complete history, physical examination, and routine diagnostic studies are performed before hospital admission. Baseline studies include a complete blood count, chest x-ray, 12-lead electrocardiogram (ECG), serum electrolytes, creatinine, blood sugar, liver function tests (bilirubin, serum glutamic-oxaloacetic transaminase, alkaline phosphatase, total protein, albumin), platelet count, prothrombin time (PT), partial thromboplastin time (PTT), fasting serum cholesterol and triglycerides, calcium, phosphorus, and pulmonary function tests in patients with chronic lung disease. Any preoperative consultations with other specialists are arranged, before admission.

   B.   Preoperative angiography. Preoperative angiography (see Chap. 6) is performed at least 24 to 48 hours before an elective operation and can be done on an outpatient basis with brief postprocedural observation and intravenous hydration. Ideally, a day's delay before the operation is allowed to be sure that renal function does not deteriorate after the contrast load from the angiogram.

   C.   Day before operation. Final preparations on the day before operation include:

   1.   The patient is typed and cross-matched for 2 to 4 units of packed red blood cells for aortic operations and typed and held for femoropopliteal reconstructions. If autotransfusion is planned, arrangements are made for its availability.

   2.   For bowel preparation, the patient receives clear liquids and a laxative (e.g., magnesium citrate, 120 mL p.o.) the evening before surgery.

   3.   Since elective arterial patients may have chronic intravascular volume depletion from diuretics and acute dehydration from the angiogram and the bowel preparation, an intravenous infusion of Ringer's lactated solution at 100 to 125 mL/h is started before surgery. Depending on individual patient requirements, such hydration may take 6 to 12 hours prior to operation. Thus, selected patients will require hospital admission on the evening prior to aortic surgery.

   4.   Skin preparation includes shaving hair in the operative field as close to the time of operation as possible to minimize bacterial colonization of the shaved areas. A shower with hexachlorophene, chlorhexidine gluconate, or povidone-iodine soap also is done as close to the time of operation as possible, usually just before the intravenous infusion is started.

   5.   Patients are instructed in deep breathing and coughing, as well as in the use of an incentive spirometer. We also teach the patient leg exercises that are used as prophylaxis against deep venous thrombosis, for stimulation of lower-extremity blood flow, and for maintenance of leg muscle tone prior to ambulation.

   6.   Preoperative prophylactic antibiotics are administered intravenously when the patient is called to the operating room. A semisynthetic penicillin or a cephalosporin is used. For patients with a history of penicillin allergy, the cephalosporins are avoided and the patient receives another antibiotic (e.g., vancomycin, 500 to 1,000 mg) with good coverage for hospital-acquired organisms.

VII.   Operative principles. The details of operative technique are beyond the scope of this handbook. Other operative atlases describe techniques for arterial reconstruction. Certain principles of intraoperative care, however, do warrant emphasis in a book on patient care.

A. Patient positioning. The patient is kept in the supine position with the electrocautery ground beneath the buttocks. The arms generally are adducted to the sides. Ischemic heels are elevated or wrapped with a soft dressing to prevent pressure sores.

B. Skin preparation. The operating room should be warmed (70°F to 75°F) during the skin preparation to reduce heat loss from the patient. The skin preparation extends from the nipples to the knees for aortofemoral reconstructions and to the toes for patients who may require an associated femoropopliteal bypass. Care must be taken to avoid pooling of the preparatory solution beneath the patient, especially in contact with the electrocautery ground. Full-thickness chemical skin burns can result from pooling and prolonged contact with the solution. After application of the antiseptic preparatory solution, the skin is covered with a plastic Steri-Drape (3M Health Care, St. Paul, MN, U.S.A.). Although Steri-Drapes (3M Health Care) may not reduce the incidence of wound infection, we recommend their use to prevent contact of graft materials with the skin, which may contaminate the graft.

C. Intraoperative monitoring. All lower-extremity arterial reconstructions are monitored with a pulse volume recorder (PVR), a similar plethysmograph, or a Doppler flow detector (see Chap. 9). As a general rule, PVR cuffs are placed one limb segment below the anticipated reconstruction site (i.e., at the calf for aortofemoral bypass and at the ankle for femoropopliteal bypass). A baseline recording is made. Additional recordings are made immediately following the arterial reconstructions and before the patient leaves the operating room. Sterile cuffs should be used in the operative field.

D. Systemic anticoagulation. Heparin is used for systemic anticoagulation while the aorta and distal arteries are clamped. Our experience has indicated that an adequate heparin dose is 3,000 to 5,000 units given intravenously 5 minutes before aortic clamping. Although monitoring of heparin effect may not be necessary, we prefer to check an activated clotting time (ACT) before and after heparinization. An ACT of 200 to 300 s is adequate for most cases. Smaller additional doses of heparin (500 to 1,000 units) are given during regional irrigation of the iliac and major femoral artery branches. Reversal of heparin is optional at the termination of the procedure. In general, heparinization with the above doses does not require reversal, since the heparin effect diminishes in about 90 minutes. However, if one chooses to reverse heparinization, ACTs are the primary method used to monitor reversal with protamine sulfate (0.5 to 1.0 mg for every 1 mg of heparin).

E. Intraoperative diuretics. Diuresis (0.5 to 1.0 mg/kg body weight) must be established prior to aortic clamping. Infrarenal aortic clamping diminishes renal cortical blood flow (see Chap. 8) which can be prevented by intravascular volume expansion and administration of the osmotic diuretic mannitol. We give 12.5 to 25.0 g mannitol just before clamping the aorta. When needed, small (10 to 20 mg) doses of furosemide are added. In addition, dopamine (2 to 3 μg/min i.v.) causes renal vasodilatation.

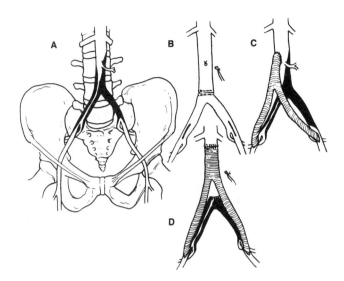

Figure 12.3.   Types of aortoiliac reconstruction. Aortoiliac endarterectomy (B) is our preferred operation for occlusive disease localized to the distal abdominal aorta and common iliac arteries (A). For aortofemoral grafting, the proximal anastamosis may be performed end-to-side (C) or end-to-end (D) (see text). (Adapted from Darling RC, et al. Aorto-iliac reconstruction. *Surg Clin North Am* 1979;59:565–579.)

F.   Proximal aortic anastomosis. Controversy continues over whether the proximal aortic graft anastomosis should be end-to-end or end-to-side (Fig. 12.3). Our experience strongly favors end-to-end aortic anastomosis. Its primary advantages are:

1.   The origin of the graft is from a higher and less diseased part of the infrarenal abdominal aorta.

2.   A better hemodynamic situation, as the aortic blood flow is directed through the graft without competitive flow from the distal aorta.

3.   A more anatomic position and better retroperitoneal coverage as a segment of infrarenal aorta is resected prior to placement of the graft. The onlay or end-to-side aortic anastomosis leaves the graft protruding anteriorly. For this reason, the end-to-side graft seems more likely to adhere to adjacent bowel and cause aortoenteric fistula.

G.   Distal anastomosis in aortofemoral bypass has a significant influence on graft patency. There are five methods of distal anastomosis (Fig. 12.4).

1.   **Type 1, anastomosis to the common femoral artery,** is preferred for patients with widely patent profunda femoris and superficial femoral arteries.

2.   **Type 2 anastomosis carries the graft onto the proximal superficial femoral artery** and is recommended when

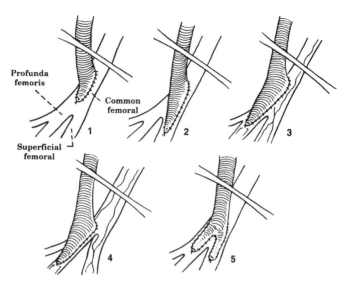

Figure 12.4. Types of femoral anastomosis for aortofemoral bypass grafts: *1*, Type 1 anastomosis to the common femoral artery; *2*, Type 2 anastomosis, in which the graft is carried onto the proximal superficial femoral artery; *3*, Type 3 anastomosis, in which the graft is carried onto the profunda femoris artery; *4*, Type 4 anastomosis, involving only the profunda femoris artery; *5*, Type 5 anastomosis, involving a patch angioplasty of both the superficial and deep femoral arterial orifices. (Adapted from Darling RC, et al. Aorto-iliac reconstruction. *Surg Clin North Am* 1979;59:565–579.)

the orifice of the superficial femoral artery is stenotic but the distal arteries and profunda femoris artery are otherwise normal.

3. Type 3 anastomosis (known as profundaplasty) carries the graft onto the profunda femoris artery and is recommended for patients with extensive superficial femoral artery occlusion. In most patients, the profunda femoris artery is of adequate diameter (3 to 4 mm) and length (15 to 20 cm) to maintain aortofemoral graft flow and perfuse the leg via collaterals.

4. Type 4 anastomosis is done only to the profunda femoris artery. It is necessary when the common femoral and superficial femoral arteries are extensively obliterated.

5. Type 5 anastomosis splits the hood of the graft to patch proximal stenoses of both the superficial femoral and the profunda femoris arteries.

H. Gastrointestinal decompression with a nasogastric tube is often necessary for 24 to 72 hours.

1. Gastrointestinal ileus may be prolonged after aortic reconstruction, especially if extensive lysis of adhesions or dissection of the duodenum is necessary. In our experience, most patients have sluggish intestinal peristalsis for 2 to 3 days after operation. Although nasogastric decompression was once used routinely for this entire period, the vast majority (90%) of patients can tolerate the removal of the nasogastric tube on the first postoperative morning. After removing the tube, we generally wait 24 to 48 hours to be certain that peristalsis is adequate before beginning a liquid diet, which is advanced to solids in the following 24 to 48 hours.

2. Appetite after aortic reconstruction usually is poor, and patients generally do not resume normal caloric intake for at least 5 to 7 days. A weight loss of 5 to 10 lb is not uncommon in the first month following surgery. Patients who have marginal nutritional status prior to operation or a complicated postoperative course may not tolerate further weight loss, and their caloric intake may require parenteral supplementation.

VIII.   Postoperative care. Despite multiple medical problems and sometimes extensive operations, most patients who undergo aortic or peripheral arterial reconstruction can expect an uncomplicated recovery if certain principles of care are followed.

A.   Initial stabilization of the patient should be done in an intensive care setting where vital signs, urine output, ECG rhythm, and respiratory status can be monitored continuously for 12 to 24 hours On arrival to the intensive care unit the patient's blood pressure, heart rate and rhythm should be checked and arterial blood gases drawn for analysis. If the patient is intubated, the ventilator settings should be adjusted after review of the initial blood gas. The criteria for extubation are discussed in Chapter 10.

After these vital functions have been stabilized, additional baseline tests may be obtained, including a portable chest x-ray to check endotracheal tube position and to ensure adequate lung expansion. In addition, a 12-lead ECG should be compared with the preoperative ECG for any changes indicative of intraoperative myocardial ischemia. Cardiac isoenzymes should be sent for study if intraoperative myocardial ischemia was detected, however routine cardiac enzymes are unnecessary. Blood also should be sent for measurement of hematocrit, serum electrolytes, blood sugar, PT/PTT, and platelet count.

Management of common early postoperative problems is outlined in Chapter 10.

B.   Fluid management must be meticulous, as many vascular patients have heart disease and do not tolerate fluid overload. A few guidelines for fluid administration should make fluid management easy.

1. Patients leave the operating room after large amounts of fluid have been given. Most of this fluid is sequestered in interstitial spaces and will remain there until it is slowly mobilized and excreted in 48 to 72 hours In addition, inappropriate secretion of antidiuretic hormone results in sodium and water retention. Therefore, postoperative fluids should be limited to about 80 mL/h (1 mL/kg body weight per hour) of 5% dextrose in half normal saline with 20 to 30 mEq potassium per liter. When needed, the rate of intravenous fluid can be increased or boluses given.

2. Some patients are cold and vasoconstricted when they arrive in the recovery area. As they rewarm and vasodilate additional fluid may be necessary, indicated by decreased urine output, low filling pressures, and tachycardia. If the hemoglobin is less than 8 g/dL or hematocrit less than 25%, packed red blood cells should be transfused. Otherwise, volume replacement may be made with a bolus (5 to 10 mL/kg of a balanced salt solution, e.g., Ringer's lactated solution).

3. When patients begin to mobilize excess fluid on the **second or third postoperative day,** maintenance intravenous rates may need to be reduced to an amount sufficient to keep veins open. If the patient is edematous and urine output has not increased, a small dose (10 to 20 mg) of furosemide may initiate a good diuresis.

C. **Pulmonary care** after extubation is discussed in Chapter 10.

D. **Wound care** requires special attention, since local infection may rapidly extend to a prosthetic graft or cause a bacteremia that could seed the graft surface. Initial dressings should be removed on the first postoperative day. If the wound is sealed, no further dressing is needed. If serosanguineous fluid is leaking from the wound, a sterile gauze dressing should be applied until the drainage stops. Lymph leaks from groin incisions may be treacherous, since infection of the deeper inguinal lymphatics may also infect an adjacent graft. Most minor lymph leaks will resolve in 3 to 5 days. If a groin lymph leak is copious and not decreased or closed in 3 to 5 days, wound exploration and reclosure should be done. Prolonged lymph leakage increases the risk of bacterial invasion of the perigraft lymphatics and may result in an early prosthetic graft infection.

E. The proper time to **ambulate** a patient after aortic or other peripheral arterial reconstruction is another controversial area. Proper timing is individualized with consideration of the following:

1. Many patients are not hemodynamically stable for 24 to 48 hours, and tachycardia with swings in blood pressure is not well tolerated. Incisional pain may also contribute to tachycardia and hypertension. Furthermore, within 48 to 72 hours, mobilization of fluid expands intravascular volume, placing additional stress on the heart. If hemodynamically labile patients attempt to ambulate before tachycardia is controlled and fluids are mobilized, they may experience myocardial ischemia. Myocardial infarction occurs most commonly on the third postoperative day.

2. If the patient has an inguinal lymph leak, it is most likely to stop if lower-extremity activity is curtailed by bed rest. Since ambulation may be delayed for 24 to 72 hours, we insist that patients perform leg exercises (flexion and extension of calf and thigh muscles) for at least 5 minutes every hour. (Figure 12.5 shows several important features of the patient's bed position and equipment.) These exercises improve venous emptying from calf muscles and are prophylaxis for deep venous thrombosis. The leg exercise also increases blood flow to the legs and consequently through any graft. Finally, these exercises help maintain leg muscle tone prior to ambulation.

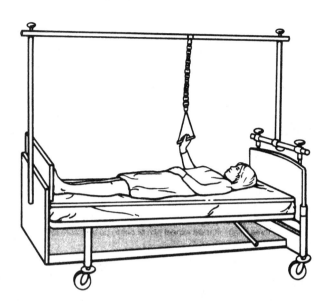

Figure 12.5.   Postoperative bed position following aortic and lower-extremity arterial reconstruction. Important features include a foam mattress to alleviate pressure sores, an overhead trapeze to assist with movement in bed, and a footboard for lower-leg exercises.

In our experience, delayed ambulation in some patients has not increased either pulmonary complications or venous thromboembolism, provided coughing, deep breathing, and footboard exercises are performed routinely.

F.   Convalescence following aortic or peripheral arterial surgery generally takes 6 to 8 weeks. However, patients often expect a quicker recovery. Therefore, we inform them that normal appetite may not return for 3 to 4 weeks, that their weight may not stabilize for 1 month or so, and that their general strength and well-being may not fully recover for 2 to 3 months. We recheck these patients in 4 to 6 weeks after discharge. The main exception is the need to check wounds and remove skin clips or sutures after early hospital discharge.

G.   Long-term success of lower-extremity arterial reconstruction and patient survival depends on many factors. For simplicity, we emphasize to the patient three things that we expect him or her to do to improve long-term success:

1.   All tobacco use must be eliminated. Although most patients will stop at the time of operation, at least 50% eventually return to some tobacco use. Those who smoke are at increased risk of graft failure and other cardiovascular events, especially myocardial infarction and stroke.

2.   Weight must be controlled with a low-fat, low-cholesterol diet. It often is helpful for a dietitian to discuss such a diet with the patient and family.

3. Physical and mental activities must be engaged in regularly. Regular exercise, such as walking, maintains cardiorespiratory conditioning and enhances lower-extremity blood flow. Keeping the mind occupied gives the patient a better sense of well-being and productivity. Many patients experience postoperative depression and need reassurance that with time their strength and well-being will improve. When indications for lower-extremity revascularization are analyzed, 60% to 70% of previously employed patients with claudication and 50% of patients presenting for limb salvage return to work. The remaining patients are often retired but resume normal daily activities in 6 to 8 weeks.

H. Postoperative outpatient checkups are the primary means to determine long-term graft patency and to detect new manifestations of cardiovascular disease at other locations. Reevaluation usually is performed 4 to 6 weeks after surgery and then at 6 months postoperatively, and then annually.

IX. Postoperative complications. Early graft-related complications following operations for lower-extremity claudication affect about 3% of patients. Late complications such as anastomotic aneurysm, graft thrombosis, or graft infection are more common, involving approximately 10% of patients. We focus here on the recognition of such complications and the principles of management.

A. Early graft-related complications

1. Hemorrhage from an arterial graft anastomosis is manifested by a groin or leg hematoma in femoral or popliteal anastomoses and shock in aortic or iliac anastomoses. Treatment is early reoperation, evacuation of the hematoma, and suture control of the bleeding site. Failure to follow this approach may result in infection of the hematoma, pseudoaneurysm formation, or death.

2. Thrombosis may be the result of a technical error at the anastomosis, a thromboembolus, or inadequate runoff to maintain graft flow. Routine perioperative vascular monitoring (see Chap. 9) should recognize thrombosis before severe ischemia occurs. Proper management includes operative reexploration and thromboembolectomy. It often also includes operative arteriography if the adequacy of runoff is questioned.

3. Infections of aortofemoral or femoropopliteal grafts were classified by **D. Emerick Szilagyi who described three grades of infection: grade I, superficial involving the skin and dermis, grade II, involving the subcutaneous and fatty tissue but not the graft, and grade III, involving the graft** (Table 12.2). This grading system has important implications related to the management of infections involving arterial reconstructions. Grade I infections can be managed with close observation, local wound care, and antibiotics, while grade II infections require opening and irrigation in the operating room. Grade III infections may lead to hemorrhage, and therefore graft removal with extraanatomic bypass is the preferred method of management.

4. Colon ischemia may affect 1% to 5% of patients who undergo aortic reconstruction for occlusive disease and usually effects the left or sigmoid colon. Ischemia may result from

Table 12.2.   Clinical classification of infection associated with arterial reconstruction

Grade	Clinical description of infection	Management
I	Involving only the skin and dermis	Local wound care and antibiotics
II	Extending into subcutaneous and fatty tissue but not the graft	Exploration and washout of the wound in the operating room
III	Graft involved in the infection	Exploration and washout of the wound with graft removal and establishment of alternative route perfusion

From Szilagyi DE, Smith RF, Elliott JP, Vrandecic MP. Infection in arterial reconstruction with synthetic grafts. *Ann Surg* 1972;176:321–333, with permission.

inferior mesenteric artery ligation, low cardiac output states and/or inadequate collateral blood flow from the superior mesenteric or internal iliac arteries. Superficial mucosal or muscularis ischemia usually causes transient diarrhea and resolves spontaneously without mortality. Late colon stricture may occur. Transmural colon ischemia will progress to bowel perforation, sepsis, and death in at least 70% of cases.

Clinical manifestations vary with the severity of ischemia. Bloody diarrhea, lower abdominal pain, and unexplained fluid requirements or sepsis suggest colon ischemia. Flexible lower-gastrointestinal endoscopy may reveal changes of patchy hemorrhage and edema or more severe signs of ulceration and pseudomembranes. Mild cases need bowel rest, antibiotics, and hydration until the diarrhea resolves. Resection of necrotic colon with formation of a colostomy is necessary in cases of severe ischemia manifest by peritonitis or sepsis.

B.   Late graft-related complications

1.   Gastrointestinal hemorrhage, especially hematemesis, in a patient who has received a prosthetic aortic graft must raise the suspicion of an aortoenteric fistula. Although the initial hemorrhage may stop and not recur for days, untreated aortoenteric fistulas eventually lead to hemorrhage and death. Therefore, such patients should be resuscitated and undergo emergency endoscopy. Aortography in cases of aortoenteric fistula is often normal and not the most helpful diagnostic test. If the source of hemorrhage is located in the stomach or duodenal bulb, appropriate therapy is instituted. However, if no gastric or duodenal lesions are evident and blood is coming from the distal duodenum, the patient should undergo emergency abdominal exploration for diagnosis and repair of a suspected aortoduodenal fistula. Repair generally requires closure of the intestine and removal of the adjacent graft with extraanatomic bypass. If graft-enteric erosion is not associated with local abscess, however, *in situ* graft replacement, bowel repair, and omental coverage of the new graft will succeed in 85% of patients.

If gastrointestinal hemorrhage is minor, a more elective evaluation may be accomplished. An indium white blood cell scan and computed tomography (CT) scan are sensitive tests for localization of an abnormality at the fistula site. A CT scan will usually show adherence of adjacent bowel to the graft with no intervening fat plane. Although arteriography seldom shows the aortoenteric fistula, the arteriogram may demonstrate a local pseudoaneurysm and provides useful anatomic information for the reconstruction. Angiography also may delineate other causes of hemorrhage, such as angiodysplasias of the intestine.

2. Chronic aortic or lower-limb graft infection may present as an aortoenteric fistula, femoral pseudoaneurysm, groin abscess, or chronically draining sinus tract (Table 12.2). Most infections of aortic prostheses originate in the groin and are commonly caused by Staphylococcus. Although infection may originate at one anastomosis, it rarely remains localized, and spreads along the perigraft plane to eventually involve the entire graft.

Sometimes the diagnosis of infection is difficult. Infections may be indolent, with negative fluid and blood cultures, no fever, and no leukocytosis. An arteriogram should be done to define the involved anatomy and an indium white blood cell scan may demonstrate the infected site. In addition, a CT scan or high-resolution ultrasound may show poor incorporation of the graft or perigraft fluid collections.

Although removal of a focally infected segment of graft may succeed in eliminating infection, resolution of many graft infections will require extraction of the entire prosthesis and an extraanatomic bypass. Putting off or limiting operations often allows a local infection to spread, and eventually life-threatening graft hemorrhage or sepsis may occur.

Patients with infected abdominal aortic grafts have discouraging 30-day and 1-year survival rates of 70% to 80% and 40% to 50%, respectively. Staged revascularization (i.e., axillofemoral bypass) followed by infected abdominal graft removal in 24 to 48 hours accounts in part for improved perioperative survival seen in recent series. Mortality is lower when a new remote revascularization precedes removal of an infected abdominal aortic graft or treatment of an aortoenteric erosion or fistula. Such a staged approach substantially reduces major amputation from 40% when graft removal precedes revascularization to 5% to 10% when the extraanatomic bypass is done first. When extraanatomic revascularization precedes removal of an infected graft, subsequent infection of the new bypass has been rare. In recent years, *in situ* reconstruction of the aorta with superficial femoral vein grafts or aortic homografts have added another therapeutic option.

3. Graft thrombosis that occurs within a few weeks to months of operation often is the result of a technical problem of graft placement or anastomosis. Graft occlusion after this time generally is caused by disease progression at or beyond the distal anastomosis. Impending graft failure may be recognized by recurrent progressive claudication or a decrease in Doppler ankle pressures, especially after exercise. Duplex ultrasound surveillance is an excellent method to detect hemodynamically significant anastomotic or graft stenoses. These warning signs are an indication for arteriography to define correctable lesions before total thrombosis occurs. Reoperations to maintain patency of failing or thrombosed aortofemoral grafts succeed in nearly 80% of patients and result in long-term limb preservation in 60% to 70%. Operative mortality for revision of femoral anastomotic problems is 1.5% in our experience.

4.   Anastomotic pseudoaneurysm occurs most frequently at the common femoral artery. The causative factors are complex and include atherosclerotic deterioration of the artery and anastomotic disruption due to tension, inadequate suture bites, infection, graft dilation, or suture deterioration. Clinically, asymptomatic anastomotic aneurysms of less than 2.5 cm may be safely followed by observation. However, large false aneurysms or symptomatic aneurysms should be electively repaired before they are complicated by thrombosis, distal emboli, or rupture.

5.   Sexual dysfunction in men following aortoiliac operations may be manifested by impaired or absent penile erection and lack of ejaculation after otherwise normal coitus. Previously normal sexual function may be altered by the interruption of preaortic sympathetic fibers, the parasympathetic pelvic splanchnic nerves, or the internal iliac artery flow. It is obvious that the surgeon must know whether any sexual dysfunction existed before surgery. If impotence is a significant problem to the patient, he may be referred to a urologist for evaluation and treatment.

6.   Spinal cord ischemia following operations on the abdominal aorta is rare and considered unpredictable. However, a recent review emphasized that the problem appears to occur in patients in whom internal iliac artery perfusion was impaired, when atheromatous embolism is evident, and when early postoperative hypotension or low cardiac output may further compromise marginal spinal cord perfusion.

SELECTED READING

Brewster DC. Current controversies in the management of aortoiliac occlusive disease. *J Vasc Surg* 1997;25:365–379.

Dawson DL, Cutler BS, Meissner MH, et al. Cilostazol has beneficial effects in treatment of intermittent claudication: results from a multicenter, randomized, prospective double-blind trial. *Circulation* 1998;98:678–686.

Dormandy JA, Murray GD. The fate of the claudicant—a prospective study of 1969 claudicants. *Eur J Surg* 1991;5:131–133.

Frangos SG, Chen AH, Sumpio B. Vascular drugs in the new mellinnium. *J Am Coll Surg* 2000;191:76–92.

Gardner AW, Poelhman ET. Exercise rehabilitation programs for the treatment of claudication pain: a meta-analysis. *JAMA* 1995;274:975–980.

Green RM, Abbott WM, Matsumoto T, et al. Prosthetic above-knee femoropopliteal bypass grafting: five-year results of a randomized trial. *J Vasc Surg* 2000;31:417–425.

Hakaim AG, Hertzer NR, O'Hara PJ, et al. Autogenous vein grafts for femorofemoral revascularization in contaminated or infected fields. *J Vasc Surg* 1994;19:912–915.

Howard G, Wagenknecht LE, Burke GL, et al. Cigarette smoking and progression of atherosclerosis. *JAMA* 1998;279:119–124.

Nevelsteen A, Wouters L, Suy R. Aortofemoral Dacron reconstruction for aorto-iliac occlusive disease: a 25-year survey. *Eur J Vasc Surg* 1991;5:179–186.

Ricco JB. Unilateral iliac artery occlusive disease: a randomized multi-center trial examining direct revascularization versus crossover bypass. *Ann Vasc Surg* 1992;6:209–219.

TransAtlantic Inter-Society Consensus Working Group. Management of Peripheral Arterial Disease: TransAtlantic Inter-society Consensus. *J Vasc Surg* 2000;31(Part 2):S54–75.

Upchurch GR Jr, Conte MS, Gerhard-Herman MD, et al. Infrainguinal arterial reconstructions with vein grafts in patients with prior aortic procedures: the influence of aneurysm and occlusive disease. *J Vasc Surg* 2000;31:1128–134.

Valintine RJ, Hagino RT, Jackson MR, et al. Gastrointestinal complications after aortic surgery. *J Vasc Surg* 1998;28:404–412.

Valentine RJ, Hansen ME, Myers SI, et al. The influence of aortic size on late patency after aortofemoral revascariztion in young adults. *J Vasc Surg* 1995;21:296–305.

Walker RD, Nawaz S, Wilkinson CH, et al. Influence of upper- and lower-limb exercise training on cardiovascular function and walking distance in patients with intermittent claudication. *J Vasc Surg* 2000;31:662–669.

Weitz JI, Byrne J, Clagett GP. Diagnosis and treatment of chronic arterial insufficiency of the lower extremities: a critical review. *Circulation* 1996;94:3026–3049.

Zieske AW, Takei H, Fallon KB, et al. Smoking and atherosclerosis in youth. *Atherosclerosis* 1999;144:403–408.

Threatened Limb Loss

Threatened limb loss is a general term that implies an acute or chronic disease process that, if left untreated, may result in amputation. The term does not specify etiology, and the underlying problem may be diabetic neuropathy, or acute or chronic arterial ischemia. The threatened limb secondary to venous obstruction, infection, or trauma is discussed elsewhere (see Chaps. 21, 22, and 24).

Prompt recognition of the signs of critical limb ischemia and prompt initiation of therapy are necessary if the limb is to be saved. The initial patient evaluation, therefore, must determine whether the patient needs emergent treatment or a less urgent diagnostic work-up. This determination is based primarily on the patient history and physical exam (see Chap. 3) supplemented by the results of noninvasive vascular tests (see Chap. 5) and radiologic studies (see Chap. 6).

In Chapter 12, we discussed the management of claudication of the lower extremities. Special attention was given to principles of aortoiliac revascularization. In this chapter, we concentrate on femoropopliteal and tibial reconstructions, which are more frequently required for limb salvage. However, since many aortoiliac bypasses also are performed as limb salvage procedures, Chapter 12 should also be reviewed for a complete overview of lower-extremity arterial revascularization.

I.   Common clinical presentations. Patients with critical limb ischemia present with one or more of the following problems:

A.   Rest pain in the lower extremity may be the first symptom of severe ischemia (grade II, category 4; Table 13.1). There are many causes of leg and foot pain in which arterial perfusion to the foot may be normal. These include diabetic neuropathy, arthritis, venous insufficiency, and causalgia-type syndromes.

Specific features suggest pain to be of ischemic origin. Ischemic rest pain is localized primarily to the forefoot below the ankle and the foot usually has dependent rubor and elevation pallor. Palpable pulses are absent. **Ischemic rest pain usually does not occur unless the patient has at least two hemodynamically significant arterial occlusive lesions.** Most individuals with rest pain will have one of two distinct anatomic patterns of occlusive disease (see Fig. 12.2, Chap. 12) that must be defined before an appropriate therapy can be selected (Fig. 13.1).

1.   Combined aortoiliac and superficial femoral arterial occlusive disease (type 2; Fig. 12.2), or

2.   A femoropopliteal arterial occlusion with distal tibial occlusive disease (type 3; Fig. 12.2).

B.   Nonhealing ulcers of the foot may also be the result of arterial ischemia (grade III, categories 5 and 6; Table 13.1). Even with arterial perfusion, healing may be prevented by infection of bone or soft tissue, pressure from improper footwear, or improper medical treatment. A good history and physical

Table 13.1. Categories of limb ischemia

Grade	Category	Clinical description	Objective criteria
0	0	Asymptomatic—no significant occlusive disease	Normal treadmill/ stress test[a]
I	1	Mild claudication	Complete treadmill test[a]; AP after test <50 mm Hg
	2	Moderate claudication	Between categories 1 and 3
	3	Severe claudication	Cannot complete treadmill test[a]; AP after test <50 mm Hg
		Subcritical limb ischemia	
		No symptoms or tissue loss	Resting AP <40 mm Hg, ankle or metatarsal PVR flat or barely pulsatile; TP <30 mm Hg
		Critical limb ischemia	
II	4	Ischemic rest pain	Resting AP <40 mm Hg, ankle or metatarsal PVR flat or barely pulsatile; TP <30 mm Hg
III	5	Minor tissue loss— nonhealing ulcer, focal gangrene and pedal ischemia	Resting AP <60 mm Hg, ankle or metatarsal PVR flat or barely pulsatile; TP <40 mm Hg
	6	Major tissue loss— extending above TM level, functional foot no longer salvagable	Same as category 5

[a] 5 min at 2 mph on a 12% incline.
AP, ankle pressure; PVR, pulse volume recording; TP, toe pressure; TM, transmetatarsal.
Adapted from TransAtlantic Inter-society Consensus (TASC) on the Management of Peripheral Arterial Disease (PAD). *J Vasc Surg* 2000;31(Part 2):S168.

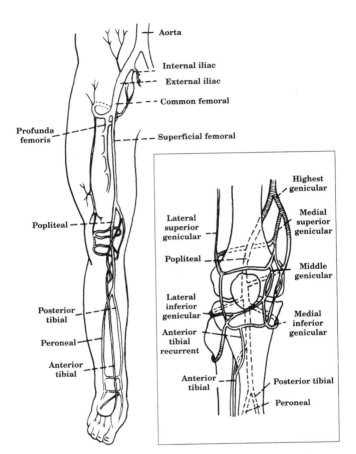

Figure 13.1. Arterial anatomy of the leg and popliteal region.

should provide information for sorting out the reasons for poor healing. The sensory neuropathy associated with long-term diabetes makes diabetic patients susceptible to **neuropathic foot ulcers.** Such patients may not feel the initial sore and therefore not present until the ulcer is deep and infected.

C. Gangrene is a classic sign of ischemia in the skin and subcutaneous tissue (grade III, categories 5 and 6; Table 13.1). Dry gangrene is characterized by a noninfected black eschar, whereas wet gangrene has tissue maceration and purulence.

D. Microemboli cause bluish, mottled spots scattered over the toes **(blue toe syndrome)**, which may be painful. They also may be mistaken for local traumatic bruises, and their true significance overlooked. Microemboli may originate from any point in the proximal arterial system, most commonly from the heart, aneurysms or ulcerated plaques.

E. Acute arterial ischemia (Table 13.2) is characterized by the sudden onset of extremity pain, pallor, paresthesia, pulselessness, and sometimes paralysis. If the patient has a history of claudication or previous lower-extremity arterial graft, the symptoms may be caused by thrombosis of a stenotic artery or the arterial graft. **If the patient previously had no symptoms of peripheral vascular disease, the acute ischemia is more likely embolic.**

II. Diagnostic evaluation. A number of diagnostic tests are available to help determine the best treatment plan for the threatened limb. Tests should be selected to provide the maximum amount of information with the minimum amount of discomfort and delay for the patient, who often is experiencing considerable pain.

A. Noninvasive vascular testing. Continuous wave Doppler and pulse volume recording (PVR) are simple yet accurate methods to determine criteria for ischemic rest pain and the likelihood of healing (see Chap. 5). Ischemic rest pain generally is associated with a Doppler ankle pressure below 35 mm Hg in nondiabetics and below 55 mm Hg in diabetics. Ischemic rest pain is unlikely when ankle pressures exceed 55 mm Hg in the nondiabetic and 80 mm Hg in the diabetic. Foot ulcers that are not infected and not associated with osteomyelitis have a favorable chance of healing if the ankle pressure is above 65 mm Hg in the nondiabetic and above 90 mm Hg in the diabetic. Ankle and forefoot PVRs that are less than 5 mm or flat predict ischemic rest pain and poor tissue healing. Toe pressures of less than 20 to 30 mm Hg are also associated with advanced ischemia. Resting supine transcutaneous oxygen (TcO_2) measurements of less than 20 to 30 mm Hg are indicative of severe ischemia, especially if forefoot TcO_2 levels fall to less than 10 mm Hg with leg elevation.

B. Plain radiograph of the bone underlying a ulcer may show signs of osteomyelitis which include bone rarefaction, periosteal elevation, and new bone formation. A bone scan or magnetic resonance imaging is indicated when osteomyelitis seems likely but a plain radiograph is negative. Bone changes may not be apparent until osteomyelitis has been active for 2 to 3 weeks.

C. Cultures and **Gram's stains** should be made of all ulcers to identify any residing organisms and histologic stain also may reveal fungi.

D. An **electrocardiogram** (ECG) is essential when arterial embolism is suspected, as atrial fibrillation is a common underlying condition. For cases in which intermittent arrhythmia is suspected, a 24-hour continuous ECG monitor (Holter) may be used.

E. An **echocardiogram** should be done as part of the diagnostic work-up for arterial embolism that may originate from the heart. The echocardiogram may reveal a diseased valve or mural thrombus.

F. Ultrasound of the abdominal aorta also should be performed in the evaluation of thromboemboli, since emboli may be shed from a thrombus in an abdominal aortic aneurysm. If a femoral or popliteal aneurysm is suspected as a result of physical examination, ultrasound is an accurate method to confirm peripheral aneurysms that also may act as the source of emboli or acute thrombosis.

Table 13.2. Categories of acute limb ischemia

Category	Description	Capillary refill	Muscle weakness	Sensory loss	Arterial Doppler	Venous Doppler
I. Viable	Not immediately threatened	Intact	None	None	Audible	Audible
II. Threatened a. Marginally	Salvageable if promptly treated	Intact, slow	None	Minimal (toes) or none	Often audible	Audible
b. Immediately	Salvageable with immediate revascularization	Very slow or absent	Mild, moderate	More than toes, associated with rest pain	Usually inaudible	Audible
III. Irreversible	Major tissue loss, amputation regardless of treatment	Absent (marbling)	Profound, paralysis (rigor)	Profound, anesthetic	Inaudible	Inaudible

Adapted from TransAtlantic Inter-society Consensus (TASC) on the Management of Peripheral Arterial Disease (PAD). *J Vasc Surg* 2000;31(Part 2):S142.

G. Arteriography remains the definitive method to delineate the exact level of arterial occlusion and to define vascular anatomy before selecting a proper intervention (i.e., thrombolysis, balloon angioplasty, or surgical revascularization). If the femoral pulses are weak or absent, an aortogram with runoff is needed. If femoral pulses are normal and the arterial occlusive disease appears localized to the leg alone, a transfemoral arteriogram of the affected leg may suffice. A femoral artery pressure study may be done to assess the adequacy of the proximal aortoiliac inflow (see Chap. 6). Contrast angiography with digital subtraction techniques can generally visualize distal tibial or plantar arch vessels. In the operating room, a sterile Doppler probe can be used to localize a tibial or pedal artery before surgical incision. Although the presence of a patent pedal arch on arteriography was once considered predictive of success for femorodistal bypass, more recent studies report reasonable patency rates and limb salvage in patients in whom the pedal arch appears absent or diseased.

H. Coagulation and **platelet function** should be analyzed in patients who present with atypical arterial thrombosis. This group includes young adults (age 20 to 40 years) with arterial occlusive disease and other individuals with recurrent arterial thromboembolism. Antithrombin deficiency has been documented as one cause of unexplained thrombosis and graft failure. In some cases of recurrent arterial thrombosis, a familial enhanced platelet aggregability has been identified. Plasminogen abnormalities should also be considered. Other coagulation defects that must be checked include protein C and protein S deficiencies, anticardiolipin antibody, lupus-like anticoagulant, homocysteine levels, and antiphospholipid antibody. Factor V Leiden is an inherited hypercoagulable condition that alone is not associated with arterial thrombosis but may play a role in arterial ischemia if present with another hypercoagulable condition.

III. Management may begin after it has been determined whether the patient has acute or chronic limb ischemia. In our experience, the following principles provide the best chance of limb salvage.

A. Acutely limb ischemia usually is caused by a thromboembolus, popliteal aneurysm thrombosis, or a sudden graft occlusion. Thrombosis of a chronic arterial stenosis may cause temporary pain, pallor, and paresthesia, but usually it does not progress to paralysis. The acute symptoms often resolve because of previously developed collateral vessels.

1. Immediate treatment should include systemic heparinization (5,000 to 10,000 units i.v., then 1,000 units/h adjusted to maintain the APTT to twice baseline, usually 70 to 100 seconds) to prevent further propagation of thrombus. If leg pain is severe, a narcotic may be administered while further tests are being arranged.

2. Initial diagnostic tests should include routine blood counts, electrolytes, glucose, and baseline coagulation studies (prothrombin time, partial thromboplastin time, and platelet count). An ECG should be done to check for atrial fibrillation and any sign of acute myocardial infarction.

Continuous wave Doppler may be used to localize the level of obstruction and record ankle pressures. Absence of arterial signals at the ankle almost always means that urgent surgical intervention will be necessary (class IIb or III ischemia; Table 13.2). If the ankle has monophasic Doppler signals and the foot has sensation and movement (class I or IIa), 2 to 3 hours may be allowed for work-up, initial therapy, and observation. If the leg does not improve during this time, immediate surgical intervention will generally be necessary.

3. An emergency arteriogram usually is performed to determine the location of the arterial occlusion as well as the inflow and outflow on either side. However, arterial exploration in the operating room should be undertaken immediately if the acute occlusion is clearly an embolus. Intraoperative arteriograms can be performed if necessary. Time is important in acute arterial occlusion, as irreversible nerve and muscle damage may occur within 6 hours.

4. The choice of operation for an acute arterial occlusion will depend on the underlying etiology. **Thromboembolectomy** with Fogarty balloon catheters is the operation of choice for thromboemboli. Thrombectomy of the femoral or iliac arteries can be accomplished through a femoral arteriotomy. A popliteal embolus should generally be extracted through a popliteal arteriotomy, so that each tibial artery may be checked for clot. Passing a catheter from the groin will not clean out all of the tibial arteries. Extracted thromboemboli should be sent for pathologic examination, as occasionally arterial tumor embolism will be the first manifestation of an atrial myxoma or other vascular tumor. After embolectomy, the patient should be continued on heparin, followed by long-term warfarin sodium (Coumadin) therapy.

If the acute arterial ischemia is caused by a graft occlusion, **regional thrombolytic therapy** may reopen the graft and reveal the cause of the occlusion (e.g., distal anastomotic stenosis, proximal inflow disease, or graft pathology or kinking). Once the cause is identified, a more focused operation or endovascular procedure (e.g., angioplasty ± stent) can be undertaken.

Bypass grafting of an arteriosclerotic occlusion of the iliac or superficial femoral artery may be necessary to salvage the acutely ischemic leg. In another example, a few seriously ill cardiac patients who are dependent on a transfemoral intra-aortic balloon assist device will develop limb-threatening ischemia. An emergency femorofemoral bypass may be necessary if the balloon must remain in place for cardiac support.

B. Chronic critical limb ischemia is usually associated with arteriosclerotic occlusive disease of the aortoiliac region, femoropopliteal segment, or distal tibial arteries.

1. Foot protection from further injury is the first order of care. The heel should be protected from pressure sores by a soft gauze pad secured with a gauze roll, **not** tape. The heels themselves should either be elevated off of the bed surface or placed in egg-crates or commercially made vascular "boots" (e.g., Rooke boot). Lamb's wool or gauze should be placed between the toes to prevent "kissing" ulcers caused by toes

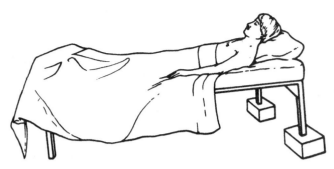

Figure 13.2.   Bed position for patient with ischemic rest pain of the lower extremity. The head of the bed is elevated 6 inches to improve arterial perfusion of the pedal circulation by gravity. Sheets are draped over a footboard to alleviate pressure on the feet.

and toenails rubbing against one another. A lanolin-base lotion should be applied daily to the foot to keep the skin soft and prevent cracking, especially over the heel. If pressure bothers the foot, bed sheets may be draped over a footboard (Fig. 13.2). Elevating the head of the bed 6 inches may relieve ischemic pain by the effect of gravity on arterial perfusion. We do not recommend so-called metal bed cradles or tents, as a patient may inadvertently abrade the lower leg or foot against the metal frame, causing skin ulceration.

2.   Preventive foot care must be taught to the patient (see Chap. 14).

3.   Local infection should be controlled before insertion of synthetic bypass grafts. Local debridement of infected toes and parenteral antibiotics should precede graft procedures by several days. Otherwise, graft infection may occur in the groin, where lymphatics may be laden with bacteria.

4.   Arteriography is discussed in Chapter 6.

5.   The choice of operation or percutaneous transluminal angioplasty depends on the location of the occlusive disease and the condition of the patient.

a.   Combined severe aortoiliac and femoropopliteal occlusive disease should be treated by bypass grafts of the aortoiliac disease. Although angioplasty ± multiple stents of diffuse aortoiliac stenoses may help initially, durability is limited to months or a few years. For extensive aortic, common and external iliac atherosclerosis, an aortofemoral bypass graft is more durable and preferable for healthier patients with longer life expectancy. When the superficial femoral artery is diseased, the femoral anastomosis of an aortofemoral graft should be carried onto the profunda femoris artery (see Fig. 12.4, Chap. 12). Long-term limb salvage will be accomplished in most patients with multilevel occlusive disease by aortofemoral bypass alone.

Approximately 20% of patients, however, will need an additional distal bypass. Determining which patients will need simultaneous aortofemoral and femoropopliteal bypasses is not easy. Preoperative factors that suggest a combined procedure is indicated are extensive below-the-knee femoropopliteal-tibial occlusions combined with open foot lesions and an ankle pressure below 30 mm Hg. In high-risk patients, extraanatomic axillofemoral or femoro-femoral bypass may be used to correct severe iliac occlusive disease.

b.   Occlusive disease of the common femoral artery, profunda orifice, and superficial femoral artery may be managed by endarterectomy and profundaplasty. Profundaplasty is most likely to succeed when (a) aortoiliac inflow is normal, (b) the distal profunda femoris artery is normal and has developed collateral pathways to the popliteal artery, and (c) the popliteal artery is patent with at least two- or three-vessel runoff. This anatomic situation is rare, so we seldom use profundaplasty as the sole operation for limb salvage.

c.   Femoropopliteal artery occlusion can be managed by bypass grafting, endarterectomy, or percutaneous transluminal angioplasty. Our method of choice is saphenous vein bypass grafting, which is superior to endarterectomy and synthetic bypass. Current synthetic choices for femoropopliteal bypass are Dacron, human umbilical vein, and polytetrafluoroethylene (PTFE). These grafts provide excellent long-term patency when the distal anastomosis is above the knee, but poorer patency is observed in below-the-knee bypasses. In a prospective randomized comparison of autologous saphenous vein to expanded PTFE grafts, primary patency of vein was clearly superior to PTFE for infrapopliteal bypass (49% versus 12% at 4 years). However, there was no significant difference in limb salvage (vein versus PTFE, 57% versus 61%). Although 2-year patency was similar for both grafts to the popliteal artery (64% to 70%), vein was superior at 5 years (vein, 68%; PTFE, 38%). Umbilical vein grafts have had a patency similar to PTFE, but manifest aneurysmal degeneration in long-term follow-up. Another option is cryopreserved vein graft, but results using cryopreserved vein have been disappointing and these are seldom used. Percutaneous transluminal angioplasty can recanalize superficial femoral artery occlusions of less than 10 cm and may be the first procedure in seriously ill patients who need limb salvage (see Chap. 6).

d.   Some poor-risk patients will have **both an iliac stenosis and a superficial femoral artery occlusion.** A combined aortofemoral and femoropopliteal procedure carries a high rate of morbidity and mortality is such patients. A safe alternative is angioplasty of the iliac stenosis followed by femoropopliteal bypass under regional (e.g., epidural) anesthesia.

e.   The most challenging group of patients who require operation for limb salvage have **severe tibial and peroneal occlusive disease.** Acceptable long-term patency (50% to 60% at 5 years) and excellent limb salvage rates

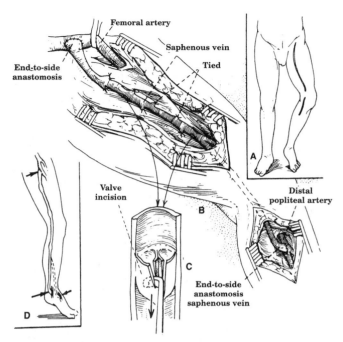

Figure 13.3. Technique of *in situ* saphenous femoropopliteal and tibial bypass grafting. A: Greater saphenous vein is exposed through one or two long incisions along the medial aspect of the thigh and calf. B: Saphenous vein is left in its natural bed. Its valves are cut with special instruments. C: Its branches are tied to prevent arteriovenous fistulas. Proximal anastomosis is made to the common femoral or superficial femoral artery, and distal anastomosis is constructed to the distal popliteal artery or to the tibial or peroneal branches. D: Long bypasses to the level of the ankle are possible by this technique.

(50% to 73% at 5 years) may be achieved by femorotibial, femoroperoneal, and pedal bypass grafts. Multisegment femorodistal occlusive disease also has been successfully treated by sequential anastomoses of a vein graft to several patent segments. **Patency of femoroinfrapopliteal vein bypasses is comparable for each tibial artery and is similar in diabetics and nondiabetics.** Whether *in situ* or reversed saphenous vein is better remains controversial.

Several factors have rejuvenated enthusiasm for *in situ* **saphenous vein bypass grafting** after its original description in 1962 (Fig. 13.3). Proponents claim a higher use of smaller veins, a lesser degree of endothelial damage, better size match at the anastomoses, improved hemodynamics, and superior early and late patency. However, similar early and late patency rates for *in situ* versus reversed infra-popliteal bypasses (1-year, 87% to 90%; 3-year, 82% to 85%; and 5-year, 77% to 85%) have been shown in several studies. Preparation of vein and the technique of anastomoses are likely more important than position of the vein. This is supported by the good results using adjuncts at the distal anastomosis of prosthetic, below-the-knee bypasses. The techniques of a **Taylor patch or Miller cuff** emphasize a long arteriotomy and placement of a cuff of vein between the prosthetic and the target arteriotomy.

Because a vein remains the best conduit for early and late patency, extra effort to obtain a suitable vein seems justified. These options include the contralateral leg vein, arm veins, composite synthetic and vein, and shorter bypasses using less vein (e.g., popliteal-tibial or tibiotibial bypasses). In our experience, vein grafts to isolated popliteal segments have been an acceptable alternative to femorodistal bypass in certain patients. These grafts have a 5-year patency similar to femorotibial bypasses (65% versus 66%, respectively). Provided that tissue necrosis is not extensive, such grafts are adequate to relieve severe ischemia, especially when a limited length of vein is available and the tibial arteries appear marginal for a distal anastomosis.

f. With an aging population, more elderly patients are presenting **with ischemic rest pain and gangrene of the foot.** Attempts to salvage such a limb may require an extended hospitalization and considerable expense. However, limb salvage is possible in 70% at 1 year and 60% at 3 years, but generally about 30% at 5 years after surgery. Successful revascularization results in lower costs than primary amputation. In patients over 80 years of age, limb salvage is comparable to younger groups, with a 3-year survival of about 50% and a limb preservation rate of 70%. Consequently, present data support an attempt at arterial reconstruction in most elderly patients with critical limb ischemia. Primary amputation is appropriate when gangrene extensively involves the forefoot and heel. Whether a failed below-knee femoropopliteal bypass changes the level of amputation depends on numerous factors, but generally an unsuccessful reconstruction does not alter final amputation level.

g.   Lumbar sympathectomy alone is not usually sufficient to salvage limbs at risk. However, relief of rest pain has been achieved when the preoperative ankle-brachial index is relatively high (i.e., >0.35). Results are less favorable when tissue necrosis is present.

h. Creation of a **distal arteriovenous fistula** as an adjunct to maintaining arterial and synthetic bypass graft patency remains controversial. The physiologic advantage of this technique is questionable and we have not embraced it.

6.   Angioscopy has been evaluated as an adjunct to *in situ* vein grafting, embolectomy, femoropopliteal bypass surgery, and laser recanalization. Clinical trials by Miller and colleagues at Harvard have supported its effectiveness, but the technology has had a limited impact so far in most practices.

IV. Perioperative care

A. Preoperative preparation. Lab tests for limb salvage cases are the same as those outlined for aortic surgery in Chapter 12. The patient should be typed and cross-matched for 2 units of packed red blood cells. Skin preparation should include the abdomen and both legs, as an opposite leg vein is occasionally explored. We recommend that a prophylactic antibiotic with good gram-positive coverage be given as the patient goes to the operating room. A first-generation cephalosporin such as cephalexin 1 g i.v. is a common choice.

B. Intraoperative care. Certain points of intraoperative patient care and surgical management deserve mention.

1. Patient positioning. Most lower-extremity arterial revascularizations are performed with the patient supine. The heels must be protected from pressure sores by elevating the calves on soft towels or placing soft pads on the heels. If PVR is being used for intraoperative monitoring of lower-extremity perfusion, the PVR cuffs should be placed at the ankles and baseline tracings should be recorded (see Chap. 9).

2. Surgical exposure. Certain features of surgical exposure facilitate performing the anastomoses and prevent postoperative wound complications.

  a. The incisions for exposure of the **great saphenous vein** must be made directly over the vein. There is a tendency to bevel the incision and bring it too far anterior to the course of the vein which results in skin flap necrosis. Leaving skin bridges along the saphenous vein harvest site may also alleviate skin flap necrosis. Some advocate subcutaneous, endoscopic vein harvest, but this technique has not achieved widespread acceptance.

  b. The **above-knee popliteal artery** can be exposed through a medial distal thigh incision going over the top (lateral) edge of the sartorius muscle and beneath the adductor magnus tendon. **Three note-worthy anatomic features are present at the adductor magnus tendon: the superficial femoral artery becomes the popliteal artery, the supreme geniculate artery (an important collateral) originates from the proximal popliteal artery, and the saphenous nerve becomes superficial.** Injury to the nerve can result in bothersome chronic leg neuralgia.

  c. The **below-knee popliteal artery** is exposed via a medial proximal leg incision. The medial head of the gastrocnemius muscle is retracted inferiorly. The popliteal vein and tibial nerve are medial and posterior to the artery. Extensive exposure of the popliteal artery may require detachment of the semimembranosus and semitendinosus muscle tendons. Insertions of the semitendinosis, gracilis and sartorius muscles form the **pes anserinus (foot of a goose)** on the medial surface of the tibia.

  d. Occasionally, the entire popliteal artery requires exposure for repair and evacuation of a popliteal aneurysm (Fig. 13.4). This exposure also allows for ligation of feeding collaterals into the aneurysm sac. Divided tendons can be

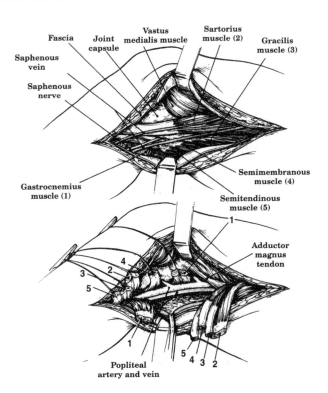

Figure 13.4. Medial approach to the popliteal artery. The saphenous nerve should be gently retracted to minimize postoperative saphenous neuralgia. Division of the medial knee tendons and medial head of the gastrocnemius muscle provides clear popliteal artery exposure with minimal morbidity. Most patients have a single great saphenous vein, although an accessory saphenous vein may be present as this illustration indicates.

anatomically reattached at the conclusion of the operation. Such an extensive exposure appears to increase postoperative leg edema but does not result in knee instability in most patients.

For focal mid-popliteal artery aneurysms or for popliteal artery entrapment, a posterior longitudinal knee incision provides excellent exposure without cutting normal tendons.

e. The **tibioperoneal trunk and proximal posterior tibial artery** can be exposed through the medial knee approach by detaching some of the soleus muscle from the tibia. Exposure of the proximal anterior tibial artery generally requires a separate anterior lateral leg incision, which is made one finger-breadth lateral to the edge of the tibia and carried 8 to 10 cm distally. The artery is located

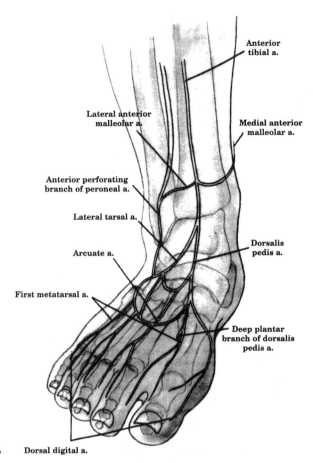

Anterior
tibial a.

Lateral anterior
malleolar a.

Medial anterior
malleolar a.

Anterior perforating
branch of peroneal a.

Lateral tarsal a.

Dorsalis
pedis a.

Arcuate a.

First metatarsal a.

Deep plantar
branch of dorsalis
pedis a.

A   Dorsal digital a.

**Figure 13.5. Anatomy of the pedal arteries. A: Dorsum of foot.
B: Plantar surface of foot. (Adapted from Gloviczki P, Bower TC,
Toomey, et al. Microscope-aided pedal bypasses is an effective and
low-risk operation to salvage the ischemic foot.** *Am J Surg*
1994;168:76–84.)

in the groove between the anterior tibial and extensor dig-
itorum longus muscles.
    f.   Bypasses can also be taken to the pedal arteries (Fig.
13.5) in select patients. The most common pedal artery for
distal anastomosis is the dorsalis pedis followed by the
common and lateral plantar arteries.
3.   Preparation of the saphenous vein. Endothelial damage during preparation of saphenous vein is an important factor in graft failure. Optimum preparation includes gentle dissection of the vein, careful ligation of side branches away from

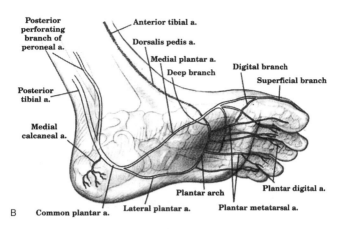

Figure 13.5.   (*Continued*)

the vein wall, minimal warm ischemic time if the vein is removed from the leg, and limited distention. Gentle dilation of the vein can be achieved with a papaverine solution (1 mL, or 30 mg, of papaverine in 9 mL of saline). Immersion of the vein in cold Ringer's lactate or blood may minimize endothelial damage.

4.   Distal arterial control can be accomplished with minimal damage to the arteries by using a **pneumatic thigh tourniquet** inflated to 300 mm Hg after the lower limb is wrapped tightly with an elastic Esmarch's bandage.

5.   Anastomotic technique should emphasize a long gentle anastomotic angle to minimize turbulence. Distal popliteal and tibial arterial anastomoses are constructed more accurately under low-power magnification. If prosthetic bypass is performed to tibial vessels, the use of a **Taylor vein patch or a Miller vein cuff** may reduce intimal hyperplasia at the distal anastomosis and improve patency.

6.   Vascular monitoring (see Chap. 9).

7.   Postoperative dressings should be applied so as not to constrict at the knee. A loosely wrapped Kerlix dressing will adequately cover the incisions and avoid the use of a large amount of tape which may cause epidermal damage.

C.   Postoperative care. Patients should remain under intensive observation for at least 6 to 12 hours after lower-extremity revascularization. It is during this immediate postoperative period that most early graft occlusions occur. Hourly checks of pedal pulses, PVRs, or Doppler ankle pressures should be made. To enhance early perioperative patency, one has several options. One is low molecular weight dextran 40 infused for the initial 24 postoperative hours. Our regimen has been 100 mL i.v. in the recovery room and 20 mL/h for one 500-mL bottle. Subsequently, patients receive aspirin, 80 to 325 mg daily, and low-dose heparin,

5,000 units subcutaneously, until discharge. Another option is low-dose intravenous heparin (300 to 500 units per hour). Long-term anticoagulation with warfarin and children's aspirin (80 mg) is often used for below-knee synthetic grafts and revision grafts to the tibial arteries.

Guidelines for postoperative laboratory tests, fluid administration, and antibiotic use are outlined in the previous chapter (see Chap. 12).

   1. Postoperative day 1. The initial dressings should be removed, and new dressings applied only if serosanguineous or lymph drainage continues. Strict bed rest is continued for any patient with a popliteal or tibial bypass. Lower-extremity footboard exercises are done every hour to increase lower-extremity arterial and venous flow. Patients must be monitored closely for perioperative myocardial and cerebral ischemia.

   2. Postoperative days 2 to 5. Bed rest for 1 to 2 days allows the early calf and foot swelling to resolve. Incisional pain is improved enough by the second or third postoperative day to allow ambulation. Some patients with more distal bypasses to the ankle or foot may require 3 to 5 days of bed rest before pedal and ankle edema has resolved enough to allow ambulation. If such patients ambulate too early, swelling may compromise tenuous incisions. Continuous epidural anesthesia followed by epidural analgesia for 24 to 48 hours has been an excellent method in our experience to keep patients comfortable. Initially, we encourage the patient to use crutches or a walker to help with weight-bearing. We discourage prolonged sitting, as this position worsens leg swelling. Many patients have lower-leg edema for 6 weeks to several months after lower-extremity revascularization. Below-the-knee support hose may alleviate this swelling.

   3. Associated amputations. Some patients require an amputation after lower-extremity arterial bypass to remove necrotic tissue present before surgery. Whether amputations should be done simultaneously with arterial reconstruction is debatable. Certainly, infected lesions or abscesses need debridement prior to grafting. Superficial dry gangrene may autoamputate after foot circulation is improved. Thus, we normally wait 5 to 7 days after arterial reconstruction to perform necessary digital or foot amputations. This time allows better demarcation of the proper amputation level. Although this has been our general approach, we have combined femoropopliteal revascularization with toe or forefoot amputations in select patients.

V. Postoperative complications
A. Early problems. As with aortoiliac reconstructions, the most common early postoperative graft-related complications in limb salvage cases are hemorrhage, thrombosis, and infection.

   1. Hemorrhage usually follows one of two patterns. In the first pattern, bleeding frequently occurs within 24 hours from the vein graft or an anastomosis. Early repair and hematoma evacuation usually do not lead to graft failure or infection. The second pattern of postoperative hemorrhage occurs from 3 to 28 days after operation and in most cases is caused by graft infection. Hemorrhage usually occurs at the proximal or distal anastomosis. These patients are at greater risk of eventual limb loss.

2. Thrombosis in the first 24 hours after operation is most often the result of a technical problem; most commonly a poorly constructed anastomosis. Other possible technical problems include graft kinking, extrinsic muscle or tendon compression, an intimal flap, or clamp injury to an artery. Causes of early thrombosis other than technical problems include inadequate outflow and inadequate vein graft size (<4 mm). Occasionally early graft thrombosis is due to a previously undiagnosed hypercoagulable condition. In our experience, the long-term prognosis of early graft failure has been poor, even if the graft is successfully opened.

3. Infection following arterial bypass or reconstruction usually occurs in the groin. Common underlying factors are obesity and fat necrosis or hematoma. The classification and management of these infections was discussed previously (see Table 12.2, Chap. 12).

4. Compartment syndrome is caused by prolonged ischemia (>8 hours) before revascularization that causes swelling of the calf muscles. Since these muscles are enveloped in fixed fascial compartments, swelling leads to myonecrosis and permanent nerve damage. The anterior compartment is most susceptible to this ischemic syndrome. The earliest clinical signs are leg pain with sensory deficits on the dorsum of the foot and weakness of toe dorsiflexion. Treatment is fasciotomy. Prophylactic fasciotomy should be considered for all cases of acute arterial ischemia in which revascularization is delayed beyond 6 to 8 hours.

5. Femoral nerve injury may occur after groin operations, especially in repeat procedures or extensive dissections of the profunda femoris artery. The injury may not be apparent until the patient tries to ambulate and discovers that they cannot extend at the knee because of quadriceps weakness. Treatment requires a flexible knee brace. Many femoral nerve apraxias will resolve in 3 to 6 months.

B. Late problems. Late postoperative graft-related complications occur in about 30% of patients who undergo arterial procedures below the inguinal ligament. The most common problem is graft thrombosis. Two main factors contribute to late graft failure. One factor is progression of atherosclerotic disease in proximal and distal arteries. However, increasing evidence documents that alterations in the vein graft may also lead to graft thrombosis. Mills and colleagues have emphasized that 10% to 15% of reversed saphenous vein grafts develop significant inflow, intrinsic graft or outflow stenosis at a mean follow-up of 2 years. The peak incidence of early hemodynamic graft failure occurs within 12 months of graft implantation. Intrinsic graft stenosis causes the majority of failures (60%). These lesions are usually focal intimal hyperplasia distributed equally at the proximal and distal anastomoses. The remaining causes are inflow failure (13%), outflow failure (9%), muscle entrapment (4%), and hypercoagulable conditions (4%).

If these vein graft alterations are detected before graft thrombosis, successful repair and long-term patency can be accomplished in 75% to 85% of cases over 5 years. **Current emphasis is on detecting failing grafts before they occlude.** Periodic reevaluation (3 to 6 months) should focus on any recurrent symptoms and objective signs of a failing graft. These signs include a 0.15 fall in the ankle-brachial pressure index. Important duplex ultrasound predictors of graft failure include a decrease in peak systolic flow velocity to less than 45 cm/s in the graft plus an increased peak systolic velocity across a stenotic area (two to three times the normal graft velocity).

When infrainguinal bypasses fail, reoperative surgery can achieve limb salvage in about 50% of patients. **Late cumulative graft patency is better for revised grafts than revised, thrombosed grafts (65% to 75% versus 5% to 15% at 5 years).** There is a significant improvement in early patency rates when a new bypass graft is inserted as compared to thrombectomy and patch angioplasty of the original graft.

SELECTED READING

Akbari CM, LoGerfo FW. Diabetes and peripheral vascular disease. *J Vasc Surg* 1999;30:373–384.

Faries PL, LoGerfo FW, Arora S, et al. Arm vein is superior to composite prosthetic-autogenous grafts in lower extremity revascularization. *J Vasc Surg* 2000;31:1119–1127.

Fujitani RM. Revision of the failing vein graft: outcome of secondary operations. *Semin Vasc Surg* 1993;6:118–129.

Green RM, Abbott WM, Matsumoto T, et al. Prosthetic above-knee femoropopliteal bypass grafting: five-year results of a randomized trial. *J Vasc Surg* 2000;31:417–425.

Hallett JW Jr, Byrne J, Gayari MM, et al. Impact of arterial surgery and balloon angioplasty on amputation: a population-based study of 1155 procedures. *J Vasc Surg* 1997;25:29–38.

Harris PL, Veith FJ, Shanik GD, et al. Prospective randomized comparison of *in-situ* and reversed infrapopliteal vein grafts. *Br J Surg* 1993;80:173–176.

How TV, Rowe CS, Gilling-Smith GL, et al. Interposition vein cuff anastamosis alters wall sheer stress distribution in the recipient artery. *J Vasc Surg* 2000;31:1008–1017.

Ihnat DM, Mills JL, Dawson DL, et al. The correlation of early flow disturbances with the development of infrainguinal graft stenosis: a 10-year study of 341 autogenous vein grafts. *J Vasc Surg* 1999; 30:8–15.

Kreienberg PB, Darling RC III, Chang BB, et al. Adjunctive techniques to improve patency of distal prosthetic bypass grafts: polytetrafluoroethylene with remote artertiovenous fistulae versus vein cuffs. *J Vasc Surg* 2000;31:696–701.

Ouriel K, Shortell CK, DeWeese JA, et al. A comparison of thrombolytic therapy with operative revascularization in the initial treatment of acute peripheral arterial ischemia. *J Vasc Surg* 1994;19:1021–1030.

Rhodes JM, Gloviczki P, Bower TC, et al. The benefits of secondary interventions in patients with failing or failed pedal bypass grafts. *Am J Surg* 1999;178:151–155.

TransAtlantic Inter-Society Consensus Working Group. Management of Peripheral Arterial Disease: TransAtlantic Inter-society Consensus. *J Vasc Surg* 2000;31(Part 2).

Veith FJ, Gupta SK, Ascer E, et al. Six-year prospective multicenter randomized comparison of autologous saphenous vein and expanded polytetrafluoroethylene grafts in infrainguinal arterial reconstructions. *J Vasc Surg* 1986;3:104–114.

Veterans Administration Cooperative Study Group. Johnson WC. Comparative evaluation of PTFE, HUV, and saphenous vein in fempop AK vascular reconstruction. *J Vasc Surg* 2000;32:267–277.

Weitz JI, Byrne J, Clagett GP, et al. AHA Medical/Scientific Statement. Diagnosis and treatment of chronic arterial insufficiency of the lower extremities: a critical review. *Circulation* 1996;94:3026–3049.

Foot Care

Foot sores can become major problems in patients with diabetes mellitus or atherosclerotic peripheral vascular disease. Serious infection and extensive tissue necrosis may complicate apparently minor foot lesions. Too frequently, the eventual outcome is amputation. Proper foot care can prevent many foot problems that threaten the lower extremity. Unfortunately, numerous patients never learn the basic principles of foot care because many physicians have received minimal formal instruction in this area. The purpose of this chapter, then, is to summarize general principles of foot care.

I. **Magnitude of the problem.** Foot problems due to diabetic neuropathy or arterial ischemia not only consume a great deal of the patient's time but also devastate financial resources if prolonged hospital care is required. Foot lesions are the primary problem of one of every five diabetics who are hospitalized. About 50% of diabetics who have one leg amputated eventually will lose the other extremity. For at least 50% to 75% of our patients with atherosclerotic peripheral vascular disease, foot lesions or rest pain are the primary indication for a vascular operation. Despite hospital care and operation in some patients, limb salvage is not achieved in 10% to 20% of cases. Amputation often is necessary in such situations. Rehabilitation after lower-extremity amputation usually takes 1 to 3 months and costs thousands of dollars. The benefits of preventing foot problems in these patients should be obvious. Fortunately, the time and cost of preventive foot care are relatively minor compared to the great expenditures incurred once a foot lesion occurs.

II. **The susceptible foot.** Certain patients with diabetes and atherosclerosis are especially susceptible to developing nonhealing foot lesions. The diabetic with **peripheral sensory neuropathy** probably is the most susceptible. Because of diminished sensation, minor foot lesions such as blisters, skin cracks, and ingrown toenails may not be noticed by the patient. Even foreign bodies that penetrate the foot may not be felt. The classic example is the diabetic who is not aware of a nail or piece of glass in the foot. Many such diabetics also have retinopathy and may not be able to see such minor lesions.

Anatomic foot deformities also predispose a person to development of foot problems, especially corns, calluses, and pressure sores. Improperly fitted shoes may cause too much pressure over certain anatomic points (Fig. 14.1). **Dry, hyperkeratotic skin,** especially over the heels, tends to crack. At the base of these cracks, subcutaneous infections often originate and undermine the skin. The result is subcutaneous soft tissue necrosis, cellulitis, or abscess, and larger nonhealing ulcers. Finally, **arterial ischemia** impedes wound healing. Minor foot ulcerations often fail to heal in patients with absent pedal pulses and dependent forefoot rubor. As indicated in earlier chapters, healing of superficial foot lesions is unlikely if ankle pressures are less than 80 mm Hg in

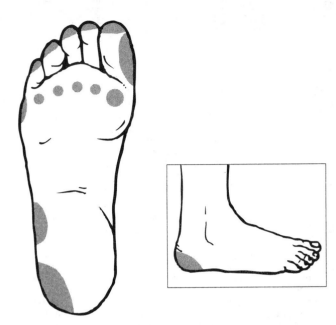

Figure 14.1.   Common locations for pressure-related ulcerations of the foot. Properly fitted footwear is an important factor in preventing pressure sores.

diabetics and 55 mm Hg in nondiabetics. Toe pressures of less than 30 mm Hg and forefoot transcutaneous oxygen (TcO_2) tensions of less than 10 to 20 torr are also predictive of slow or no healing.

III.   Prevention. Each physician who cares for patients with diabetes and vascular disease is responsible for educating these patients in proper foot care. The principles of proper foot care are easily learned by most people. We have found a printed booklet of general directions for foot care to be especially helpful for outpatients. The physician or office nurse should explain specific instructions and demonstrate proper care of foot lesions to both the patient and the patient's family. A family member often is the best physician's assistant in detecting and treating minor foot problems at home.

Additional professional home care may be provided by a visiting nurse. Telecommunication allows visiting medical personnel to use digital cameras to photograph ulcers and transmit them immediately via computer technology to physicians at the central medical facility. The images can be reviewed instantaneously with the field personnel, and suggestions for wound care can be made without the patient leaving the home.

Prevention of serious foot problems may be discussed conveniently under the following general categories: daily foot care, footwear, exercise, and first aid treatment.

A. Daily foot care

1. Washing. The feet should be washed daily with warm (never hot) water and a mild soap. Feet should not be soaked. Soaking tends to macerate skin and may cause burns if the patient has a sensory neuropathy and the water is too hot. After washing, the foot should be thoroughly dried, especially between the toes, where moisture promotes fungal infections.

2. Inspection. The foot should be examined for cuts, blisters, ingrown toenails, discolored skin, and cracks. In particular, the heel and spaces between the toes should be checked, since lesions are commonly overlooked in these locations. If the patient has poor vision, a family member or friend should inspect the foot. A physician should be notified of any problems.

3. Moisturizing the skin. Dryness leads to cracking of the skin. Therefore, daily application of a moisturizing lotion to the foot, especially the heel, is essential to good foot care. A few examples are lanolin, Eucerin, Nivea, Alpha Keri, Vanicream, and Vaseline Intensive Care lotion. These lotions should not be applied between the toes, since they may cause excess moisture and thus promote fungal infection.

4. Foot powder. An antifungal powder such as Desenex should be applied between the toes if foot perspiration is excessive or "athlete's foot" is suspected. Common signs of fungal infection are itching, small blister formation, and skin scaling between the toes or on the sole of the foot.

5. Toenails. Toenails should be cut or filed straight across, never shorter than the end of the toe. If nails are cut shorter than the lateral nail groove, they tend to become ingrown. The best time to trim nails is after a foot bath, when the foot is clean and the nail usually is softer. A podiatrist should cut thick nails or ones that split easily.

6. Corns and calluses. Corns and calluses are the result of friction and pressure from footwear. They usually occur over bony prominences. A podiatrist or physician should care for them. An improperly treated corn or callus often results in an ulcer and infection that involves underlying bone (osteomyelitis). Patients should be cautioned not to trim them and not to apply plasters or chemicals to remove them.

7. Toe care. If one toe is causing pressure on another, a small piece of lamb's wool or absorbent gauze between the toes may prevent a pressure ulcer.

8. Avoidance of trauma. Foot protection should be worn at all times. Excessive heat from heating pads, hot packs or soaks, and heating lamps must be avoided, particularly if peripheral neuropathy is present. Adhesive tape is not recommended, since it may denude superficial skin. If tape is necessary, paper tape is preferred.

B. Footwear

1. Patients with peripheral neuropathy and arterial ischemia should never go barefoot!

2. Feet should be kept warm and dry with **socks or stockings.** Woolen socks are best in cold weather and cotton socks when it is warm. Nylon socks or hose that cause excess perspiration should be avoided. Clean socks should be worn each day.

3.   Shoes should fit comfortably and allow plenty of room for the toes. Many diabetics prefer specially made footwear. Soft, spacious athletic shoes often are adequate. Other specially made footwear are also available for diabetics and can be purchased at most shoe stores affiliated with medical centers (e.g., Darco products). Women should avoid pointed shoes that cramp the toes. New shoes should be broken in gradually to avoid blisters.

C.   Exercise. Exercise promotes the development of collateral circulation and maintains normal venous and lymphatic flow by the musculovenous and lymphatic pumping mechanism.

1.   Walking is the safest exercise for the feet, provided shoes fit properly.

2.   Patients should be encouraged to walk daily. If they have intermittent claudication, they should be instructed to walk slowly, rest when claudication occurs, and then resume walking. They should be encouraged to gradually increase their walking distance each week.

3.   Ambulation and dependency of the extremity should be curtailed when foot sores are present. Dependency leads to swelling that impedes healing and the resolution of infection.

D.   First aid treatment. When the patient first notices a foot sore, he or she should begin certain types of first aid. Even if the lesions seem minor, the patient should be encouraged to promptly notify his or her physician, who generally should inspect the problem and prescribe definitive therapy. Procrastination on the part of the patient often results in inappropriate self-treatment of a foot problem and a consequent complication.

1.   Foot lesions or injuries should be washed with warm water and mild soap. **Injuries should not be soaked for prolonged periods, especially in hot solutions that may macerate or burn tissue.** The foot should be carefully dried.

2.   In general, strong topical antiseptic solutions such as iodine should not be used. An ointment such as bacitracin may be applied to the lesion.

3.   The best dressing is simply a clean gauze bandage secured with a roll of gauze or paper tape.

4.   The next step of treatment should be examination by a physician.

IV.   Definitive treatment. Definitive treatment of foot problems may require the efforts of the primary physician, podiatrist, or surgeon. When the patient with a foot problem is first seen, several basic questions must be considered. First, what is the likelihood that the foot problem is curable and will not lead to limb loss? Second, what is appropriate therapy? Finally, can this therapy be accomplished on an outpatient basis or is hospitalization necessary?

A.   Likelihood of healing. We generally rely on several sources of information to predict the likelihood of healing: physical examination, noninvasive vascular tests (Doppler ankle or toe pressures, forefoot TcO_2 tensions, and/or pulse volume recordings [PVRs]), and bone studies (radiograph or bone scan).

1.   Small (<2 cm in diameter) superficial skin ulcers, corns, calluses, and ingrown toenails detectable by **physical examination** alone usually heal or are manageable without amputation. Exposed bone at the base of any lesion generally indicates osteomyelitis, even if the radiograph appears normal. Such lesions are unlikely to heal without some type of amputation. Lesions in an area of dependent rubor or ischemic rest pain also seldom heal. A continuing problem is predicting which foot ulcers will heal when pedal pulses are not palpable. An absent femoral pulse and dependent forefoot rubor generally indicate that an open foot lesion is unlikely to heal without surgical intervention.

2. Noninvasive vascular tests provide some predictive value in the healing of foot lesions. Noninfected foot ulcers may heal in patients with good femoral pulses but absent distal pulses when ankle pressures are greater than 65 mm Hg in the nondiabetic and 90 mm Hg in the diabetic. PVRs at the ankle of greater than 15 mm are favorable for healing. In our experience, flat or severely diminished (<5 mm) forefoot PVRs generally correlate with nonhealing. Favorable Doppler pressures or PVRs do not ensure healing, but they at least suggest that initial treatment may be conservative. TcO_2 measurements are also helpful in determining whether ulcers are primarily neuropathic or ischemic. TcO_2 forefoot levels of less than 40 mm Hg suggest ischemia. When TcO_2 is 20 to 30 mm Hg at rest and drops to less than 10 mm Hg with foot elevation, a foot lesion is unlikely to heal unless a revascularization procedure is performed.

3. The use of **radiologic studies** to detect bony change of osteomyelitis should be considered for patients with ulcers over bones. Plain radiograph may not show signs of osteomyelitis for at least 2 to 3 weeks. These signs include bony rarefaction, local periosteal elevation, and new bone formation. A bone scan or magnetic resonance imaging may be a more sensitive indicator in equivocal cases.

B. Principles of treatment

1. Corns and calluses are pressure-induced lesions. Corns represent a traumatic keratosis or overgrowth of the epidermis. They generally occur over a bony prominence (e.g., at the dorsal aspect of the fifth toe). They are conical in shape, the base being superficial and the apex deep, and press against deeper structures. Calluses are flat keratoses that generally occur on the bottom of the foot over bony prominences. Poorly fitted footwear often is the cause of corns and calluses. The danger of these lesions is infection, which may occur beneath them where a bursa or space may form between the superficial keratosis and underlying bone.

Optimum treatment for corns begins with removing the **superficial** corn surface with a scalpel or similar cutting instrument. Care must be taken not to cut into the deep vascular layer of the corn, which may not heal. After removing the cornified layer, a U-shaped felt pad may be applied behind the corn to alleviate local pressure that originally caused the corn. These pads disperse local pressure. Footwear should be changed to ensure no pressure on the corn. Calluses also should be managed primarily by redistributing pressure with inlay pads.

2. Ingrown toenails (onychocryptosis) may be complicated by infection. Three basic types of lateral nail problems occur and threaten the diabetic and vascular patient with serious infection and gangrene.

    a. The **incurved** or simple inverted nail curves into the lateral nail groove, causing tenderness and pain with ambulation. To force the lateral nail edge forward and prevent it from digging into the toe pulp, any debris must be cleared from beneath the leading edge of the nail and then cotton must be gently packed beneath the nail edge. If cotton is simply packed along the lateral nail groove, the incurved nail will worsen as the packing pushes the nail down.

    b. An **ingrown nail** is the result of not trimming the nail straight across and leaving a sharp, jagged lateral edge on the nail. This pointed spicule of nail is called a **shard.** Shards tend to penetrate the lateral nail groove and cause infection, so they should be removed. Infection at a shard location may be treated with warm boric acid soaks for 20 to 30 minutes every 4 hours. A broad-spectrum oral antibiotic [e.g., cephalexin, or Keflex (Dista Products Company, Indianapolis, IN, U.S.A.)] may be needed if local infection is present.

    c. Hypertrophic ungualabium represents an overgrowth of chronic granulation tissue over the lateral nail plate. Hypertrophic ungualabium may follow any incurved or ingrown nail or partial excision of the nail. The hypertrophic tissue tends to grow over the lateral nail edge, making local infection more difficult to clear. Proper treatment may require partial or complete removal of the nail and antibiotics for cellulitis.

3. Minor foot ulcers (superficial, <2 cm in diameter, and with no exposed bone) should receive the same daily hygiene described above (see Section III.A). For established clean lesions, bacitracin ointment and a small dry gauze dressing applied twice daily may be used. For ulcers with necrotic debris or crusting, wet-to-dry saline dressings changed four times a day are most useful, and one should clean up and debride the lesion. Sharp debridement should be done by a physician and be limited to necrotic tissue. If the ulcer has a dry eschar, callus around the ulcer edge should be trimmed to allow adequate drainage of moisture or pus from beneath the eschar. Otherwise, pus may be trapped beneath the eschar and cause deeper infection and abscess. Dakin's antiseptic solution (diluted sodium hypochlorite) with gauze packs may be used to debride particularly dirty wounds or necrotic fat or fascia. Since Dakin's antiseptic solution may damage normal skin, its use should be reserved for patients with foot pulses. Dilute acetic acid solution 0.25% (vinegar) on gauze dressings three to four times a day is also effective in cleaning contaminated diabetic foot wounds, especially those with Pseudomonas species.

4. Large heel ulcers (>2 cm in diameter) often extend into subcutaneous fat and are extremely difficult to resolve. If possible, a clean dry eschar, which can be protected with a gauze pad, should be obtained. Vigorous debridement to bleeding subcutaneous fat frequently results first in deeper extension of the tissue necrosis and eventually in exposure of the calcaneus and osteomyelitis. These large heel ulcers may eventually lead to amputation, especially in diabetics with neuropathy.

5. Foot cellulitis is apparent by local swelling, erythema, tenderness, and warmth. Such infection may spread rapidly in diabetics. Optimum treatment includes strict bed rest, leg elevation, and administration of antibiotics. Before starting the patient on antibiotics, a Gram's stain and culture of foot ulcers should be done. An oral cephalosporin (e.g., cephalexin, 250 to 500 mg p.o. q6h) usually is effective for local cellulitis **without** diffuse forefoot involvement, lymphangitic spread, or fever. These signs of more extensive infection are an indication for parenteral therapy with broad-spectrum antibiotics. In general, antibiotics effective against anaerobes are unnecessary and probably should be withheld until specific anaerobes are identified. Foot soaks are not recommended, since they contribute nothing to the above therapy and only introduce more bacteria.

6. Foot abscesses require urgent and generous incision and drainage. In general, they require emergency hospitalization. Multiple small incisions with infected tunnels do not heal well. Gauze packing is preferable to rubber drains, since packing debrides better.

C. Hospitalization. Hospitalization obviously is indicated for foot lesions complicated by cellulitis, abscess, or sepsis. If conservative therapy has not begun to heal other minor foot ulcers after 3 weeks, the patient should be considered for an arteriogram and arterial reconstructive procedure, or an amputation.

ACKNOWLEDGMENT

Special credit for this chapter must be given to the Joslin Diabetic Clinic, Boston, where so many of these principles of foot care originated.

SELECTED READING

Akbari CM, Logerfo FW. Diabetes and peripheral vascular disease. *J Vasc Surg* 1999;30:373–384.

Cina C, Katsamouris A, Megerman J, et al. Utility of transcutaneous oxygen tension measurements in peripheral arterial occlusive disease. *J Vasc Surg* 1984;1:362–371.

Dillon RS. Successful treatment of osteomyelitis and soft tissue infections in ischemic diabetic legs by local antibiotic injections and the end-diastolic pneumatic compression boot. *Ann Surg* 1986;204: 643–649.

Kozak GP. *Management of diabetic foot problems.* Philadelphia: Saunders, 1995.

Laing P. Diabetic foot ulcers. *Am J Surg* 1994;167(suppl 1A):31S.

Levin ME, O'Neal LW, eds. *The diabetic foot,* 3rd ed. St. Louis: Mosby, 1988.

Mueller MP, Wright J, Klein SR. Diabetes and peripheral vascular disease. In: Veith FJ, Hobson RW II, Williams RA, et al., eds. *Vascular Surgery,* 2nd ed. New York: McGraw–Hill, 1994:514–522.

Amputations

Amputation must be planned and conducted with the same meticulous care given to arterial reconstructions. Otherwise, the patient faces poor amputation healing and a long hospitalization. The therapeutic goals of an amputation should be control of ischemic pain or infection and wound healing. Specific rehabilitation goals vary widely depending on the amputation level and the functional capacity of the patient. All rehabilitation, however, should be focused on gaining maximal functional capacity from the amputation, whether walking significant distances or simple weight-bearing to allow independent transfers.

This chapter is limited to amputations performed on patients with peripheral arterial occlusive disease and diabetes mellitus.

I. Preoperative care

A. Patient acceptance. When the necessity of an amputation becomes apparent to the surgeon, he or she must help the patient accept the operation. If the patient is experiencing pain, he or she usually will accept the amputation. It is especially important to discuss the need for amputation and the plan for rehabilitation with the patient's family. In addition, we ask the amputation rehabilitation service to evaluate the patient before the operation. In most cases, upper-extremity and some lower-extremity strengthening exercises will be initiated before amputation is performed.

B. Medical stabilization. Except when the infection is life-threatening, we prefer a period of wound care and intravenous antibiotics prior to amputation in cases of cellulitis. Management of the infected foot is described in Chapter 14.

Occasionally, an elderly patient who is toxic from an ischemic, infected foot will present in diabetic coma, with dehydration and electrolyte imbalance, acute myocardial infarction, acute congestive heart failure, or digitalis toxication. Emergency amputation in such patients has a high mortality rate. Ideally, the medical condition of such patients should be stabilized before operation. A valuable adjunct in preparation of these critically ill patients for amputation has been a technique called **selective physiologic amputation.** It involves local hypothermia, with tourniquet occlusion just above the level of infection. The technique has been carefully investigated in a large number of patients and should be familiar to surgeons who treat such severely ill patients.

The following technique is recommended for selective physiologic amputation in patients who need urgent amputation but are so critically ill on admission that they could not tolerate operation:

1. The extent of gangrene or infection is determined and the site for physiologic amputation is chosen. Generally, this is done below the knee, and the subsequent definitive surgical amputation can be done above or below the knee, depending on tissue condition. Seventy percent of patients who are initially treated by cryoamputation of the foot can undergo a successful below-knee amputation.

2. Tissue distal to the selected site is wrapped in sheet wadding, and a soft rubber tourniquet is applied proximal to the infected or necrotic tissue to occlude arterial supply. Local infiltration anesthesia may be used at the tourniquet site. However, this area usually is already numb, and local anesthesia unnecessary. This tourniquet must be secure, since accidental release could shower the systemic circulation with acidotic debris and bacteria.

3. One-inch thick blocks of dry ice are wrapped in towels and placed around the extremity no higher than 3 inches **below** the tourniquet. These dry ice packs may be held in place by a rubber sheet or pad. The dry ice is replaced every 8 hours.

4. The duration of physiologic amputation may be hours to days; the average duration is about 3 days, with a range of 9 hours to 15 days.

5. Physiologic amputation should be reserved for patients who are desperately ill from both gangrene or infection and life-threatening medical problems. In our experience, this technique is seldom necessary but is highly effective in the rare patient who requires intensive medical stabilization before amputation.

II. Amputation level. Selecting a proper amputation level is based primarily on clinical examination and knowledge of the extent of arterial occlusive disease in the individual patient. Pulse volume recordings (PVRs), segmental limb pressures, and transcutaneous oxygen (TcO_2) tensions are helpful but not infallible (see Chap. 5). Our data also suggest that a TcO_2 tension value of at least 40 mm Hg measured on the skin flap of the proposed level of amputation is predictive of success. An amputation site-to-chest TcO_2 ratio of greater than 0.59 is also associated with a high likelihood of healing. Final judgment must be based on the following clinical criteria:

A. Active infection controlled.
B. Good-looking skin at amputation site.
C. No dependent rubor proximal to the level of amputation.
D. Venous filling time of less than 20 seconds.
E. No pain proximal to the amputation level.

III. Operative technique. The following principles of operative technique are crucial to the success of single-digit amputations, transmetatarsal amputations (TMAs), below-knee amputations (BKAs), and above-knee amputations (AKAs). Gentle handling of tissues and careful hemostasis are the two critical prerequisites to primary healing.

A. Single-digit amputation. The skin incision for single-digit amputation should be made at a 90-degree angle to avoid beveling. The medial and lateral skin flaps should be left long and then trimmed if necessary. The proximal phalanx should be divided through the shaft of the bone and not through the joint. A single-layer closure is made with interrupted simple sutures. A soft, bulky dressing is applied.

B. Ray amputation. Infection involving the metatarsal head precludes the performance of a simple toe amputation. In these cases, extension of the amputation to excise the metatarsal head (Ray amputation) accomplishes removal of all necrotic or infected tissue. The incision for the Ray amputation is a raquet-type of incision with the vertical component on the dorsum of the foot over the metatarsal to be resected. The circular incision is around the toe to be removed with the metatarsal head. The intact specimen of the Ray amputation should include the toe, the metatarsal phalangeal joint, and the metatarsal head. All tendon remnants should be excised as proximally as possible and vertical mattress sutures (monofilament) used to approximate the deep tissue and skin layers.

C. Transmetatarsal amputation can provide excellent results, especially in diabetics who have neuropathic toe ulcers. A strongly positive forefoot PVR or TcO_2 tensions of greater than 40 torr are the best noninvasive predictors of success. Several aspects of the technique warrant emphasis. The plantar flap should be cut 1 cm from the web space and not undercut. The dorsal incision should be slightly curved and carried from side of the foot to the other, just distal to the anticipated line of bone transection at the midportion of the metatarsal shafts. Care must be taken to avoid retracting the plantar and dorsal flaps. The cut should be carried directly through the tendons to the metatarsal shafts which are divided with an oscillating saw with a small blade. A single-layer closure is carried out with no subcutaneous stitches, and the forefoot is splinted for 3 to 5 days. A problem area of wound healing often is the mid-dorsal flap. If a small area of necrosis occurs here, the TMA may be salvaged by careful local debridement of the necrosis and placement of a small gauze wick. The primary advantage of a transmetatarsal amputation is its excellent function with minimal disability. The transmetatarsal amputation avoids the **equinus and equinovalgus deformities** inherent in more proximal forefoot amputations with take the insertions of the muscle which dorsiflex the foot.

D.   Other mid-foot and forefoot amputations. The **Lisfranc amputation** is a forefoot disarticulation between the tarsal and metatarsal bones and is a proximal extension of the transmetatarsal amputation. **Chopart's amputation** is a forefoot disarticulation at the talo-navicular and calcaneocuboid joints (within the tarsals). These amputations preserve a weight-bearing stump on which to transfer but offer little in hopes of meaningful ambulation and are rarely required in patients with ischemic tissue loss of the foot.

E.   Syme amputation. The Syme amputation divides the talar-tibial joint and does not require healthy plantar skin distally. The ideal indication for the Syme amputation is a distal forefoot infection that involves the distal plantar skin rendering it unacceptable as a flap for a more distal forefoot amputation. This amputation is technically demanding and necessitates good posterior tibial artery perfusion to the heel flap and results in a stump that is useful for short periods of weight-bearing only.

F.   Below-knee amputation (BKA) is preferable to an AKA, as rehabilitation requires less energy when the knee joint is preserved. In addition to the above criteria for amputation level, a BKA generally will not be appropriate when either temperature demarcation or ischemic lesions extend above the ankle. A flexion contracture at the knee in a bedridden patient is also a relative contraindication to a BKA. In this setting, the amputation stump is be chronically forced into the bed which results in poor wound healing and stump breakdown. We prefer a long posterior myocutaneous flap, which is cut about 1 inch longer than the anterior-posterior diameter of the proximal calf. The anterior edge of the tibia should have a 45-degree bevel to keep it from protruding. The fibula is cut 1 inch shorter than the tibia. The muscle and enveloping fascia of the calf are approximated with interrupted absorbable sutures, and the skin is closed with interrupted nylon sutures. The skin should not be handled with tissue forceps at any time. The stump is carefully padded with fluffed gauze bandages, and a rigid posterior plaster splint is applied and left undisturbed for 5 days. This period of immobilization prevents any disturbance of the closure, reduces edema, and maintains the knee in extension so that knee contracture is minimized. We do not usually drain these BKA's.

G. Through-knee amputation. The through-knee amputation or knee disarticulation is used rarely but may be useful in patients who have infection which precludes creation of the flaps necessary to cover a BKA. The advantages of the through-knee amputation are retention of a long and powerful muscle-stabilized lever arm and improved stump proprioception and potential for improved prosthetic control. After disarticulation of the knee joint, the weight bearing surface of the femoral condyles is cut approximately 1.5 cm above the condylar ends and the femoral margins contoured. This surface is then stabilized with the patellar and biceps tendons as well as the medial hamstrings sutured to the intracondylar notch. The wound is typically closed using a long anterior flap.

H. Above-knee amputation is seldom necessary if the below-the-knee skin condition is good and a good femoral pulse is present. As much thigh length as possible should be preserved when an AKA is done. The end of the femur will migrate to the lateral edge of the amputation stump unless some step is taken to fix it in the mid-portion of the stump. This can be accomplished by placing several mattress sutures between the vastus lateralis and the biceps muscle just lateral to the femur. As with any amputation, the skin must be closed with a gentle technique. Fluffed bandages are applied to the incision and are held in place with a stockinette secured by benzoin painted on the proximal thigh.

I. Management of failed femorodistal grafts. When synthetic bypass grafts to the knee or leg fail, a BKA or AKA is often necessary. The amputation frequently cuts across the thrombosed graft. If the graft is infected prior to amputation, it must be completely removed to prevent the persistence of a septic focus in the lower limb, especially if the graft is attached to a more proximal aortofemoral graft. Likewise, an amputation site that becomes infected and contains an old thrombosed graft end is unlikely to heal until all the prosthetic material is removed.

J. Ischemic amputation sites. Occasionally, an AKA stump will become ischemic with rest pain, necrotic edges, or gangrene. Such ischemia prevents healing and must be corrected by improving profunda femoris perfusion. Otherwise, the

**Table 15.1.   Postamputation results,
rehabilitation, and energy expenditure**[a]

Primary healing	75%
Eventual healing	80%
Mortality	7–10%
Rehabilitation with prosthesis	
Conventional techniques[b]	65%
Immediate postoperative prosthesis	87%
Average time from amputation to rehabilitation	
Conventional techniques	133 days
Immediate postoperative prosthesis	31 days
Energy expenditure (% increase compared to controls)	
Below-knee amputation	9–25%
Above-knee amputation	25–100%
Bilateral below-knee amputation	40%

[a] These data are averages from a large number of surgical series.
[b] Conventional techniques include a delay of several weeks for primary wound healing before fitting a prosthesis.
Adapted from Malone JM. Lower-extremity amputation. In: Moore WS, ed. *Vascular surgery*, 5th ed. Orlando: Grune & Stratton, 1998:844–885.

patient faces a higher AKA or hip disarticulation. The attendant mortality rate of higher amputation is nearly 30%.

IV.   Postoperative care (Table 15.1). We have found that certain guidelines improve primary wound healing and facilitate early postoperative physiotherapy and eventual rehabilitation. The immediate postsurgical prosthesis has been under investigation for more than two decades and has been reported to be highly successful and to accelerate rehabilitation. This method has merits, but we caution that it must be used by individuals who are skilled in its use. Otherwise, the following principles of postoperative care generally will give good results.

A.   Primary dressing and splint. The primary dressing and splint are left intact for the first 5 to 7 days and are not removed unless the patient has fever of unclear etiology. At this point, the initial dressing is removed, and the amputation site is inspected. If it is healing satisfactorily, a new plaster pylon cast is applied and changed every 7 to 10 days. After about 3 weeks, the amputation stump is ready for suture removal and progression toward a temporary prosthesis.

B.   Physiotherapy. A physical therapist should see the patient on the first postoperative day. Upper-extremity strengthening exercises can be continued at that time. If the condition of the patient allows, quadriceps-strengthening exercises are also initiated. Between the seventh and fourteenth postoperative days, the patient begins using a wheelchair. Crutch-walking usually is begun between the tenth and fourteenth day.

C.   Suture removal. Sutures are left intact for at least 3 weeks.

D.   Prosthesis fitting. Measurements and fitting for a prosthesis usually are done 4 weeks after operation, unless the immediate postoperative fit is being used.

E. Rehabilitation. During the first postoperative week, long-term rehabilitation plans are discussed with the patient and his or her family. They are assisted in selecting a rehabilitation center that is well qualified and convenient to their home. These arrangements must be initiated early, since they often require 7 to 14 days to confirm.

SELECTED READING

Ayoub MM, Solis MM, Rogers JJ, et al. Thru-knee amputation: the operation of choice in non-ambulatory patients. *Am Surg* 1993;59: 619–623.

Durham JR. Lower extremity amputation levels: indications, determining the appropriate level, technique and prognosis. In: Rutherford RB, ed. *Vascular surgery*. Philadelphia: W.B. Saunders, 2000: 2185–2213.

Dwars BJ, van den Brock TAA, Rauwerda JA, et al. Criteria for reliable selection of the lowest level of amputation in peripheral vascular disease. *J Vasc Surg* 1992;15:536–542.

Hallett JW Jr, Byrne J, Gayari MM, et al. Impact of arterial surgery and balloon angioplasty on amputation: a population-based study of 1155 procedures. *J Vasc Surg* 1997;25:29–38.

Houghton AD, Taylor PR, Thurlow S, et al. Success rates for rehabilitation of vascular amputees: implications for preoperative assessment and amputation level. *Br J Surg* 1992;79:753–755.

Miller N, Dardik H, Wolodiger F, et al. Transmetatarsal amputation: the role of adjunctive revascularization. *J Vasc Surg* 1991;13: 705–711.

Nehler MR, Whitehill TA, Bowers SP, et al. Intermediate-term outcome of primary digit amputations in patients with diabetes mellitus who have forefoot sepsis requiring hospitalization and presumed adequate circulatory status. *J Vasc Surg* 1999;30:509–517.

Patel KR, Chan FA, Clauss RH. Functional foot salvage after extensive plantar excision and amputations proximal to the standard transmetatarsal level. *J Vasc Surg* 1993;18:1030–1036.

Ubbink DT, Spincemaille GH, Reneman RS, et al. Prediction of imminent amputation in patients with non-reconstructible leg ischemia by means of microcirculatory investigations. *J Vasc Surg* 1999;30: 114–121.

Valentine RJ, Myers SI, Inman MH, et al. Late outcome of amputees with premature atherosclerosis. *Surgery* 1996;119:487–493.

Weaver FA, Modrall JG, Baek S, et al. Syme amputation: results in patients with severe forefoot ischemia. *Cardiovasc Surg* 1996;4: 81–86.

Winburn GB, Wood MC, Hawkins ML, et al. Current role of cryo-amputation. *Am J Surg* 1991;162:647–650.

Aneurysms and Aortic Dissection

Management of aneurysms and aortic dissection requires an understanding of natural history, diagnosis, and treatment options. In recent years, these options have changed dramatically with development of endovascular techniques. **Despite these changes, the best results continue to follow carefully planned elective treatment before complications of rupture, thrombosis, or embolism occur.** The contrast in mortality between elective (2% to 5%) and ruptured abdominal aortic aneurysm (AAA) repair (50% to 70%) remains one of the most striking examples of the importance of early recognition and proper treatment of these diseases.

Aortic dissections are a commonly encountered degenerative disease of the aorta, which are distinctly different from aortic aneurysms. This chapter will focus on the natural history, diagnosis and management of aneurysms and aortic dissections. The hemodynamics of aneurysms are discussed in Chapter 1. Chapter 3 outlines the initial physical evaluation, and Chapter 6 describes appropriate radiologic tests.

ABDOMINAL AORTIC ANEURYSM

I. **Epidemiology.** During the past 30 years, the incidence of AAAs has tripled. This is attributed to both increased detection with the use of ultrasound and computed tomography (CT) and an aging population. The rising incidence has been tenfold for small AAAs (<5 cm), while the incidence for larger aneurysms has increased by a factor of two. Small aneurysms account for about 50% of all recognized AAAs, an important epidemiologic finding given the uncertainty surrounding the appropriate management of small AAAs.

II. **Natural history.** Aortic aneurysms are a disease of the elderly diagnosed in the sixth and seventh decades of life. As many as 20% of patients with an AAA have a family history of aortic aneurysm. The expansion rate of AAAs is 2 to 3 mm per year and increases as the aneurysm enlarges. Twenty percent of aneurysms expand at a rate of more than 4 mm per year, while 80% grow at a slower pace. Importantly, cigarette smoking increases the expansion rate of AAAs.

Rupture remains the most threatening outcome of an AAA and is related directly to aneurysm diameter. Although this concept is not controversial, experts continue to debate the size at which an aneurysm should be repaired. For years, AAAs greater than 6 cm in diameter were considered appropriate for elective repair. Subsequent autopsy studies revealed that even small aneurysms (4 to 5 cm) could rupture, which resulted in a more aggressive approach to small AAAs.

More recent data from population-based studies of living patients have indicated that rupture risk escalates when the AAA exceeds 5 cm in size (Figs. 16.1 and 16.2). Rupture risk

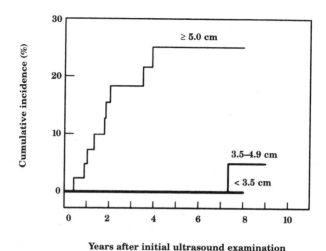

Figure 16.1.   Cumulative incidence of rupture of abdominal aortic aneurysms according to the diameter of the aneurysm at the initial ultrasound examination. (From MP Nevitt, DJ Ballard, JW Hallett Jr. Prognosis of abdominal aortic aneurysms: a population-based study. *N Engl J Med* 1989;321:1009–1014, with permission.)

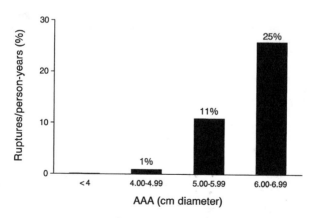

Figure 16.2.   Rupture risk of abdominal aortic aneurysm (*AAA*) per year for size diameter. (From Reed WW, Hallett JW Jr, Damiano MA, et al. Learning from the last ultrasound: a population-based study of patients with abdominal aortic aneurysm. *Arch Int Med* 1997;157:2064–2068, with permission.)

for small (<5 cm) AAAs is approximately 1% per year, 5% to 10% per year for medium-sized (5 to 7 cm) AAAs, and at least 10% to 25% per year for large (7 cm) AAAs. As many as one-half of small AAAs will require elective repair over a 5-year follow-up. Nearly all small AAAs that eventually rupture have enlarged to over 5 cm in diameter. Unfortunately, the frequency of ruptured AAA remains high despite an increase in elective repairs. This is due to the fact that at least 50% of patients with a ruptured AAA are unaware of the aneurysm until the day of rupture. Such patients obviously never had the opportunity of elective repair.

Other less common outcomes of AAAs include embolic complications and rupture into the vena cava resulting in aortocaval fistula. In a few cases, aneurysms may become infected and present as a pulsatile abdominal mass accompanied by fever and bacteremia. Rarely, an aneurysm will erode into the intestine, presenting as gastrointestinal bleeding from an aortoenteric fistula.

III.   Indications for operation

   A.   In low-risk patients, an AAA of 5 to 6 cm in diameter is an indication for elective repair. For high-risk individuals, we generally defer operation until the aneurysm shows enlargement, usually to more than 6 cm, or until a smaller aneurysm becomes tender or symptomatic. Smaller aneurysms may need to be simultaneously repaired in patients who undergo aortofemoral bypass for aortoiliac occlusive disease. **The prospective randomized United Kingdom Small Aneurysm Trial did not show a survival advantage for early repair of small AAAs (4.0 to 5.5 cm) compared to observation. However, surveillance is important as nearly two-thirds of small AAAs eventually required surgical repair.**

   B.   A less common but more urgent indication for surgical repair is evidence of **peripheral emboli.**

   C.   Emergency repair is indicated for all patients with a known aneurysm that has become **tender** or is associated **with abdominal or back pain.** These patients should be hospitalized and considered to have a symptomatic aneurysm, although their abdominal symptoms may be nonspecific at first and their initial vital signs may be normal.

   D.   Patients with **ruptured aneurysms** and shock should be taken directly to the operating room for resuscitation and operation. In addition, there are now reports of treating ruptured AAAs by endovascular stent grafts, an option that may become more available with the evolution of this technique.

IV.   Preoperative evaluation. The preoperative evaluation for an elective AAA should define the size and extent of the aneurysm, associated medical risks, and associated vascular disease. Diagnostic tests should be selected so that information is not duplicated and costs are minimized.

   A.   Size and extent. The reliability of abdominal exam to detect and size an AAA is poor enough that a more accurate diagnostic test is necessary. The simplest and least expensive test to diagnose and measure an AAA is ultrasound. Measurement of the anterior–posterior diameter is more accurate than the transverse diameter, reliably measuring the aneurysm within 3 to 4 mm. Ultrasound is also a favored method follow AAA diameter over time.

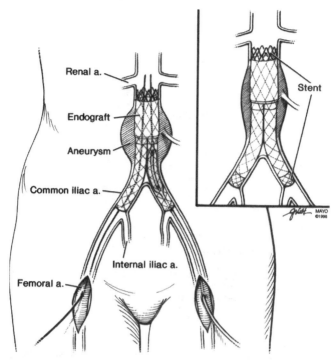

Figure 16.3. Clinical trials are examining the feasibility, safety, and durability of stented intraluminal grafts passed retrograde from a femoral artery surgical exposure into abdominal aortic aneurysms and secured by expandable metallic stents.

Although some surgeons prefer routine CT or magnetic resonance imaging (MRI) scanning of a suspected AAA, these imaging modalities cost more than ultrasound and should be reserved for aneurysms in which elective repair is proposed. A common indication for CT scanning of an AAA is anatomic evaluation for an endovascular stent graft (Fig. 16.3). In this setting a CT scan assesses **(a) the diameter of the proximal AAA neck, (b) the relationship of the AAA neck to the renal arteries (length of neck), (c) the tortuosity (angle) of the aneurysm neck and iliac arteries, and (d) the diameter of the iliac arteries as attachment sites for bifurcated stent grafts.** In addition, CT scanning is essential when a suprarenal or thoracoabdominal aneurysm is suspected. One must remember that CT scan may overestimate the size of an aneurysm because the measurements are made perpendicular to the body axis and may be distorted if the aorta is tortuous (see Fig. 6.2, Chap. 6).

B. Aortography. Arteriography is not reliable for determining the aortic aneurysm diameter as luminal thrombus obscures the outer limit of the wall. Some experts favor routine aortography to detect unrecognized multiple renal arteries, mesenteric artery stenoses, or pelvic arterial occlusive disease. However, if certain clinical criteria are considered, aortography can be used selectively prior to AAA repair. Such criteria include:

1. Decreased peripheral pulses or symptoms of lower extremity claudication indicating arterial occlusive disease.
2. Poorly controlled hypertension or renal insufficiency, indicating renal artery occlusive disease.
3. Suprarenal, or thoracoabdominal aortic aneurysms that require delineation of renal, visceral, and intercostal arteries involved by the aneurysm.
4. Symptoms of intestinal ischemia or a high-pitched epigastric bruit, suggesting visceral artery disease.
5. A suspected horseshoe kidney on ultrasound, CT scan, or excretory urogram (associated with multiple renal arteries).
6. Preparation for endovascular stent graft placement.

One or more of these criteria is present in 30% to 50% of patients with an AAA. Currently, gadolinium-enhanced magnetic resonance aortography provides excellent aneurysm imaging in most patients.

   C.   Medical risks. Most significant medical risks can be detected by history and physical examination. Many patients with AAAs are hypertensive, and 35% to 50% have obvious coronary artery disease. A cardiologist should evaluate patients with a past history of myocardial infarction, angina pectoris, chronic congestive heart failure, chronic arrhythmias, or significant heart murmurs. In our experience, preoperative stabilization of cardiac disease and careful perioperative cardiac care contribute to a low elective operative mortality (2% to 3%). Preoperative pulmonary function tests are not done routinely but are indicated for patients in whom the history and physical exam suggest significant dyspnea.

   A more aggressive approach to elective AAA repair for elderly patients and patients with increased cardiac or pulmonary risk has been advocated by some. Endovascular stent grafts offer an option that may be safer for these high-risk patients. Obviously, such patients must be carefully selected and treated by an experienced anesthesia and surgical/endovascular team. Under these conditions, AAA repair on high-risk patients can be accomplished with an operative mortality of 5% to 7%. If not repaired, 30% to 50% of these high-risk patients die of AAA rupture.

   Patients with significant coronary artery disease should undergo myocardial revascularization before elective aneurysm repair. About 5% of AAA patients will have angina requiring preoperative coronary revascularization before AAA repair. For 85% of such patients, surgical revascularization will be necessary while 15% can be adequately treated with coronary angioplasty. Those patients who undergo coronary artery bypass grafting need 6 to 8 weeks of recovery before aneurysm surgery, although earlier repair may be indicated in those with very large (>7 cm) AAAs. In contrast, AAA repair can usually proceed within 7 to 10 days after coronary angioplasty. In those patients with obstructive pulmonary disease preoperative optimization of pulmonary function should be attempted (see Chap. 7).

D. Associated vascular disease. Approximately 10% of AAA patients have an **asymptomatic carotid bruit.** In our practice, these patients undergo noninvasive carotid studies to define hemodynamic significance of the bruit. Patients with bilateral high-grade (80% to 99%) carotid stenoses may undergo elective repair of one side before aneurysm repair. However, patients with symptomatic or large aneurysms (>7 cm) should undergo AAA repair without delay for cerebrovascular surgery. The risk of perioperative stroke with asymptomatic carotid disease is relatively low.

V. Preoperative preparation. The preoperative preparation for **elective** AAA repair is the same as described previously for aortic reconstruction for occlusive disease (see Chap. 12). If autotransfusion is to be used, arrangements for the equipment and technician should be confirmed well before the time of surgery. The routine use of rapid intraoperative autotransfusion has allowed 70% to 80% of patients to undergo open AAA repair without transfusion of banked blood.

VI. Management of a ruptured aneurysm. Although endovascular stent grafts have been applied in select ruptured AAAs, the standard of care remains emergent open surgical repair. The key to successful management of a ruptured AAA is expeditious movement of the patient to an operating room. Delay in the emergency or radiology departments often results in deterioration and death from hemorrhage.

Operative mortality for a ruptured AAA has remained unchanged in the past 20 years. Only 50% of patients with a ruptured AAA who arrive at the hospital will be discharged alive. Factors predicting poor outcome or death are profound shock, cardiac arrest (need for CPR), preexisting cardiac or renal disease, and technical complications during the operation. Several factors, however, can enhance the likelihood of survival for a patient with a ruptured AAA:

A. Rapid transport. Patients with suspected AAA rupture should be transported rapidly to a hospital, where a surgical team should be waiting for assessment and resuscitation. An operating room should be readied as the patient arrives.

B. Resuscitation. Initial resuscitation should include two large-bore (14 or 16 gauge) intravenous lines, a nasogastric tube, and a Foley catheter. Blood should be typed and cross-matched for multiple units of packed red blood cells. Ringer's lactate solution is effective in initial volume expansion. If the patient is in shock prior to the availability of cross-matched blood, emergency release type O negative blood should be given. **Blood pressure should be maintained at a level to support urine output and mental status and not necessarily a normal value.** Systolic blood pressure of 100 mmHg is adequate if the patient is awake with good urine output. Use of inotropic agents, vasopressors and volume to achieve a **normal** blood pressure may actually worsen the situation by causing more bleeding.

If available, a rapid autotransfusion device should be set up in the operating room. Arterial and central venous lines can be placed and prophylactic antibiotics administered in the operating room.

C.   Accurate diagnosis. If the diagnosis of ruptured AAA is in question and the patient is hemodynamically stable, an abdominal CT scan or ultrasound should be considered. An electrocardiogram (ECG) should also be performed to rule out acute myocardial infarction.

D.   Immediate operation. A patient who presents with syncope or shock and a known AAA (or pulsatile abdominal mass) should be taken directly to the operating room. If a patient presents with syncope or shock but does not have a known AAA, then a brief abdominal ultrasound is preferred in the emergency department. This exam is used only to confirm the presence or absence of an aneurysm and not signs of rupture.

E.   Temperature control. Cold kills! Patients with a ruptured AAA and shock become hypothermic quickly. Those with a body temperature below 33°C develop capillary leak syndrome necessitating more volume, manifest a diffuse coagulopathy, and slip suddenly into life-threatening cardiac arrhythmias. The three useful means of preventing hypothermia are **(a) warming the operating room to 70°F to 80°F before the patient arrives, (b) using the Bair Hugger warming tent over the upper thorax and head, and (c) use of high volume, counter-current warming infusing systems for all administered intravenous fluids.**

F.   Aortic control. Since blood pressure can crash with induction of anaesthesia, the abdomen and groins should be prepped, and the operating team ready when the patient is anesthetized. A midline incision from xyphoid to pubis is the most direct approach. If the retroperitoneal hematoma if massive, initial aortic control should be gained by compression or clamping of the aorta at the diaphragm (Fig. 16.4). In many patients, however, the aorta can be clamped below the renal arteries. At this site care must be taken to avoid injury to the duodenum and left renal vein. Rarely, a patient with multiple prior abdominal operations may need a left thoracotomy for initial aortic clamping. Prior to clamping, mannitol (25.0 g) is given as a diuretic and free-radical scavenger. Low-dose intravenous dopamine (2 to 3 µg/kg/min) may also be useful for its vasodilatory effect on the renal and mesenteric circulations.

G.   Anticoagulation. Administration of heparin during ruptured AAA repair may be problematic. If the patient is hypothermic and in shock, a coagulopathy may already exist. On the other hand, lower extremity thrombosis is not uncommon during ruptured AAA repair. Consequently, smaller systemic doses of heparin (2,500 to 3,000 units) or regional administration of heparin into the iliac arteries may decrease lower-extremity thrombosis.

H.   Assessing limb and vital organ perfusion. Lower-extremity perfusion must be assessed **before** leaving the operating room. This can be achieved by palpating pulses, listening for Doppler signals at the feet, or by using calf plethysmographic pulse wave forms. If thrombosis is suspected, a Fogarty thromboembolectomy catheter should be passed immediately.

Likewise, the colon should be inspected for viability. If questionable, intravenous fluoroscein (2 ampules) can be given and the bowel inspected with a Wood's lamp. When the abdomen is

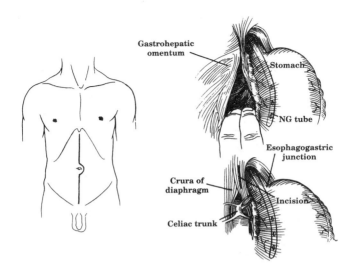

A

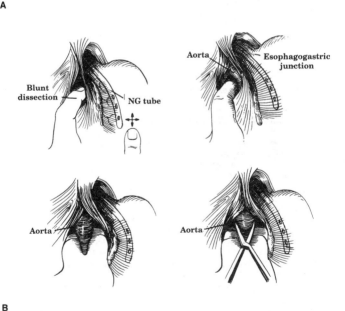

B

Figure 16.4.   **Supraceliac aortic clamping is useful for large ruptured abdominal aortic aneurysms and huge retroperitoneal hematomas that obscure the proximal aneurysm neck at the renal level.** *NG*, nasogastric. (By permission of the Mayo Foundation.)

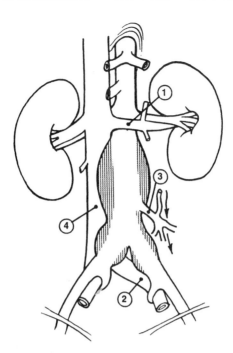

Figure 16.5.   Anatomic trouble spots in abdominal aortic aneurysm exposure. (*1*) The left renal vein or one of its branches (left renal lumbar, gonadal, or adrenal) may be injured during exposure of the aneurysm neck, especially with ruptured aneurysms. In 5% of cases, the left renal vein lies posterior to the aorta and may be injured in any attempt to encircle the proximal aorta for control. (*2*) The common iliac veins are usually adherent to the iliac arteries and may be injured during dissection. (*3*) The inferior mesenteric artery should be ligated on or within the aneurysm sac to avoid ligation of critical collateral vessels from the marginal artery of Drummond. (*4*) Dissection of the aneurysm sac from the vena cava is usually unnecessary.

massively distended, a tight primary closure may compromise renal or visceral perfusion. In such instances, a prosthetic-based delayed closure of the abdomen should be considered. The prosthetic can be removed and primary fascial closure accomplished when abdominal edema has improved.

   VII.   Aneurysm repair and Stent graft therapy. The following principles describe AAA repair and summarize endovascular stent graft therapy or abdominal aortic aneurysms (Fig. 16.3).

   A.   Open aneurysm exposure (Fig. 16.5) is obtained through a midline incision. We have found that, although transverse abdominal incisions or lateral extraperitoneal abdominal incisions may be used, they may make proximal aortic control of high aneurysms difficult. Flank incisions also limit exposure of the right distal iliac arteries. For aneurysms that extend nearly to the renal arteries, exposure is facilitated by division of the left renal vein, leaving the adrenal and gonadal veins as outflow for the left kidney. Another alternative is extensive mobilization the left renal vein by division of the adrenal, gonadal, and lumbar branches.

B.   Limited dissection of the lateral and posterior aneurysm is done to minimize blood loss and operative time. After proximal and distal clamping, the graft is sutured inside the aneurysm sac after all the thrombus has been removed from the aneurysm **(Creech technique).** If the duodenum is densely adherent to the AAA **(inflammatory aneurysm),** we do not dissect the duodenum free from the aneurysm but attempt to work around it. If infection is suspected, the aneurysm should be cultured and completely excised. Maintaining blood flow to the left colon via the inferior mesenteric artery or hypogastric arteries is essential to preventing colonic ischemia following abdominal aortic reconstruction.

C.   Retroperitoneal coverage of the graft should be completed using the aneurysm sac to wrap or separate the graft from the intestine. If this is not done, the intestine, especially the duodenum, may adhere to the graft and cause an eventual aortoenteric fistula.

D.   Endovascular grafting introduced by Parodi et al. (Fig. 16.3), is an option for elective treatment of AAAs. This therapy involves the transfemoral passage of a balloon-expandable, synthetic graft (straight or bifurcated) into the aorta after surgical exposure and control of the femoral arteries. The graft is positioned and deployed below the renal arteries using intraoperative flouroscopy and contrast angiography. This technique faces potential limitations. Specifically, inability to pass the device through diseased or tortuous iliac arteries, peripheral embolism of plaque, and an inadequate length of normal caliber aorta below the renal arteries **(length and diameter of neck).** In addition, aneurysms of the iliac vessels complicate deployment of bifurcated grafts. Inadequate proximal or distal attachment results in a leak into the AAA sac **(endoleak)** or graft migration. Currently, endograft placement is feasible in 30% to 50% of patients and evolution of this technology is likely to occur that will expand its applicability.

VIII.   Concurrent intraabdominal disease. In general, we prefer not to combine elective AAA surgery with other intraabdominal procedures that could be safely postponed. However, certain circumstances have led us to combine aneurysm repair with other procedures.

A.   Asymptomatic gallstones usually are left alone. Cholecystectomy is performed when **gallbladder disease** is apparent—that is, when the patient has had recent symptoms of cholecystitis, the gallbladder appears chronically inflamed, multiple small stones are present, or common duct stones are palpable. The rationale for cholecystectomy in the latter group is prevention of postoperative cholecystitis, which is associated with a high mortality rate.

B.   Severe peptic ulcer disease that is not well controlled by medication may be an indication for a highly selective vagotomy that does not open the gastrointestinal tract.

C. Severe reflux esophagitis that is not controlled medically may be managed by some type of fundoplication.

D. Renal tumors may require nephrectomy at the time of AAA repair.

E. Colon or bladder tumors present the dilemma of whether they should be resected before or after aneurysm repair. If a tumor is found incidentally during elective aneurysm repair, we manage the aneurysm first and return 3 to 6 weeks later to resect the tumor. If both the tumor and the aneurysm are known preoperatively, we address the more pressing problem first. For example, an obstructing colon tumor would be relieved before repair of a smaller (4 to 6 cm) aneurysm. Occasionally, we encounter the combination of a tender aneurysm and a nearly totally obstructive colon tumor, such that both diseases may require correction at the same operation. Normally, graft contamination can be avoided if the retroperitoneum is completely closed before the bowel resection. **When feasible, an endovascular stent graft obviates these dilemmas.**

F. Benign prostatic hypertrophy (BPH) requiring transurethral prostatic resection (TURP) or **prostatic cancer** requiring prostatectomy plus iliac node dissection is a common problem in patients with aortoiliac aneurysms. If the BPH has caused urinary retention and/or infection, a TURP should be considered before AAA repair. When a prostatectomy for cancer is indicated, we tend to repair the aneurysm first if it is 5 cm or larger and do the iliac node sampling simultaneously. The prostatectomy is delayed until the patient has recovered from the AAA repair. **Endovascular stent grafts again change the options in these clinical scenarios.**

IX. Postoperative care. General principles of postoperative care are summarized in Chapter 10, and specific discussion of care following aortic surgery is present in Chapter 12.

X. Postoperative complications. Early postoperative complications include cardiac or respiratory dysfunction, bleeding, ulceration of the gastrointestinal tract, renal failure, and postoperative psychosis (see Chap. 10). In addition, graft thrombosis, and limb and colon ischemia occur in the early postoperative period. Aortoenteric fistula, graft infection and sexual dysfunction are complications seen in the later postoperative period (see Chap. 12).

Endovascular stent grafts have their own unique postoperative complications. The most problematic is an endoleak at either the proximal or distal deployment sites **(type I endoleak).** Every effort should be made to eliminate this leak during the initial procedure. Continued aneurysm filling by lumbar or mesenteric arteries **(type II endoleak)** maintains pressure in the aneurysm sac **(endotension)** and requires immediate or delayed embolization. Other poststent complications include limb kinking and occlusion, iliac artery rupture, femoral artery injuries, and peripheral atheroembolism. Despite these potential complications, conversion to an open surgical procedure is rare (<5%).

XI. Long-term follow-up. The most important factor in long-term survival of patients following AAA repair is coronary heart disease. Patients with clinically evident heart disease have a decreased late survival rate (50% at 5 years and only 30% to 40% at 10 years). In contrast, patients without evident coronary disease have a 70% to 80% 5-year survival and a 50% 10-year survival. Although less common than cardiac morbidity, stroke affects 5% of AAA patients at 5 years and 10% at 10 years. Late graft complications (e.g., thrombosis, infection, anastomotic aneurysms) affect 3% to 5% of patients following AAA repair. Although these problems can occur any time, they tend to appear relatively late (i.e., 5 to 15 years after graft placement). **Finally, about 5% to 10% of patients will eventually develop another aortic aneurysm in the chest or upper abdomen.**

After AAA repair, patients should be rechecked every 2 to 3 years for graft patency and anastomotic pseudoaneurysm as well as for the development of femoral or popliteal aneurysms. Because coronary artery disease is a leading cause of death in these patients, we recommend that those with symptomatic coronary disease be followed by an internist or cardiologist.

Since endoleaks remain a continual late threat for stent grafts, these patients require closer periodic graft surveillance for the remainder of their lives. Initially, this surveillance is frequent (6 to 8 weeks postprocedure) and then at least every 6 months. Endoleaks are present in about 15% to 20% at 1 year, and surgical conversion is necessary in approximately 3% per year. Usually AAAs shrink after stent graft placement when there is no endoleak. Nonetheless, rupture risk is still 1% per year and does not appear to correlate with the presence of endoleak. Stent graft kinking or occlusion is more common than with surgical grafts and affecting 3% to 5% of patients per year of follow-up.

All graft-related complications considered, grafts placed at open aneurysm repair have fewer late problems than current stent grafts. **This fact should be discussed frankly with patients before electing an endovascular procedure, especially in relatively healthy patients with longer life expectancies.**

THORACOABDOMINAL AORTIC ANEURYSM

Thoracoabdominal aortic aneurysm (TAA) is defined as simultaneous aneurysm involvement of the thoracic and abdominal aortic segments. TAAs represent less than 10% of degenerative aortic aneurysms and are classified based on a scheme reported by E. Stanley Crawford (Fig. 16.6). Natural history data on TAAs reveals a negligible rupture risk for aneurysms less than 4 cm. In contrast, 5-year rupture risk is nearly 20% for TAAs between 4 and 6 cm and 33% for those larger than 6 cm. Therefore, the threshold for repair should be 6 to 7 cm in healthy patients or patients with symptomatic aneurysms.

I. Preoperative evaluation. In addition to history and physical exam, an abdominal CT scan and contrast aortography are necessary in patients having TAA repair. Preoperative arteriographic localization of the great radicular artery **(Adamkiewicz)** is felt by some to be useful in avoiding perioperative spinal cord ischemia. This artery arises from a T_9 to T_{12} intercostal artery in 75% of patients and is the main blood supply to the anterior spinal artery. Currently, we do not perform routine angiography for intercostal artery localization, but rely on intraoperative techniques to reduce spinal cord ischemia.

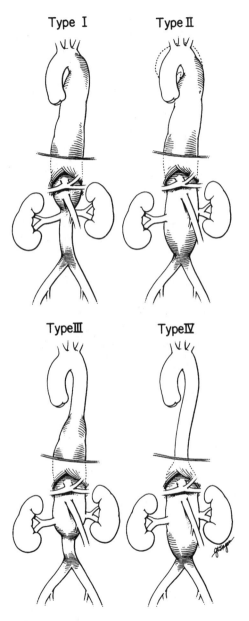

Figure 16.6.   Crawford classification of thoracoabdominal aortic aneurysms. (From Crawford ES, Crawford JL, Safi HJ. Thoracoabdominal aortic aneurysms: preoperative and intraoperative factors determining immediate and long-term results of operations in 805 patients. *J Vasc Surg* 1986;3:389–404, with permission.)

II.   Operative principles. The operative approach to TAA follows one of two distinct methods: (a) **clamp-and-sew** with adjuncts used to minimize end organ ischemia or (b) **distal aortic perfusion with sequential clamping** of the graft. Both use a left thoracoabdominal approach, and the choice is influenced by the experience of the surgical, anesthesia and intensive care teams. The following are adjuncts used individually or together during TAA repair to reduce morbidity.

A.   Distal aortic perfusion is achieved with left atrial to femoral artery bypass utilizing a Bio-Medicus pump (Medtronics, Minneapolis, MN, U.S.A.). This technique provides distal perfusion during aortic graft placement and may benefit the heart by unloading the left ventricle during cross-clamp.

B.   Regional spinal cord hypothermia (mean 26°C) using an epidural catheter with infusion of cold saline reduces the metabolic rate and demand of the spinal cord. Temperature and pressure may be monitored simultaneously with a separate intrathecal catheter.

C.   Cerebrospinal fluid drainage improves perfusion pressure of the spinal cord when pressure is greater than 10 to 15 cm H_2O. This technique is commonly used perioperatively and for 1 to 3 days following the operation.

D.   Renal cooling. Direct application of ice and infusion of renal preservation solution (4°C lactated Ringer's with mannitol and methylprednisolone) into the renal artery after opening the aorta reduces local metabolic demands and stimulates diuresis.

E.   In-line mesenteric shunting. After performance of the proximal anastomosis an arterial perfusion catheter is placed from the proximal graft to the celiac or superior mesenteric artery ostia. This allows prograde, pulsatile perfusion to the viscera while the remainder of the graft is being placed.

III.   Postoperative course. Mortality of TAA repair averages 10% but is much higher in urgent or ruptured cases. Other factors that increase morbidity are operative time of more than 5 to 6 hours, prolonged cross-clamp time, hypothermia (<35°C), and blood loss of more than 2 to 3 L.

Respiratory failure is the most common complication following TAA repair (25% to 45%). Risk factors are active smoking, baseline pulmonary disease, and division of the phrenic nerve during thoracoabdominal exposure. The incidence of **spinal cord ischemic complications** ranges from 4% to 16% in large series following all types of TAA. This can be as high as 30% in patients with extensive type I and II TAA. **Renal failure** can be expected in 5% to 20% of patients following TAA repair and increases the risk of mortality nearly tenfold. A survival of 60% at 5 years can be expected following elective TAA repair with cardiac events representing the leading cause of death. Rupture of another aneurysm accounts for 10% of late deaths emphasizing the importance of lifelong aneurysm surveillance.

AORTIC DISSECTION

Dissection is a common vascular catastrophe affecting the aorta and is distinct from degenerative aneurysms. Dissection results from an aortic defect which allows a false lumen between the

DeBakey Type I Type II TypeIII

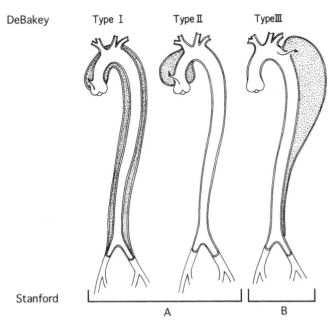

Stanford

A   B

Figure 16.7. Classifications of aortic dissection.

intima and adventitia to form. The **DeBakey classification** of aortic dissection includes types I and II, which involve the ascending aorta, and type III, which involves only the descending aorta (Fig 16.7). The **Stanford classification** includes type A, involving the ascending aorta, and type B, involving only the descending aorta. Complications of dissection include aortic valve insufficiency, aneurysm formation, aortic rupture and visceral, renal or peripheral ischemia.

   I.   Preoperative evaluation. Aortic dissections present as tearing chest or back pain in patients between the age of 50 and 70 years. A history of hypertension is present in 80% to 90% of patients. The physical exam should be mindful of cardiac, visceral, or peripheral findings from the dissection. Initial diagnostic tests should include an EKG and chest radiograph. The diagnosis of dissection can be made by spiral CT scan, MRI, or transesophageal echocardiography. The diagnostic test of choice should be expeditious in patients in whom dissection is suspected. Contrast aortography is generally helpful if dissection is confirmed and an operation planned.

   II.   Management. A critical initial step in the management of aortic dissection is decreasing the mean arterial pressure and contracting force of the heart. This is achieved with intravenous beta-blockade with or without the use of sodium nitroprusside. Nearly all patients with dissections involving the ascending aorta (DeBakey, types I and II; Stanford type A) require emergent surgery to prevent death from cardiac tamponade or aortic regurgitation with heart failure. This involves replacement of the ascending aorta and aortic valve via a median sternotomy. DeBakey type III or Stanford type B dissections can be managed medically with surgery via a left thoracoabdominal approach reserved for the 10% to 40% of patients who develop complications of the dissection (distal ischemia, aortic rupture, aneurysm formation, or pain).

III. Postoperative course. Patients with Stanford A dissections have a higher likelihood of death in the first 24 to 48 hours after onset than patients with Stanford B dissections. However, the operative mortality of Stanford B dissections is higher (30% to 50%) should an operation become necessary because of failure of medical management. Stanford A dissections carry an operative mortality of approximately 10% to 15%. A 5-year survival of 75% to 85% exists in patient who leave the hospital alive following aortic dissection.

FEMORAL ARTERY ANEURYSM

Femoral artery aneurysms (FAAs) usually are found in male patients who have aneurysmal disease of the abdominal aorta and or the popliteal arteries. The more common complications of FAAs are thrombosis, and distal embolization and less commonly rupture. Approximately 30% of FAAs present as a surgical emergency. Therefore, elective surgical repair is warranted in most cases.

I. Preoperative evaluation. Because the majority of patients with FAAs will have an associated AAA or popliteal artery aneurysm, the preoperative evaluation must include careful palpation of the abdominal aorta and popliteal arteries Ultrasound of the abdominal aorta and the popliteal space adds to the physical exam. An arteriogram of the involved femoral artery and distal runoff should be done to delineate involvement of the profunda femoris and superficial femoral arteries.

II. Operative principles. Three factors govern the choice of operation for common FAAs: (a) location of the origin of the profunda femoris artery, (b) patency of the superficial femoral artery, and (c) patency of the aneurysm itself.

A. In **type 1 FAAs** in which the profunda femoris orifice is distal to the aneurysm and all vessels are patent, the simplest and most successful repair is a vein or synthetic graft interposition for the resected aneurysm.

B. In **type 2 FAAs,** the profunda femoris arises from the aneurysmal sac. We cannot overemphasize the importance of **maintaining patency of the profunda femoris when such aneurysms are repaired.** In most instances, such aneurysms are resected and an interposition graft is carried out to the superficial femoral artery. A small side-arm graft then is constructed to the profunda femoris artery.

C. When the superficial femoral artery is **chronically occluded,** it is ligated and an end-to-end anastomosis of the graft to the profunda femoris artery is performed.

IV. Postoperative follow-up. After FAA repair, patients should be followed annually. Duplex ultrasound is an ideal method to monitor grafts and to discover other aneurysms. Newly discovered aneurysms of the abdominal aorta or popliteal arteries should be corrected as indicated.

POPLITEAL ARTERY ANEURYSMS

Popliteal artery aneurysms (PAAs) seldom rupture but instead present with limb-threatening ischemia in the majority of cases. Ischemia results from acute thrombosis of the PAA or chronic embolization of debris into the tibioperoneal circulation. Alternatively, PAAs present as a mass behind the knee which may obstruct the popliteal vein, or compress the tibial nerve. Popliteal aneurysms at greatest risk for thromboembolic events have three characteristics: **(a) size greater than 2 cm, (b) intraluminal thrombus seen on ultrasound, and (c) decreased pedal pulses indicating compromised runoff from thromboembolism or atherosclerosis.**

I.   Preoperative evaluation. Like patients with FAAs, these patients must be carefully examined for other aneurysms, especially in the aortoiliac location. Preoperative angiography should show not only the location of the PAA but also delineate the below-the-knee runoff. The presence of a patent distal popliteal artery or an adequate posterior or anterior tibial artery is the most important determinant of successful repair for PAAs.

II.   Operative principles. The preferred surgical treatment for a smaller (3 cm) PAA has been proximal and distal ligation of the aneurysm combined with a reverse saphenous vein bypass. The aneurysm is usually exposed through a medial knee incision although a posterior knee exposure works well for focal popliteal aneurysms. The posterior popliteal approach avoids cutting any tendons. Consequently recovery is easier than after a medial knee incision with any tendon repair. When possible, the aneurysm should not be resected, since this dissection can injure the popliteal vein. Larger aneurysms should be opened, the thrombus removed, and a portion of the sac resected to prevent compressive symptoms from the mass effect of the aneurysm.

When thromboembolism has occluded the infrapopliteal outflow acutely, two methods may help reestablish distal flow. One is regional thrombolytic therapy used preoperatively or smaller regional doses instilled directly into the tibial arteries at the operating table. The second is retrieval of thrombus by a Fogarty thromboembolectomy catheter.

Occasionally chronic infrapopliteal thromboembolism and/or atherosclerosis will have occluded the tibial runoff and left an unfavorable anatomic situation for a bypass. If the ankle-brachial index is 0.35 or higher and the only symptom is rest pain, a lumbar sympathectomy may help avert the need for amputation.

Although endovascular stent grafts have been placed in popliteal artery aneurysms, continual knee flexion and activity are problematic and limit long-term patency.

III.   Postoperative follow-up. Patients surgically treated for PAAs should be reevaluated annually. Ultrasound is the ideal test to monitor any popliteal graft and to check for associated aneurysms of the aortic, femoral, and opposite popliteal artery.

SELECTED READING

Cambria RP, Davison JK, Carter C, et al. Epidural cooling for spinal cord protection during thoracoabdominal aneurysm repair: a five-year experience. *J Vasc Surg* 2000;31:1093–1102.

Clouse WD, Hallett JW Jr, Schaff HV, et al. Improved prognosis of thoracic aortic aneurysms: a population-based study. *JAMA* 1998; 280:1926–1929.

Coselli JS, Plestis KA, La Francesca S, et al. Results of contemporary surgical treatment of descending thoracic aortic aneurysms: experience in 198 patients. *Ann Vasc Surg* 1996;10:131–137.

Cronenwett JL, Johnston KW. The United Kingdom small aneurysm trial: implications for surgical treatment of abdominal aortic aneurysms. *J Vasc Surg* 1999;29:191–194.

Diwan A, Sarkar R, Stanley JC, et al. Incidence of femoral and popliteal artery aneurysms in patients with abdominal aortic aneurysms. *J Vasc Surg* 2000;31:863–869.

Finlayson SRG, Birkmeyer JD, Fillinger MF, et al. Should endovascular surgery lower the threshold for repair of abdominal aortic aneurysms? *J Vasc Surg* 1999;29:973–985.

Hallett JW Jr. Management of abdominal aortic aneurysms. *Mayo Clin Proc* 2000;75:395–399.

Hallett JW Jr, Marshall DM, Petterson TM, et al. Graft-related complications after abdominal aortic aneurysm repair: reassurance from a 36-year population-based experience. *J Vasc Surg* 1997;25: 277–286.

Lowell RC, Gloviczki P, Hallett JW Jr. Popliteal artery aneurysms: the risk of nonoperative management. *Ann Vasc Surg* 1994;8:14–23.

Nevitt MP, Ballard DJ, Hallett JW Jr. Prognosis of abdominal aortic aneurysms. *N Engl J Med* 1989;321:1009–1014.

Porter JM, Abou-Zamzam AM Jr. Endovascular aortic grafting: current status. *Cardiovasc Surg* 1999;7:684–688.

Reed WW, Hallett JW Jr, Damiano MA, et al. Learning from the last ultrasound: a population-based study of patients with abdominal aortic aneurysm. *Arch Int Med* 1997;157:2064–2068.

Safi HJ. How I do it: thoracoabdominal aortic aneurysm graft replacement. *Cardiovasc Surg* 1999;7:607–613.

Seelig MH, Oldenburg WA, Hakaim AG, et al. Endovascular repair of abdominal aortic aneurysms: where do we stand? *Mayo Clin Proc* 1999;74:999–1010.

U.K. Small Aneurysm Trial Participants. Mortality results for randomised controlled trial of early elective surgery or ultrasonographic surveillance for small abdominal aortic aneurysms. *Lancet* 1998;352:1649–1655.

U.K. Small Aneurysm Trial Participants. Health service costs and quality of life for early elective surgery or ultrasonographic surveillance for small abdominal aortic aneurysms. *Lancet* 1998;352: 1656–1660.

White GH, Yu W, May J, et al. Endoleak as a complication of endoluminal grafting of abdominal aortic aneurysms: classification, incidence, diagnosis and management. *J Endovasc Surg* 1997;4: 152–168.

Renovascular Hypertension

Renal artery disease is being recognized increasingly as a contributing cause to hypertension and progressive renal insufficiency in adults, especially in the elderly with generalized atherosclerosis. Recent renal artery investigations at the time of coronary angiography reveal renal artery stenoses in up to 20% to 30% of patients with coronary atherosclerosis. Currently, the appropriate management of the renal artery disease is nothing less than controversial.

One controversy revolves around the natural history of renal atherosclerosis. A second centers on appropriate indications for renal balloon angioplasty and stenting. A third focuses on which patients should undergo surgical revascularization, which can be one of the most technically difficult of all vascular operations. In most cases, such procedures are performed to correct a renal artery stenosis causing renovascular hypertension or chronic renal insufficiency. Other less common lesions include aneurysms, emboli, traumatic lesions, and arteriovenous fistulas. This chapter summarizes general principles of diagnostic evaluation, indications for angioplasty or operation, surgical options, operative techniques, and perioperative care associated with renal artery reconstruction.

The options for managing renovascular disease continue to expand. Advances have recently been made in medical, radiologic, and surgical management. Antihypertensive medications such as angiotensin-converting enzyme (ACE) inhibitors and calcium channel blockers are allowing better control of severe hypertension caused by renal artery stenosis. Radiologists have become active in performing percutaneous transluminal balloon dilatation + stenting of renal artery lesions. Surgical options also have increased. *Ex vivo* renal reconstruction, renal autotransplantation, and finer anastomotic technique done under magnification have allowed the vascular surgeon to correct difficult renal artery problems that previously resulted in nephrectomy.

I. Renin–angiotensin system. To logically manage renovascular hypertension, one must review the relationship of the kidney to blood pressure control. By adjusting sodium and water retention, the kidney helps maintain blood pressure through regulation of extracellular fluid. A decrease in blood volume or an obstruction of a renal artery lowers renal blood flow. Baroreceptors in the juxtaglomerular apparatus detect decreases in renal blood flow and respond by releasing the enzyme **renin.** Renin cleaves a plasma globulin called angiotensin I, forming the vasoconstricting peptide **angiotensin II.** Angiotensin II increases blood pressure by stimulating adrenal release of aldosterone, by causing vasoconstriction, and by exerting an antidiuretic, antinatriuretic action on the kidney. The result is sodium and water retention which expands extracellular fluid volume and increases blood pressure. Research has identified a hormone, **atrial natriuretic peptide** (ANP), that inhibits renin secretion, and opposes the vasoconstrictive action of angiotensin II. ANP is a natriuretic and vasorelaxant peptide secreted by the atria.

II. Diagnostic evaluation. Approximately 5% to 15% of patients with arterial hypertension have a treatable renal artery stenosis. This association occurs more often in hypertensive children and young adults, who more commonly have aortic coarctations, congenital renal artery stenoses, or fibromuscular dysplasia than older patients. Elderly adults with diffuse atherosclerosis are also at higher risk for renal artery disease. However, history, physical examination, and routine laboratory tests do not usually allow differentiation between renovascular and essential hypertension. Other diagnostic tests are necessary to delineate the etiology.

A. Screening tests. Historically the test for renovascular hypertension was an intravenous pyelogram (IVP) showing delayed function in the affected kidney. However, the IVP has a sensitivity of approximately 75% and consequently may miss some patients with significant renal artery stenosis. Recently, **duplex ultrasonography** has assumed a more prominent role in screening for renal artery disease. However, ultrasound is limited by requiring a fasting patient, a skilled ultrasonographer, and a dedicated period of time (45 to 60 minutes). Another option used commonly is **magnetic resonance angiography** with gadollium enhancement. Although improving rapidly in quality, MR angiograms may still provide limited clarity in some patients. Furthermore, they are relatively expensive, and are not always technically possible. Nonetheless, we prefer to use MR angiography to screen patients with suspected renovascular disease with elevated serum creatinines before a contrast angiogram for either angioplasty or surgical planning.

Two other functional tests for renovascular hypertension are the **captopril test** and **captopril renal scanning.** The captopril test involves oral administration of captopril, an ACE inhibitor, after baseline measurement of plasma renin activity and blood pressure. Renovascular hypertension should be suspected when the postcaptopril plasma renin level is excessively high. Some studies indicate that the sensitivity of this test approaches 100%, with a specificity of 90%. However, the test is less accurate in the presence of renal failure. Criteria for a positive captopril renal scan include a reduction in glomerular filtration rate and a delay in the time to peak clearing of the radionuclide.

B. Arteriography. The cornerstone of diagnosis remains arteriographic demonstration of stenotic lesions in one or both renal arteries. We generally recommend an arteriogram when one or more of the following indications exist in a hypertensive patient:

1. Hypertension poorly controlled by adequate medical therapy.
2. Hypertension of recent origin with recent progression.
3. Hypertension in a child, adolescent, or young adult.
4. Hypertension associated with a localized epigastric bruit.
5. Possible renovascular etiology suggested by the IVP, duplex scan, renal scan, or MR angiogram.
6. Rising serum creatinine.

The arteriogram should include (a) an abdominal aortogram, (b) selective renal artery injections in different planes, and (c) a celiac artery injection with a lateral view if the splenic or hepatic arteries are to be used for splenorenal or hepatorenal bypass.

C.   Renin determination. The presence of a renal artery stenosis on an arteriogram does not establish its functional importance. A comparison of renin determinations of venous samples taken from each renal vein and the inferior vena cava above and below the renal veins is helpful in establishing hemodynamic significance of a renal artery stenosis. Since an ischemic kidney will produce more renin, a renal vein ratio of at least 1.5:1.0 should be present if the stenosis is to be considered hemodynamically significant. One exception to this rule occurs when definite collateral vessels have developed. Positive renal vein renins generally predict a favorable response to correction of renal artery stenosis.

Certain aspects of renal vein renin determination must be emphasized if meaningful results are to be obtained. Antihypertensive medications and unrestricted sodium intake are two factors that may affect renal vein renin assay. For example, beta-blockers can suppress renin output. The result is false nonlateralization of the renal vein renins. Likewise, sodium intake may also reduce renin output.

Probably the most practical current method to stimulate a difference in renal vein renins is captopril administration (25 mg p.o.) after baseline renins are collected. Renal renin levels are recollected 30 minutes after captopril. A 30-minute post-captopril renal venous ratio of 3 or greater enhances the likelihood that hypertension will respond to surgical or angioplasty treatment of a renal artery stenosis. Despite the predictive value of renal vein renins, their use in everyday clinical practice has diminished in recent years.

III.   Indications for invasive intervention. There are four main indications for a renal artery intervention, either surgical or endovascular.

A.   Renovascular hypertension is by far the most common indication. A renal vein renin ratio of 1.5 from the affected kidney is predictive of improvement or cure in about 75% of cases. Success also depends on the etiology of the renal artery disease and the age of the patient. The best surgical or angioplasty results have been reported in younger patients (<50 years old) with fibromuscular dysplasia or focal atherosclerotic lesions. Long-term relief or cure of hypertension occurs in at least 90% of such patients. In contrast, patients with renal artery disease and generalized atherosclerosis may have less satisfactory improvement. Although most patients with advanced renal atherosclerosis will not be cured, their blood pressure can usually be controlled with less medication. Consequently, 70% to 80% of such patients will be improved clinically (i.e., diastolic pressures < 90 mm Hg).

Despite nonlateralizing renins, operation or angioplasty ± stenting may be indicated if the clinical picture and arteriographic lesion suggest a high likelihood of renovascular hypertension.

In certain situations, initial treatment should be angioplasty. The primary example is the patient with fibromuscular renal disease of the main renal artery. Percutaneous transluminal balloon angioplasy is initially successful in 80% to 90% of these patients. Angioplasty also provides satisfactory dilation in some patients where the fibromuscular dysplasia extends into the first renal artery branches.

Finally, controversy continues over whether patients with renovascular hypertension should be managed medically until hypertension can no longer be easily controlled by antihypertensives. Recent evidence indicates that renal function continues to deteriorate in about 40% of patients with atherosclerotic renal artery stenosis under good medical control of hypertension. Deterioration is more likely in patents with bilateral renal stenoses or stenosis to a solitary kidney. Consequently, medically treated patients must have their blood pressure, serum creatinine, and glomerular filtration rate followed every 3 to 6 months.

B.   The preservation of renal function by renal artery surgery or angioplasty is receiving increased attention. Patients who are most likely to benefit from invasive therapy to preserve renal function often are difficult to select. Certainly, consideration should be given to patients with severe bilateral renal stenoses or a severe stenosis of a solitary functioning kidney (prior nephrectomy, nonfunctioning contralateral kidney, or total renal artery occlusions). Progressive renal deterioration may be indicated by decreasing kidney size, despite little angiographic change in the appearance of the renal artery stenoses and minimal change in serum creatinine.

Several surgeons have encouraged a more aggressive approach to revascularization of functioning kidneys with proximal renal artery occlusion. Such kidneys may retain significant function by collateral blood flow. No single factor predicts salvage of a kidney with a chronic renal artery occlusion. Although kidneys less than 9.0 to 9.5 cm in length have poorer results, successful revascularization has been achieved in smaller kidneys. Other predictors of renal salvage have been rich perihilar collateral circulation, distal renal artery reconstitution, and biopsy evidence of intact viable glomeruli. However, biopsy is subject to random sampling. In experienced hands, the best approach to such patients appears to be surgical exploration with either renal artery reconstruction if a viable kidney is present or nephrectomy if salvage is not possible.

The role of balloon angioplasty + stenting in preserving renal function in cases of severe bilateral renal artery stenoses is debatable. Although serum creatinine may be stabilized, improvement has been rarely documented after angioplasty. Because angioplasty does not affect adjacent ulcerative atherosclerosis, small atheroemboli may continue to shower the kidneys and slowly deteriorate parenchymal function. In contrast, surgical transaortic endarterectomy removes both the renal atheroma and adjacent aortic disease.

C.   Surgical correction of aneurysmal or occlusive disease of the aorta may necessitate preservation of a main or accessory renal artery. Accessory renal arteries less than 2 mm in size can usually be ligated without significant loss of renal function.

D.   Other renal artery problems requiring renal artery reconstruction include aneurysms, emboli, dissections, traumatic lesions, and arteriovenous fistulas. Renal artery aneurysms generally should be repaired when they are associated with hypertension and they appear causative. Other indications for repair may be distal emboli arising from an aneurysm thrombus, increasing diameter size greater than 1.5 to 2.0 cm, and actual rupture. Rupture of a renal artery aneurysm appears more likely during pregnancy. Therefore, women with renal aneurysms in the childbearing period should be considered for elective aneurysm repair. A renal artery embolus should be suspected in any patient with conditions predisposing to arterial emboli who develops acute flank pain. Renal arteriovenous fistulas are difficult surgical problems, especially when they are in the renal parenchyma. Intrarenal arteriovenous fistulas may be treated by transcatheter steel coil occlusion accomplished under fluoroscopic control by a vascular radiologist.

IV.   Surgical options. Preservation of a functioning kidney is the primary goal of any renal operative procedure. Nephrectomy is done only when no other method of saving a good kidney appears possible. A wide variety of autogenous and synthetic graft materials are available for renal artery reconstruction. Endarterectomy is another alternative. Figures 17.1 and 17.2 illustrate our preferred methods of renal artery revascularization. Autogenous grafts, such as those from the saphenous vein or another artery, are preferable to synthetic materials. Factors that generally increase the risk of operative morbidity and mortality are azotemia (creatinine >3 mg/dL), complex or bilateral renal revascularizations, past myocardial infarction, compromised ventricular function, aortic aneurysm repair, and diffuse vascular disease.

V.   Preoperative preparation. Before renal artery revascularization, blood pressure and renal function must be stabilized as much as possible.

A.   Blood pressure. Most of these patients have significant hypertension, which increases the risk of myocardial and cerebrovascular events. Generally, blood pressure will improve with hospitalization and bed rest, sometimes allowing a reduction in antihypertensive medications. We try to stop diuretic therapy 24 to 48 hours prior to the operation so that chronically contracted intravascular volume can expand. Beta-blockers should not be abruptly stopped since discontinuation may result in tachycardia and myocardial ischemia.

B.   Renal function. About one-third of patients undergoing renovascular surgery have chronic renal insufficiency (creatinine >2 mg/dL). Several factors can cause deterioration in their creatinine clearance prior to hospitalization and during preoperative evaluation.

1.   Vigorous diuretic therapy can cause intravascular volume contraction and prerenal azotemia.

2.   ACE inhibitors must be administered cautiously, if at all, in patients with bilateral renal artery stenoses or a solitary kidney with a high-grade stenosis. ACE inhibitors disturb renal blood flow autoregulation, probably by decreasing efferent arteriolar resistance, which must be maintained to

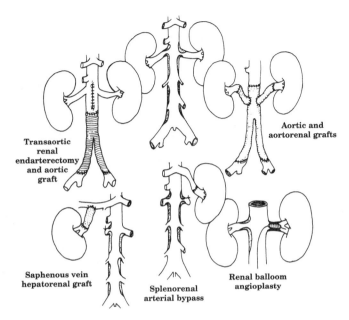

Figure 17.1.   Options for renal revascularization for atherosclerotic disease.

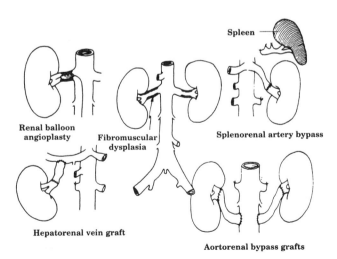

Figure 17.2.   Options for renal revascularization for fibromuscular disease.

provide an adequate perfusion gradient to the glomerulus. Worsening serum creatinine is frequently due to these drugs, which are being used increasingly for hypertension and congestive heart failure. We stop them in all patients with elevated serum creatinine. Generally creatinine will return to lower levels in 5 to 7 days.

3.   Another frequent cause for an acute rise in serum creatinine is **angiographic contrast nephrotoxicity.** Multiple consecutive studies such as an intravenous digital subtraction arteriogram followed by a standard transfemoral renal, carotid, or coronary arteriogram can quickly worsen renal function. One must keep in mind that many computed tomography (CT) scans are also done with intravenous contrast. After all contrast studies are completed, we generally observe the serum creatinine level for at least 24 hours before proceeding with any renal surgery. If creatinine rises, we delay operation until the azotemia has resolved for at least 1 to 2 days.

VI.   Operative principles

A.   Incisions. Proper operative exposure is one of the most important aspects of renal artery surgery. A midline xiphoid-to-pubic bone incision provides good access. An upper transverse or subcostal incision may be used but does not provide as good exposure of the distal aorta or iliac system. A left splenorenal arterial anastomosis can be constructed through a low, left thoracoabdominal incision (bed of the 10th rib) or a left subcostal incision.

B.   Proximal renal lesions. For central lesions, the midline retroperitoneum is opened over the aorta. On the left side, the renal vein can be mobilized by ligation and division of the **adrenal, gonadal, and left reno-lumbar branches of the left renal vein.** On the right side, the vena cava must be mobilized and retracted to expose the proximal right renal artery.

C.   Middle or distal lesions. For middle or distal lesions, on the right side, the duodenum must be reflected by a Kocher maneuver to expose the distal right renal artery. On the left side, the splenic flexure of the colon can be mobilized in a similar fashion.

D.   Renal protection. Several steps must be taken for renal protection:

1.   Intravenous hydration with a balanced salt solution (e.g., Ringer's lactated solution, 100 to 125 mL/h) is started 8 to 10 hours before surgery.

2.   Heparin (5,000 units) is given intravenously before clamping the renal artery.

3.   Mannitol (12.5 to 25.0 g) is administered early in the procedure. If a good diuresis is not achieved, 20 to 40 mg of furosemide is used.

4.   The kidney may be cooled with 200 to 300 mL of a renal perfusate if anticipated renal ischemic time is greater than 45 minutes We use a combination of 1 L of Ringer's lactated solution, 18 g mannitol, 20 mg heparin, and 500 mg methylprednisolone (Solu-Medrol, Pharmacia & Upjohn Company, Bridgewater, NJ, U.S.A.), chilled to 3°C in saline slush.

5.   Low-dose (2 to 3 μg/kg/min) dopamine causes renal vasodilatation, which may help minimize vasomotor nephropathy. We start dopamine intravenously in the operating room before renal artery clamping and continue it for at least 12 to 24 hours.

E. Type of anastomosis. The proximal anastomosis is constructed first. Then, the distal anastomosis is made end-to-end by the spatulation technique. The suture material usually is 6-0 or 7-0 polypropylene. For an especially difficult anastomosis, the suture line is interrupted. Low-power magnifying loops and a high-intensity headlight are essential in most renal artery reconstructions.

F. Intraoperative assessment of graft patency. The simplest method to ascertain blood flow is the examination of the graft or renal artery with a sterile continuous-wave Doppler. Biphasic signals should be present. Recently, intraoperative duplex ultrasonography has provided a relatively quick and reliable method to detect technical problems after renal artery grafting or endarterectomy. Significant problems are detected in about 10% of reconstructed arteries. Most of these problems are correctable and lead to results similar to those of patients with normal intraoperative ultrasound studies.

VII. Postoperative care. In the immediate postoperative period, intravascular volume must be carefully maintained to ensure adequate urine output. It may require use of a Swan–Ganz pulmonary artery catheter to monitor filling pressures in patients with significant cardiac disease. Low-dose dopamine is continued for renal vasodilation, and dobutamine is administered to patients with marginal cardiac output (<3 L/m^2). Generally, we strive to maintain a urine output of 1 mL/kg/h. Some patients have a massive diuresis (>200 mL/h) and require urinary replacement (0.5 mL of crystalloid per milliliter of urine) for 12 to 24 hours. Diuretics are usually not necessary in the first 24 hours. When a question arises about the early patency of the reconstruction, we obtain a renal scan. Before discharging the patient from the hospital, the surgeon should consider ordering a renal scan or an arteriogram to document the patency of the reconstruction at that point. Any subsequent recurrence of hypertension or deterioration of renal function requires a repeat ultrasound and/or angiographic study. Percutaneous transluminal angioplasty may be performed on an anastomotic stenosis in an attempt to salvage a failing graft. Reoperation of stenotic or thrombosed renal grafts can achieve a successful result in more than 50% of patients.

VIII. Renal balloon angioplasty. Chapter 6 discusses the results of balloon angioplasty for selected renal artery stenoses caused by fibromuscular dysplasia and atherosclerosis. Physicians who treat hypertension must be informed about this technique and understand which patients are the optimal candidates. **A recent randomized trial of renal angioplasty versus medical management for atherosclerotic renal-artery stenosis found little advantage of angioplasty over antihypertensive-drug therapy at 12 months follow-up.** Despite this lack of evidence for aggressive use of renal angioplasty, the tendency to balloon dilate renal artery stenosis associated with hypertension has increased in recent years.

IX. Quality of life. A major issue in treating renovascular hypertension and renal insufficiency is whether the side effects of medical therapy or the risks of surgical revascularization are worse than the disease itself. Certain antihypertensives (e.g., certain beta-blockers) cause enough lethargy, sexual dysfunction, and sleep disorders for 15% to 20% of patients to withdraw themselves from therapy. Likewise, patients with renovascularly related renal failure that leads to chronic dialysis have only a 50% to 60% chance of normal activity and work. These discouraging results compare to a 75% to 90% chance of improved blood pressure and 90% chance of avoiding chronic dialysis after properly conducted renovascular operations. Operative mortality ranges from 2% to 3% for patients without azotemia to 5% to 7% for those with a serum creatinine level greater than 2 mg/dL.

SELECTED READING

Cambria RP, Brewster DC, L'Italien GJ, et al. The durability of different reconstructive techniques for atherosclerotic renal artery disease. *J Vasc Surg* 1994;20:76–87.

Canzanello VJ, Textor SC. Noninvasive diagnosis of renovascular disease. *Mayo Clin Proc* 1994;69:1172–1181.

Chabova V, Schirger A, Stanson AW, et al. Outcomes of atherosclerotic renal artery stenosis managed without revascularization. *Mayo Clin Proc* 2000;75:437–444.

Chaikof EL, Smith RB 3rd, Salam AA, et al. Ischemic nephropathy and concomitant aortic disease: a ten-year experience. *J Vasc Surg* 1994;19:135–148.

Dean RH, Tribble RW, Hansen KJ, et al. Evolution of renal insufficiency in ischemic nephropathy. *Ann Surg* 1991;213:446–455.

Hallett JW, Textor SC, Kos PB, et al. Advanced renovascular hypertension and renal insufficiency: trends in medical comorbidity and surgical approach from 1970 to 1993. *J Vasc Surg* 1995;21:750–760.

Izzo JL Jr, Black HR, eds. *Hypertension primer.* Dallas: America Heart Association, 1993.

Stanley JC, Zelenock GB, Messina LM, et al. Pediatric renovascular hypertension: a thirty-year experience of operative treatment. *J Vasc Surg* 1995;21:212–227.

Stanley JC. The evolution of surgery for renovascular occlusive disease. *Cardiovasc Surg* 1994;2:195–202.

Van Jaarsveld BC, Krijnen P, Pieterman H, et al. The effect of balloon angioplasty on hypertension in atheroclerotic renal-artery stenosis. *N Engl J Med* 2000;342:1007–1114.

Weibull H, Berquist D, Bergentz SE, et al. Percutaneous transluminal renal angioplasty versus surgical reconstruction of atherosclerotic renal artery stenosis: a prospective randomized study. *J Vasc Surg* 1993;18:841–852.

Zierler RE, Bergelin RO, Isaacson JA, et al. Natural history of atherosclerotic renal artery stenosis: a prospective study with duplex ultrasonography. *J Vasc Surg* 1994;19:250–258.

Intestinal Ischemia

Intestinal ischemia comprises a small portion of all peripheral vascular problems. Although aortic atherosclerosis may involve the origins of the mesenteric arteries, intestinal collateral blood flow usually is adequate enough to prevent symptomatic, chronic intestinal ischemia. Likewise, arterial emboli can obstruct mesenteric arteries, but more commonly they flow by the visceral vessels and lodge in the leg arteries. Consequently, these anatomic and hemodynamic features make intestinal ischemia less common than chronic claudication or acute ischemia of the lower extremities.

For several reasons, acute or chronic intestinal ischemia remains one of the most challenging problems of peripheral vascular surgery. Failure to recognize that a patient has some form of intestinal ischemia is one of the main reasons for poor results. Patients often are operated on too late to salvage the ischemic intestine or, many times, to save the patient's life. Even when intestinal ischemia is recognized and treated expediently, many patients still succumb because of serious underlying medical problems. The best surgical results have been achieved in patients with chronic intestinal angina who undergo intestinal revascularization before severe weight loss or acute thrombosis occurs.

In this chapter, we emphasize early recognition of intestinal ischemia. **Delay in diagnosis represents one of the primary failings in the care of these patients.**

MESENTERIC ARTERY ANATOMY

Certain anatomic features of the mesenteric circulation determine symptoms and influence management of intestinal ischemia (Fig. 18.1). Although the three major mesenteric arteries supply specific territories, they normally intercommunicate by excellent collateral channels. These collaterals enlarge when a proximal mesenteric artery is stenotic or occluded. The primary collateral pathways between the celiac and superior mesenteric arteries are via the gastroduodenal artery to the pancreaticoduodenal arteries that connect with the superior mesenteric artery. The inferior mesenteric artery has two main sources of collateral flow when it is obstructed (Fig. 18.2). The middle colic branch of the superior mesenteric artery connects around the transverse colon to the marginal artery of Drummond, a continuation of the left colic branch of the inferior mesenteric artery. The inferior mesenteric artery also receives collateral flow via the middle hemorrhoidal artery, a branch of the internal iliac artery. These abundant collateral channels for mesenteric circulation explain the clinical observation that **intestinal angina usually does not occur until at least two of the three main mesenteric arteries have severe occlusive disease.**

CLINICAL PRESENTATION

Intestinal ischemia is classified as either chronic or acute. However, the presentations may overlap, since chronic intestinal stenosis can progress to acute thrombosis and intestinal infarction.

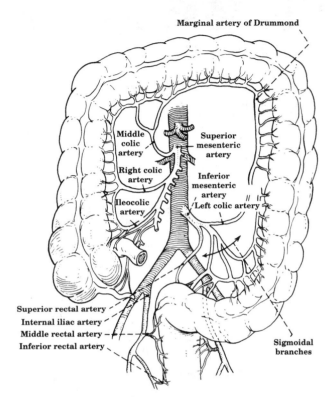

Figure 18.1.   Anatomy of the colonic arterial supply. When the inferior mesenteric artery is diseased or occluded by atherosclerosis, viability of the left colon may depend on collateral flow from the superior mesenteric artery via the marginal artery of Drummond.

I.   Chronic intestinal ischemia often eludes early diagnosis because the chronic abdominal pain is attributed to some more common gastrointestinal (GI) disorder. Frequently, the patient has undergone a negative diagnostic evaluation of the gallbladder, liver, and entire GI tract. Because of progressive weight loss, some patients are mistakenly thought to have cancer. Certain clinical features, however, should raise suspicion of chronic intestinal ischemia.

  A.   Classically, the **chronic abdominal pain** is intermittent and postprandial. It usually is localized to the epigastrium and is a dull ache or colic that begins 30 to 60 minutes after eating and may persist for a few hours. Patients may have associated abdominal bloating or diarrhea.

  B.   Involuntary weight loss eventually occurs because the patient associates eating with pain. Consequently, a "food fear" develops. Oral intake often is modified until liquids become the primary nutrient.

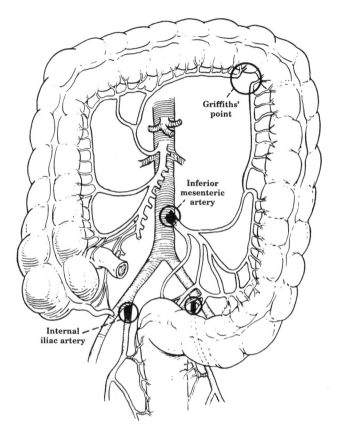

Figure 18.2.   Critical arterial inflow points for the left colon. If occlu-sive disease or operative reconstruction obliterates flow through both internal iliac arteries and the inferior mesenteric artery, the colon may become severely ischemic. Colonic ischemia is more than likely in this situation if the superior mesenteric-inferior mesenteric collateral connections are not developed or injured at Griffiths' point.

C.   Physical findings of chronic intestinal ischemia are lim-ited primarily to **weight loss** and an **abdominal bruit.** Since the weight loss usually is insidious over several months and many patients with atherosclerosis have abdominal bruits, the significance of these nonspecific findings often is overlooked when the patient initially presents.

D.   Chronic intestinal ischemia should be suspected in any adult who has chronic abdominal pain, progressive weight loss, other signs of generalized cardiovascular disease, and a nega-tive work-up for more common GI disorders.

II.   Acute intestinal ischemia has three main etiologies: thrombosis of an arterial stenosis, embolism, and non-occlusive small-vessel insufficiency. Although the initial symptom for all these etiologies is abdominal pain, the clinical setting often suggests the most likely underlying cause. The frequency of each etiology may vary among medical centers, but generally acute intestinal ischemia is caused by thrombosis in 40% of cases, embolism in another 40%, and intestinal hypoperfusion in 20% of cases.

   A.   Severe generalized abdominal pain that is disproportionate to the physical findings remains the classic presentation of acute intestinal ischemia. Nausea, vomiting, or diarrhea may follow shortly after the onset of symptoms. Although the abdomen may have diffuse tenderness, bowel sounds may be heard and peritoneal signs usually are absent. The only early laboratory abnormality may be an elevated white blood cell count (usually >18,000). When these findings are made, the clinician must suspect acute mesenteric ischemia and undertake steps to alleviate it. Aggressive radiologic and surgical intervention at this point can salvage the ischemic intestine in about 50% of such patients.

   If intestinal ischemia remains unrecognized, physical findings will change as intestinal necrosis develops. Bloody diarrhea may occur, although often it is not present. Hypovolemia becomes evident as fluids are sequestered in the ischemic intestinal wall and surrounding tissues. Fever, peritoneal signs, and shock occur as sepsis becomes established. When intestinal ischemia has advanced to this point, the likelihood of salvaging the ischemic intestine and the critically ill patient is less than 15% to 20%.

   B.   The clinical setting and the patient's past medical history usually suggest the probable etiology of acute intestinal ischemia. If chronic intestinal angina preceded acute symptoms, thrombosis of a mesenteric artery stenosis is the most likely etiology. Emboli should be suspected when atrial fibrillation is present or if the patient has had previous cerebral or lower-extremity thromboembolism. Nonocclusive, mesenteric ischemia occurs in the setting of low cardiac output. The most common predisposing conditions for nonocclusive, mesenteric ischemia are myocardial infarction, congestive heart failure, renal or hepatic disease, or any major operation that leads to hypovolemia or hypotension in a patient with atherosclerosis. This type of nonocclusive, acute mesenteric ischemia is being recognized more commonly.

DIAGNOSTIC TESTS

   When acute or chronic intestinal ischemia is suspected, the most reliable diagnostic method is arteriography. **Early angiographic diagnosis is the most important principle of successful management of acute intestinal ischemia.** An arteriogram with lateral views of the aorta to show the mesenteric artery origins is the definitive method. The angiographic catheter also has become an important route for delivering vasodilating drugs and thrombolytic agents to the mesenteric circulation.

   The evaluation of possible chronic mesenteric ischemia usually includes other diagnostic tests before angiography is done—commonly endoscopy or barium studies of the upper and lower GI tract. Abdominal ultrasound and computed tomography (CT) scanning may also reveal hepatobiliary disease or occult tumors such as cancer of the pancreas or lymphoma of the retroperitoneum.

Duplex scanning can scan mesenteric blood flow patterns, allowing noninvasive determination of stenosis and changes in flow before and after a test meal. The use of velocity wave form parameters that can discriminate between normal subjects and those with visceral artery stenosis should reduce both the incidence of missed diagnosis and unnecessary angiography. The extent of diagnostic work-up for patients presenting with chronic abdominal pain obviously must be individualized.

MANAGEMENT

Treatment of intestinal ischemia also can be organized into the two broad categories of chronic and acute ischemia.

I.   Chronic intestinal ischemia can be relieved only by correction of the occlusive lesions. There is no effective medical therapy. Surgical correction has been the most common technique, although balloon angioplasty has also been successful.

A.   One aspect of perioperative care, **nutritional repletion,** deserves special emphasis. Since chronic intestinal ischemia leads to progressive weight loss, some patients are chronically malnourished and have no nutritional reserves for a major abdominal operation. We strongly recommend that such catabolic patients receive parenteral nutrition before and after elective surgery. In general, one should not delay mesenteric artery surgery for prolonged nutritional repletion but proceed expeditiously to intestinal revascularization before the patient with progressive chronic ischemia suffers an acute catastrophic bowel infarction.

B.   There are two basic surgical options for mesenteric revascularization: bypass grafting or endarterectomy. Over the years, different authors have preferred one technique to the other. Either supraceliac or infrarenal aortomesenteric bypass grafting is the procedure of choice for most patients. The optimum method of mesenteric revascularization, however, depends highly on the number of vessel occlusions and the condition of the abdominal aorta in each patient. Transaortic endarterectomy has also been successful for multiple visceral occlusive lesions at the origins of the mesenteric arteries. Combined infrarenal aortic replacement and Dacron bypasses to mesenteric arteries appears to be the technique of choice when severely symptomatic infrarenal aortic occlusive or aneurysmal disease coexists with chronic intestinal ischemia. However, combining mesenteric revascularization and aortic replacement carries a high mortality rate (10% to 20%) in these cachectic patients. In contrast, limiting the operation to some type of aortomesenteric grafting or endarterectomy alone minimizes mortality (3% to 5%).

Regardless of which method of revascularization is selected, early relief of intestinal angina is achieved in about 90% of patients. In our reported experience, the best long-term results have been obtained by revascularization of at least two occluded or stenotic vessels. In most patients this combination has included both the celiac and superior mesenteric arteries. Symptoms recurred in 10% of patients who underwent complete revascularization, in 25% who had two of three occlusive lesions corrected, and in 50% who had a single vessel revascularized. Since revascularization of a single mesenteric occlusion offers relief to most patients, complete revascularization must be weighed against the patient's overall condition, prognosis, and other technical factors.

Chronic or acute intestinal ischemia also may be the iatrogenic result of sacrificing the inferior mesenteric artery at the time of infrarenal aortic grafting. Revascularization of the inferior mesenteric should be performed when the superior mesenteric artery is occluded and a large (>3.5 to 4.0 mm) inferior mesenteric artery is present.

Another less common form of chronic mesenteric ischemia is median arcuate compressions and stenosis of the celiac axis. Some extrinsic compression of the celiac axis by the median arcuate ligament is common in women, but most experts question its functional importance. Certainly, a celiac stenosis may be critical when occlusive disease of the superior mesenteric and inferior mesenteric arteries is present also. Division of the median arcuate ligament with either patch angioplasty of the celiac stenosis or an interposition graft may alleviate symptoms.

II.   Successful management of **acute intestinal ischemia** must begin with arteriography to define the mesenteric anatomy. Optimal therapy for acute mesenteric ischemia cannot be determined unless the clinician knows whether the problem is thrombotic, embolic, or hypoperfusion-related.

A.   **Thrombosis** usually is apparent on the arteriogram by obstruction of the superior mesenteric artery at its origin from the aorta. Systemic heparin is indicated to prevent clot propagation.

Emergency abdominal exploration should be undertaken to assess bowel viability and to revascularize the obstructed artery. Resection of a nonviable intestine without revascularization of the remaining small bowel is associated with a high incidence of further intestinal infarction and death. Generally the bowel should be revascularized before intestinal resection. An exception to this rule is resection before revascularization when a segment of intestine is grossly gangrenous or perforated. A single aortomesenteric bypass is sufficient in these seriously ill patients. When bowel contamination is present, a vein graft is preferable to a synthetic material.

Clinical judgment of intestinal viability may be enhanced by fluorescein examination of the GI tract. The test is performed by injection of 2 ampules (1,000 mg) of sodium fluorescein through a peripheral vein and immediate examination of the bowel under an ultraviolet Wood's light in a darkened operating room. A viable bowel has a smooth or uniform fluorescence. A nonviable bowel has decreased, patchy, or no fluorescence. When it appears that the bowel may survive, it may be left alone and a second-look operation should be performed within 24 hours to reassess the intestinal viability. **Second-look operations should be routine if any bowel had questionable viability at the initial operation.** Approximately half of such patients will have ischemic bowel that needs resection at the second-look procedure.

B.   **Emboli** usually lodge a few centimeters beyond the origin of the mesenteric artery at the level of the first jejunal branches. Standard therapy remains identical to the management of thrombosis, except the embolus usually is removed by a mesenteric artery arteriotomy and Fogarty catheter thromboembolectomy. Sometimes a vein patch or a bypass graft is needed if significant arterial stenosis is also present. Although thrombolytic therapy may reopen a thrombosed mesenteric artery, operative inspection of the bowel for viability is still mandatory in our experience.

C. Nonocclusive mesenteric ischemia generally is seen in critically ill patients who have low cardiac output. They often are poor risks for any surgery and many times are so labile that transport to the angiographic suite is a major undertaking in itself. Their arteriograms show peripheral mesenteric vasoconstrictions but no large-vessel occlusions. Noninvasive ischemic colitis appears to be mediated primarily by a remarkable sensitivity of the colonic vasculature to the renin–angiotensin axis.

The best results with this group of patients have been achieved by measures to improve cardiovascular hemodynamics and to vasodilate the peripherally constricted mesenteric vasculature. The recommended splanchnic vasodilator therapy is a papaverine infusion of 30 to 60 mg/h through an angiographic catheter positioned in the superior mesenteric artery. If a vasopressor is needed to increase blood pressure, dopamine would be the drug of choice, since it reduces renal and mesenteric vascular resistance.

SELECTED READING

Howard TJ, Plaskon LA, Wiebke EA, et al. Nonocclusive mesenteric ischemia remains a diagnostic dilemma. *Am J Surg* 1996;171: 405–408.

Johnston KW, Lindasy TF, Walker PM, et al. Mesenteric arterial bypass grafts: early and late results and suggested surgical approach for chronic and acute mesenteric ischemia. *Surgery* 1995;118:1–7.

Mateo RB, O'Hara PJ, Hertzer NR, et al. Elective surgical treatment of symptomatic chronic mesenteric occlusive disease: early results and late outcomes. *J Vasc Surg* 1999;29:821–832.

McAfee MK, Cherry KJ Jr, Naessens JM, et al. Influence of complete revascularization on chronic mesenteric ischemia. *Am J Surg* 1992; 164:220–224.

Moneta GL, Lee RW, Yaeger RA, et al. Mesenteric duplex scanning: a blinded prospective study. *J Vasc Surg* 1993;17:79–86.

Murray SP, Stoney RJ. Chronic visceral ischemia. *Cardiovasc Surg* 1994;2:176–179.

Perko MJ, Just S, Schroeder TV. Importance of diastolic velocities in the detection of celiac and mesenteric artery disease by duplex ultrasound. *J Vasc Surg* 1997;26:288–293.

Rhee RY, Gloviczki P, Mendonca CT, et al. Mesenteric venous thrombosis: still a lethal disease in the 1990s. *J Vasc Surg* 1994;20: 688–697.

Taylor LM, Moneta GL. Intestinal ischemia (basic data underlying clinical decision-making in vascular surgery). *Ann Vasc Surg* 1991; 5:403–406.

Thomas JH, Blake K, Pierce GE, et al. The clinical course of asymptomatic mesenteric arterial stenosis. *J Vasc Surg* 1998;27:840–844.

Zelenock GB. Visceral occlusive disease. In: Greenfield LJ, ed. *Surgery: scientific principles and practice*, 2nd ed. Philadelphia: Lippincott–Raven Publishers, 1997:1764–1779.

Upper-Extremity Arterial Disease and Vasospastic Disorders

In the spectrum of peripheral vascular diseases, upper-extremity arterial problems, including vasospastic disorders, are relatively uncommon. When pain, numbness, coldness, or ulcers involve the fingers or hand, patients generally seek early medical attention. Such symptoms restrict many normal activities and quickly raise the patient's fear of permanent loss of hand function.

The underlying causes of arm ischemia and vasospastic disorders are diverse. For simplicity, they may be organized into the broad groups of emboli, atherosclerotic or aneurysmal occlusions, trauma, and small-vessel arterial occlusive disease. In the initial patient evaluation, the clinician must determine which broad group the patient fits into (see Chap. 3). Then diagnostic tests can be selected to define the specific underlying etiology. This chapter emphasizes principles of management after a clinical diagnosis is established.

COMMON CLINICAL PRESENTATIONS

Although the etiologies for upper-extremity arterial ischemia, including vasospastic disorders, are multiple, the clinical presentations are relatively few.

I. **Raynaud's phenomenon** is simply a description of a clinical presentation or syndrome that suggests vasospasm. The underlying causes are numerous (Table 19.1). Certain clinical features help differentiate Raynaud's phenomenon from other vasospastic disorders, such as acrocyanosis and livedo reticularis (Table 19.2).

A. Raynaud's phenomenon defines an **episodic** constriction of the small arteries and arterioles of the extremities. The episodes generally are initiated by cold exposure or emotional stimuli. The symptoms of acrocyanosis and livedo reticularis are constant, although they increase with cold exposure.

B. The phenomenon usually follows a definite **sequence of color** in the digits and hand: pallor, cyanosis, and rubor. The pallor occurs when small arterioles close and skin perfusion is minimal. As cutaneous flow begins to resume, it is sluggish, and blood desaturation leads to cyanosis. Finally, cutaneous flow resumes with a hyperemic phase causing skin rubor. Some patients will not demonstrate all these color changes. Attacks usually are accompanied by numb discomfort of the fingers. Pain generally is not severe unless ulcerations are present. In contrast, acrocyanosis occurs mainly in women and is characterized by continuous bluish discoloration of the hands and occasionally of the lower extremities. Livedo reticularis also is a continuous vasospastic condition consisting of a mottled or reticulated reddish blue discoloration of the lower extremities and occasionally of the hands.

Table 19.1. Diverse etiologies of Raynaud's phenomenon

Systemic diseases or conditions
  Collagen vascular diseases (e.g., scleroderma)
  Cold hemagglutination or cryoglobulinemia
  Myxedema
  Ergotism
  Macroglobulinemia

Nerve compressions
  Carpal tunnel syndrome
  Thoracic outlet syndrome

Occupational trauma
  Pneumatic hammer operation
  Chain saw operation
  Piano playing
  Typing

Arterial occlusive disease

Table 19.2. Differentiation of vasospastic disorders

Characteristics	Raynaud's phenomenon	Acrocyanosis	Livedo reticularis
Sex	Primarily women (70–80%)	Primarily women (90%)	Men or women
Age	Young adults (15–35)	Young adults (15–35)	Any age
Color change	Pallor, cyanosis, rubor	Diffuse cyanosis	Mottled cyanosis or rubor
Location	Fingers, toes, sometimes face	Usually hands, sometimes feet	Usually legs, sometimes arms
Duration	Intermittent	Continuous	Continuous
Effect of cold exposure	Increased symptoms	Increased symptoms	Increased symptoms
Skin ulceration	Occurs when collagen vascular disease (e.g., scleroderma) is present	None	Rare

C. The phenomenon is **localized** to the fingers, toes, and occasionally nose and ears. Attacks are limited most commonly to the upper extremities and rarely involve only the toes.
D. The chance of ulceration or gangrene of the tips of the digits depends on the underlying etiology.

1. Raynaud's disease is the term applied to Raynaud's phenomenon that has no clear association with any systemic disease. It rarely results in tissue necrosis. Raynaud's disease usually occurs in young females (70% of cases). It has been suggested that, before the diagnosis of Raynaud's disease is made, the following strict criteria should be met:

a. Bilateral, symmetric Raynaud's phenomenon is present.

b. No large arterial occlusions are evident.

c. Slight or no gangrene or trophic changes apparent.

d. Symptoms present for a long period, usually 2 years, without evidence of any other systemic disease associated with Raynaud's phenomenon.

2. Raynaud's phenomenon is the term applied when a local or systemic disease appears to be the precipitating factor. Gangrene or ulceration of digits is more common in these patients, especially when they have scleroderma. Scleroderma is the most common collagen vascular disease associated with Raynaud's phenomenon. Raynaud's phenomenon is the initial symptom in 30% of cases and eventually affects 80% of patients with scleroderma. The other common rheumatic diseases associated with Raynaud's phenomenon include mixed collagen vascular disease (80%), systemic lupus erythematosus (30%), dermatomyositis/polymyositis (20%), and rheumatoid arthritis (10%). It must be remembered that Raynaud's phenomenon may exist for years before some underlying systemic collagen vascular or immunologic disease is diagnosed.

3. Acrocyanosis is not associated with skin ulceration. **Livedo reticularis** may occur with ulcerations, generally when some systemic disease (e.g., periarteritis nodosa) is present or atherosclerotic microembolism is evident.

II. Tissue necrosis includes gangrene and nonhealing ulcerations. It is not uncommon for patients to mistake microemboli or small ulcers of the fingers for inconsequential bruises or sores of the finger, not recognizing their more serious etiology. If Raynaud's phenomenon precedes the onset of tissue necrosis, other symptoms and signs of underlying systemic disease should be sought. In the absence of Raynaud's phenomenon, evidence of large-vessel occlusive disease, emboli, or small-vessel arterial occlusive disease associated with occupational trauma must be sought.

A. Large-vessel occlusive disease of the arm usually is localized to the subclavian or axillary arteries. These lesions may be arteriosclerotic and, most commonly, the origin of the left subclavian artery is involved. A less common etiology of proximal upper-extremity arterial occlusion is thrombosis of an axillary artery aneurysm caused by years of crutch use (e.g., by patients with poliomyelitis). Chronic subclavian artery trauma related to thoracic outlet syndrome also may eventually lead to vessel occlusion. Extensive acute deep venous thrombosis of the arm can cause venous gangrene, which may be initially mistaken for arterial insufficiency. Finally, postmastectomy irradiation of the axillary area can result, eventually (10 to 20 years later), in radiation-induced axillary-subclavian arterial stenosis.

B.   Emboli to the digits may originate from the heart or the subclavian artery. In severe arm ischemia secondary to emboli, the heart is the place of origin in about 50% of cases, while the other 50% of emboli are shed from the subclavian or axillary arteries. The proximal upper-extremity arteries may develop atherosclerotic ulcerative plaques or aneurysms that shed emboli. Poststenotic subclavian aneurysms associated with thoracic outlet compression or axillary aneurysms caused by prolonged crutch use also may cause embolism to the hand. Embolic or acute arterial ischemia can also be caused by thrombus shed from the anastomotic site of an occluded axillo-femoral bypass graft.

C.   Small-vessel arterial disease associated with occupational hand trauma may cause severe hand ischemia. Occupations involving repetitive vibration or percussion of the fingers or hand predispose some individuals to spasm, thrombosis, or aneurysms of the ulnar, radial, palmar, or digital arteries. The ulnar artery is especially susceptible to local trauma over the hypothenar eminence, where it is fairly superficial and easily compressed against the underlying pisiform and hamate bones. The term **hypothenar hammer syndrome** has been applied to this form of posttraumatic digital ischemia. Activities that may lead to hand ischemia are pneumatic hammer, lathe, or chain saw operation; riveting; and less strenuous activities such as piano playing and typing. In industry, the term **vibration-induced white finger** has been applied to post-traumatic digital ischemia.

Rapid onset of hand ischemia has also been seen with small-vessel occlusion caused by hypersensitivity angitis. This etiology should be suspected when no large-vessel occlusion is present and no systemic diseases are identified.

III.   Arm claudication is an unusual presentation of arm ischemia in our experience. In general, exertional arm fatigue is more commonly caused by neurologic compression at the cervical spine or thoracic outlet. Because of excellent collateral channels around the shoulder, subclavian occlusive disease often is asymptomatic or mildly symptomatic (Fig. 19.1). However, active adults, especially manual laborers, may experience forearm claudication from subclavian or brachial artery stenosis.

DIAGNOSTIC TESTS

Patient history and physical examination provide most of the information necessary to diagnose the general type of upper-extremity arterial disease (see Chap. 3). The following tests may be done to confirm the clinical impression, to identify underlying etiologies, and to monitor therapy.

I.   Doppler velocity flow detection. The Doppler system is a simple means for auscultating arm arterial flow when pulses are not palpable. The axillary, brachial, radial, ulnar, palmar, and digital arteries can easily be checked for flow. Biphasic or triphasic arterial sounds are normal, while monophasic dampened signals suggest significant obstruction. Upper-arm and forearm

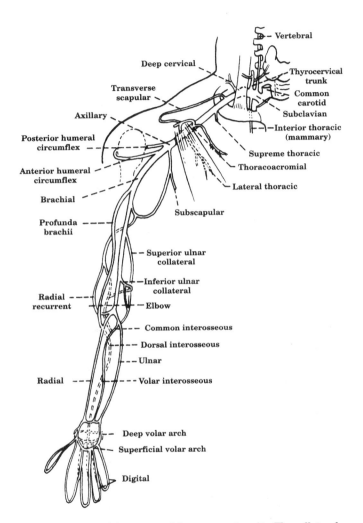

Figure 19.1. Arterial anatomy of the upper extremity. The collateral circulation of the arm is well developed, and consequently proximal large-vessel occlusion seldom results in distal extremity necrosis and amputation.

blood pressures can be measured with a routine blood pressure cuff and the Doppler unit. In cases of suspected arm claudication, baseline brachial pressures should be obtained and then a drop in pressure after arm exercise for 2 to 5 minutes should be observed.

II. Digital plethysmography or laser Doppler flow patterns may be helpful in the evaluation of digital ischemia and vasospastic disorders. Flat or severely diminished (<5 mm) pulse volume recordings (PVRs) confirm severe digital flow reduction and are predictive of poor healing when ulcers are present. The digital PVRs or laser Doppler flow measurements can be repeated to assess digital blood flow improvement after treatment, especially after alpha-blockade or sympathectomy.

III. Duplex ultrasonography provides excellent visualization of most upper-extremity arterial segments. The main limitations are the proximal subclavian arteries, especially on the left, and sometimes segments of the subclavian artery under a bulky clavicle.

IV. Arteriography. Arteriography is most helpful when large-vessel occlusion is obvious. In such cases, arteriography defines the location of the occlusion and shows the runoff to the forearm and hand. Transfemoral arteriography is recommended, since the catheter can be positioned to demonstrate the origin of the subclavian artery or be manipulated into the arm when distal runoff is of greatest interest. Arteriography is not necessary to diagnose vasospastic disorders but may be necessary to rule out any large-vessel ulcerative lesions when Raynaud's phenomenon is complicated by finger ulcers. Arteriography must show the entire upper-extremity vasculature from its origin (innominate on the right and subclavian on the left) to the digital arteries. **Failure to obtain complete upper-extremity arteriography is a common reason for a missed diagnosis (e.g., digital occlusions due to an ulcerated atheroma in the proximal subclavian artery).**

V. Digital temperature recovery time can help establish the diagnosis of Raynaud's phenomenon. The physiologic principle behind the test is simple, and the technique of the test also is fairly easy. Digital cutaneous blood flow is linearly related to digital skin temperature over a wide range. Normally, digital skin temperature recovers to normal within 10 to 15 minutes after cold exposure. In contrast, digital skin temperature in patients with Raynaud's phenomenon does not recover for at least 20 to 25 minutes after cold stimulus. The accuracy of the test is improved when the following guidelines are followed for measuring the digital temperature recovery time:

A. The patient should sit in a warm (24°C ± 2°C), quiet room for at least 30 minutes before the test.

B. Baseline digital pulp temperatures are taken with a thermistor probe.

C. The hand is immersed in an ice-water mixture for 20 seconds, removed, and dried.

D. Digital temperatures are checked every 5 minutes for 30 to 45 minutes.

E. A temperature-time graph can be constructed to show the digital temperature versus recovery time.

F. Controls for a particular laboratory should be established for comparison.

VI.   Systemic disease work-up. Since systemic diseases so often underlie vasospastic disorders and upper-extremity ischemia, a number of screening laboratory tests should be considered. A platelet count should be done, since thrombocytosis can mimic Raynaud's phenomenon. An elevated sedimentation rate should raise suspicion of a systemic illness. Since serum protein abnormalities may be associated with vasospasm, a serum protein electrophoresis should be performed and cryoglobulins, macroglobulins, and cold agglutinins should be checked. Basic immunologic tests should include antinuclear antibody, rheumatoid factor, and lupus erythematosus tests. If scleroderma is suspected, a skin biopsy in an affected area may confirm the diagnosis or a barium esophagogram may reveal characteristic esophageal dysfunctions.

MANAGEMENT

In our experience, these guidelines have provided the best assurance of relieving upper-extremity ischemia, including vasospastic disorders. Where there are areas of controversy, we offer several different points of view.

I.   Vasospastic disorders
A.   Raynaud's disease usually can be satisfactorily managed by nonoperative methods. Tissue necrosis rarely is a problem; consequently, the patient needs assurance that loss of fingers or their function is not likely to occur if the following guidelines are observed.
  1.   Avoidance of any tobacco use and protection from cold exposure are the fundamentals of initial treatment. Tobacco leads to vasoconstriction, a fact that can be documented by comparing baseline digital PVRs to tracings taken immediately after the patient smokes several cigarettes. The basics of protection from cold exposure include warm gloves and footwear during cold weather and gloves when working with the refrigerator. Maintaining core body temperature by wearing warm clothing over the trunk also helps. For many patients, these simple measures are enough.
  2. When vasospasm is not satisfactorily relieved by these simple measures, several **medical options** are available and are usually effective. The best results are obtained with drugs that diminish sympathetic neuromuscular transmission and new calcium-entry-blocking agents. Recently the drug of choice has been nifedipine, 10 mg p.o. t.i.d. For some patients, the long-acting nifedipine (XL tablets, 30 to 60 mg daily) causes fewer side effects. The most common side effects include headache, dizziness, palpitations, flushing, and edema. Another vasodilator that may help in severe cases is Doxazosin, an alpha-blocker.
  3.   Thermal biofeedback has demonstrated excellent results in patients in whom anxiety and stress play a major role in the initiation of vasospastic attacks. After biofeedback training, 80% to 90% of patients can avert an attack of Raynaud's phenomenon, and some can actually increase skin temperature as much as 4°C.
  4. The role of **surgical or thoracoscopic sympathectomy** for Raynaud's disease is limited. Few patients should need sympathectomy, since conservative management con-

trols symptoms in at least 80% of patients. Reasonable candidates for sympathectomy are those patients whose vasospastic attacks are becoming progressively debilitating, especially when trophic or ulcerative changes have occurred. Approximately 50% to 60% of such patients with primary Raynaud's phenomenon and no underlying systemic collagen vascular or immunologic disease will have improvement after sympathectomy, although the initial results may not last more than 3 to 6 months. For reasons that are not clear, sympathectomy for lower-extremity symptoms is more effective than that for arm symptoms.

B.   Raynaud's phenomenon secondary to underlying systemic disease often is a more difficult problem to manage than Raynaud's disease. Tissue necrosis with exceptionally painful digital ulcers can be a chronic problem. The fundamentals of therapy remain avoidance of tobacco, protection from cold, and calcium channel blockers. Sympathectomy is far less effective than it is for Raynaud's disease. In fact, only 20% to 30% of patients with scleroderma and Raynaud's phenomenon improve after sympathectomy, so we rarely recommend sympathectomy in these patients. Good results for digital ulceration have been reported with upper-extremity digit sympathectomy performed with an operating microscope. This procedure should be done by an experienced hand surgeon.

C.   Acrocyanosis does not lead to tissue loss, so treatment is directed at relieving cold-induced symptoms. The conservative management described for Raynaud's disease usually is sufficient.

D.   Livedo reticularis also is manageable in most cases by conservative treatment. Digital ulceration may occur when livedo reticularis is associated with periarteritis nodosa, lupus erythematosus, or cholesterol embolization. In such cases, sympathectomy should be considered, although results have been variable.

E.   Cold hypersensitivity may be seen after recovery from frostbite. The affected area may become bluish and have an associated burning pain with even mild cold exposure. The problem seems to be a variant of reflex sympathetic dystrophy (sympathetically maintained pain). Initially, the medical treatment described for Raynaud's disease should be undertaken. For severe cases, regional sympathectomy may provide lasting relief, especially if it is done before pain becomes chronic.

II.   Threatened limb loss. Although vasospastic disorders may cause ulcerations of the tips of the digits, the hand and arm seldom become ischemic. Severe hand ischemia usually is associated with large-artery occlusions, emboli, or trauma.

A.   Acute ischemia generally requires emergency surgical intervention. The history and physical examination usually will identify the probable cause. If there is a delay for medical stabilization and arteriography, we administer heparin systematically to the patient to prevent thrombus propagation. Patients who develop brachial artery occlusion after cardiac catheterization should undergo immediate brachial thrombectomy and repair under local anesthesia. Although the patient's hand may initially be relatively asymptomatic, a chronic brachial artery

occlusion can cause bothersome arm claudication in active individuals. Thus, early brachial thrombectomy and repair are
preferable to delayed surgery, can be accomplished at minimal
risk under local anesthesia, and achieve return of distal pulses
in 98% of patients.

B.   Emboli usually can be successfully extracted with Fogarty embolectomy catheters. Thromboemboli lodged in the subclavian axillary segment generally are approached through an
infraclavicular pectoral muscle-splitting incision. More distal
forearm clots are more completely removed by brachial artery
cutdown. Although distal digital and small-vessel clots have
been irretrievable by Fogarty catheters, adjuvant thrombolytic
agents may be helpful in selected patients with recent thrombosis. In many such cases, however, the distal thrombosis is relatively chronic. Thrombolytic therapy does not help much when
the clots are older than a few days. Emboli originating from
proximal subclavian ulcerative lesions will require endarterectomy or grafting to remove the source of the emboli.

C.   Large-artery occlusion generally will require bypass
grafting, replacement, or reimplantation. Proximal subclavian
obstructions may be bypassed by vein, autogenous artery (e.g.,
hypogastric), or synthetic grafts. A carotid-to-subclavian bypass
or reimplantation of the subclavian artery into the common
carotid artery are two options. Subclavian artery thrombosis secondary to thoracic outlet syndrome will require resection of the
first rib and any cervical rib in conjunction with arterial repair.
However, axillary and subclavian **vein thrombosis** secondary
to thoracic outlet compression can be alleviated by thrombolytic
infusions and anticoagulation followed by first rib resection. The
timing of the first rib resection is controversial with some surgeons proceeding immediately to rib resection after thrombolysis. However, we generally prefer to anticoagulate the patient
with warfarin for 6 to 8 weeks while the thrombogenic vein surface heals and then do the rib resection. Thrombosed axillary
aneurysms usually are replaced with saphenous vein grafts.
Saphenous vein also is the best graft material for brachial,
radial, and ulnar revascularization.

III.   Arm claudication. As discussed above, incapacitating
arm claudication is fairly uncommon because of the rich collateral
blood flow to the arm. For the few patients who need revascularization, the surgical options described above for threatened limb
loss are also applicable to relieve claudication. Success also may
be achieved by balloon angioplasty of proximal subclavian and
axillary stenoses.

LONG-TERM PROGNOSIS

The long-term prognosis for most arterial problems of the upper
extremity is good. Nonoperative treatment is successful in many
patients. Therefore, unless the viability of the extremity is acutely
threatened, a period of conservative treatment and observation
should be followed. The patients with the worst prognosis generally are those with Raynaud's phenomenon secondary to progres-

sive collagen vascular disease or those with extensive distal small-vessel occlusion secondary to recurrent emboli or thrombosis.

SELECTED READING

Fugitani RM, Mills JL. Acute and chronic upper extremity ischemia. I. Large vessel arterial occlusive disease. In: Porter JM, Taylor LM, eds. *Basic data underlying clinical decision making in vascular surgery.* St. Louis: Quality Medical Publishing, 1994:159–165.

Machleder HI. Vascular disease of the upper extremity and the thoracic outlet syndromes. In: Moore WS, ed. *Vascular surgery: a comprehensive review*, 5th ed. Philadelphia: Saunders, 1998:613–625.

Mills JL, Fugitani RM. Acute and chronic upper extremity ischemia. II. Small vessel arterial occlusive disease. In: Porter JM, Taylor LM, eds. *Basic data underlying clinical decision making in vascular surgery.* St. Louis: Quality Medical Publishing, 1994:166–170.

Wigley FM, Flavahan NA. Raynaud's phenomenon. *Rheum Dis Clin North Am* 1996;22:765–781.

Specific Venous Problems

Varicose Veins

Varicose veins are one of the most common vascular problems seen in office practice. They affect about 15% of the adult population. Most varicose veins are the result of a congenital or familial predisposition that leads to loss of elasticity in the vein wall and the absence or incompetence of venous valves. These primary varicosities generally progress downward in the greater saphenous system. Secondary or acquired varicosities occur when the venous valves have been damaged by trauma, deep venous thrombosis, or inflammation. Prolonged standing and obesity make all leg varicosities more symptomatic. The basic pathophysiology and natural history of varicose veins are summarized in Chapter 2. A description of the initial lower-extremity venous examination is found in Chapter 4. This chapter focuses on the principles of medical and surgical therapy.

I. Clinical presentation. The most common complaints of patients with varicose veins are their unsightly appearance and aching or heaviness of the legs after prolonged standing. Symptoms may not correlate well with the degree of anatomic defect. Occasionally, a patient will abrade a varicosity, which may cause a rather impressive hemorrhage. A more common complication of varicose veins is superficial thrombophlebitis, which may cause considerable pain and disability but rarely leads to pulmonary embolism. Long-standing varicose veins may also result in chronic ankle induration, stasis dermatitis, and occasionally leg ulcerations.

A. For the **initial history,** patients should be asked specifically about prior leg trauma, bone fractures, phlebitis, and bleeding or ulceration of the varicosities. In addition, they should be asked about previous treatment, including vein stripping, injection therapy, and support stockings.

B. On **physical examination,** both legs should be inspected with the patient standing in good lighting. The varicosities (location and size) should be described in the medical record. The clinician should palpate for fascial defects that indicate sites of incompetent communicating veins with the deep venous system. The femoral triangle and the lower abdomen should be palpated to rule out any masses compressing the leg veins. The Trendelenburg test should be performed to determine whether the proximal greater saphenous vein and valves are incompetent and the primary source of venous reflux distending the varicosities. Of course, incompetence of the greater or lesser saphenous veins can be confirmed by Duplex ultrasound. Perforating veins can also be localized by ultrasound.

C. One unusual variant of varicose veins occurs with the **Klippel–Trenaunay syndrome,** which appears to be a fetal developmental abnormality. The result is maintenance of microscopic arteriovenous communications in the upper or lower limb. The classic clinical triad includes (a) hemangiomas, (b) hypertrophy of soft tissue and bone with overgrowth of the extremity, and (c) varicose veins. Because of the benign course of this disease, the majority of these patients do not have surgery and do well with conservative therapy. Occasionally, a more aggressive operative approach may be necessary in patients with large, symptomatic varicosities, especially if hemorrhage or ulceration has occurred.

II.   Medical treatment

A.   The majority of patients with varicose veins can be managed initially by nonoperative treatment. The patient should be instructed to **avoid (a) prolonged standing, (b) prolonged sitting, (c) obesity, and (d) constricting garments.** They also are instructed to do the following:

1. Shower or bathe in the evening.
2. Apply well-fitted, below-the-knees support stockings (20 to 30 mm Hg) before ambulating in the morning. Above-the-knee heavy support stockings generally are not necessary, since the majority of symptoms from varicose veins occur below the knee, where venous pressure is highest. Women with varicose veins may receive adequate support from a variety of high-quality sheer panty hose with graduated pressure from the ankle to waist. Several companies that specialize in venous hosiery currently offer such panty hose [e.g., Sigvaris (Ganzoni and Cie, AG, St. Gallen, Switzerland), Jobst (Beiersdorf–Jobst Inc., Charlotte, NC, U.S.A.), and Medi (Medi USA Inc., Whitsett, NC, U.S.A)].
3. Elevate the feet and legs for 10 to 15 minutes whenever possible.
4. Walk to improve the musculovenous pump of the calf.
5. Avoid trauma to varicose veins.

These simple measures will alleviate the heavy, aching leg feelings that bother most patients with varicose veins.

B.   Sclerotherapy is the injection of a sclerosing agent into the varicose vein to damage its endothelium and thus cause an aseptic thrombosis, which organizes and closes the vein. We use sclerotherapy as primary treatment for less extensive varicose veins and spider vein clusters. In contrast, sclerotherapy is not durable treatment for large (8 to 12 mm) varicosities that cascade down the entire lower extremity from a completely incompetent greater saphenous vein. The reaction from sclerotherapy may make subsequent surgical stripping of large varicosities more difficult. Sclerotherapy probably is also useful to obliterate small residual varicosities that persist after great saphenous stripping and ligation of perforating veins. Over a long follow-up period, surgery improves or cures about 80% of patients with varicose veins, while injection therapy succeeds in one-third of patients followed for 5 years.

The essentials of safe and effective sclerotherapy are as follows:

1.   Veins that should **not be injected** include those in the lower one-third of the leg and ankle, particularly those arising from incompetent ankle perforators; veins on the foot; veins in fat legs where perivenous reactions may cause painful fat necrosis; and veins in the areas of postphlebitic stasis dermatitis.

2. No more than 0.5 mL of the sclerosant (sodium tetra-decyl sulfate 3%, hypertonic saline, or morrhuate sodium) should be used in any one injection site. A small-gauge (size 25, 26, or 30) needle is used to inject four to six locations at one injection session.

3. The injection is done while the patient is reclining, not standing. The sclerosant is retained in the vein segment by compressing it above and below the injection site for about 1 minute. The injection is stopped if the patient complains of severe local pain, since this suggests extravasation of the sclerosant outside the vein.

4. A compressive elastic bandage is applied and the patient is actively ambulated immediately. This ambulation helps the musculovenous pump of the calf wash out any sclerosant that may have leaked into the deep venous system. The exact time the compressive bandage remains in place is variable, but usually 1 week is sufficient for an average injection in the small vein.

III. Surgical treatment. Varicose veins of the great and small saphenous systems can be cured by proper stripping and ligation of incompetent communicating veins.

A. Indications for operation. The best surgical candidates are active, healthy patients who are not overweight. Severe aching varicosities, varicose vein hemorrhage, or superficial thrombophlebitis are indications for operation. Some patients simply desire removal of the varicose veins for cosmetic reasons. Occasionally, primary varicose veins lead to leg ulcers.

B. Preoperative preparation. The area of skin preparation includes the groin as well as the lower extremity. Before operation, the varicose veins are marked with an indelible felt-tipped pen or other nontoxic dye while the patient stands. The sites of suspected perforators are marked with an X. The surgeon or surgeon's assistant should do this marking and be sure that the patient agrees with the veins to be removed. The best time for marking is immediately before operation. After being marked, the patient should wear pajama pants or have a sheet placed between the lower extremities to prevent ink marks rubbing off onto the opposite leg. Unless the patient has had a history of thrombophlebitis, prophylactic low-dose heparin is not used.

C. Operative technique. Several technical features of vari-cose vein surgery deserve emphasis. The operation is, in part, a cosmetic procedure; therefore, skin incisions should be small (0.5 to 1 cm). The stab-avulsion technique has become popular, but the surgeon must be certain that the varicosity is removed completely. It is easy with this technique to miss significant seg-ments of varicosities if one does not understand the technique

The next controversy is whether to strip the entire greater saphenous vein or only the portion in the thigh. This decision depends on whether the below-knee greater saphenous vein is varicose. If it is, we prefer to strip the vein from the groin to the ankle. If one does this stripping properly, injury to the saphenous nerve is unlikely. At the ankle, the great saphenous vein should be exposed medially and slightly inferior to the medial malleolus, so that the branches extending onto the foot

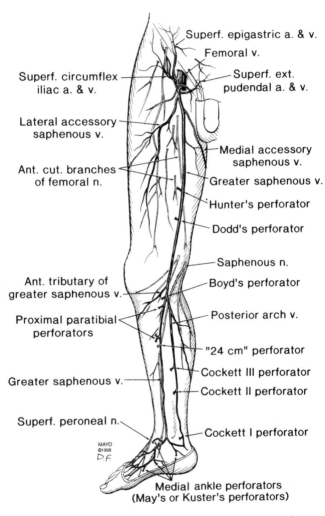

Figure 20.1.   Anatomy of the greater saphenous veins and perforators. The enlarged vein of the saphenofemoral region demonstrates the major proximal branches of the saphenous vein, which should be ligated and divided during ligation and stripping of the great saphenous veins.

can be ligated accurately or removed. Each tributary at the proximal saphenofemoral junction (usually five or six) should be ligated carefully. A meticulous search must be made for accessory greater saphenous veins, which are not uncommon. Perforators are ligated at the fascial level (Fig. 20.1). Finally, skin incisions are closed with fine, interrupted sutures (e.g., 4-0 nylon). Some surgeons prefer interrupted adsorbable subcuticular sutures. Steri-Strips may be applied to complete this plastic closure following the stab-avulsion technique. Compressive gauze bandages are applied with an elastic wrap from the toes to the groin.

Some surgeons strip only the evident varicose veins and preserve the greater saphenous trunk. This approach is reasonable if the greater saphenous vein is competent. Competency should be confirmed by preoperative Duplex ultrasound if one selects to leave the greater saphenous trunk intact. However, most patients with large, symptomatic lower-limb varicose veins have a diffusely incompetent greater saphenous vein from the groin to the leg.

D. Postoperative care. At the surgeon's discretion, the patient is discharged on the day of operation or the next morning, depending on the extent of groin and lower-limb dissection and early postoperative pain. Most simple vein surgery is currently outpatient. For the first postoperative night, the patient is kept on bed rest with the operated leg elevated. The next morning, the dressings are removed and a new below-the-knee elastic bandage is applied. The patient should ambulate every 2 hours for 5 to 10 minutes, beginning on the first postoperative day.

In general, these patients do not have much postoperative pain. Below-the-knee elastic support is continued until the patient is rechecked in the office in 1 week. For some patients, this support is continued for several more weeks to alleviate mild leg swelling and dependent heaviness that may follow lower-extremity venous surgery.

SELECTED READING

Bergan JJ. New developments in the surgical treatment of venous disease. *Cardiovasc Surg* 1993;1:624–631.

Dwerryhouse S, Davies B, Harradine K, et al. Stripping the long saphenous vein reduces the rate of reoperation for recurrent varicose veins: five-year results of a randomized trial. *J Vasc Surg* 1999;29:589–592.

Evans CJ, Allan PL, Lee AJ, et al. Prevalence of venous reflux in the general population on duplex scanning: the Edinburgh vein study. *J Vasc Surg* 1998;28:767–776.

Gloviczki P, Yao JST, eds. *Handbook of venous disorders.* New York: Chapman and Hall, 1996.

Jacob AG, Driscoll DJ, Shaughnessy WJ, et al. Klippel–Trenaunay syndrom: spectrum and managment. *Mayo Clin Proc* 1998;73: 28–36.

Jiang P, van Rij AM, Christie R, et al. Recurrent varicose veins: patterns of reflux and clinical severity. *Cardiovasc Surg* 1999;7: 332–339.

Labropoulos N, Mansour MA, Kang SS, et al. New insights into perforator vein incompetence. *Eur J Vasc Endovasc Surg* 1999;18: 228–234.

Noel AA, Gloviczki P, Cherry KJ, et al. Surgical treatment of venous malformations in Klippel–Trenaunay syndrome. *J Vasc Surg* 2000; 32:840–847.

Samson RH, Yunis JP, Showalter DP. Is thigh saphenectomy a necessary adjunct to high ligation and stab avulsion phlebectomy? *Am J Surg* 1998;176:168–171.

Wakefield TW, Greenfield LJ. Venous physiology and disorders of the superficial and deep veins. In: Greenfield LJ, ed. *Surgery: scientific principles and practice*, 2nd ed. Philadelphia: Lippincott–Raven Publishers, 1997:1935–1944.

Venous Thromboembolism

The current clinical approach to venous thromboembolism is remarkable for recent progress in prevention, diagnosis, and treatment. A better understanding of the pathophysiology of acute deep venous thrombosis (DVT) and pulmonary embolism (PE) has resulted in more aggressive preventive measures. The limitations of the physical examination in accurate diagnosis of venous thromboembolism have culminated in the development of noninvasive methods to detect DVT and document PE. Finally, clinical trials continue to define optimal treatment regimens. The details of prevention, diagnosis, and treatment are still debated. However, certain principles of care are generally accepted. These fundamental concepts are the focus of this chapter.

I. Prevention. Several prophylactic measures may decrease the incidence of venous thromboembolism, especially in sick patients at bed rest. These preventive measures may be organized conveniently around Virchow's etiologic triad for venous thrombosis: stasis, hypercoagulability, and vein injury.

A. Stasis. Prolonged immobilization of the lower extremities is perhaps the single most important event that precedes acute DVT. At bed rest, blood tends to pool in large, valveless venous sinuses of the calf muscles. The soleus venous plexus normally drains anteriorly into the tibial veins. Consequently, if the body is supine, blood pools in the calf muscles unless these muscles contract to empty the calf veins. ^{125}I-labeled fibrinogen studies show that calf vein thrombosis often begins while the patient is supine on the operating table.

Venous stasis in the calf may be prevented by elevation and intermittent or continuous mechanical compression of the leg. Simply elevating the leg 15 to 20 degrees improves emptying of major leg veins but may not completely empty the soleus venous sinuses. Likewise, graduated compression stockings may hasten flow in the tibial veins but not completely empty the soleus plexus, where clots often begin. Generally we do not use them in patients with arterial occlusive disease since the compression may worsen ischemic skin. Several studies have confirmed that intermittent pneumatic leg compression reduces postoperative DVT, especially in urologic and neurosurgical patients. Although effective, pneumatic boots are somewhat cumbersome and expensive. Finally, one of the simplest, yet most effective, methods of preventing calf vein stasis is to have the patient exercise the legs (plantar flexion) against a footboard for 5 minutes every hour. This exercise not only promotes venous flow but actually may enhance fibrinolytic activity, which clears small clots.

We generally take the following approach to mechanical prevention of venous stasis in patients undergoing major vascular operations. At the time of operation, the operating table is placed at 15 degrees of the Trendelenburg position to hasten deep venous emptying. After surgery, patients do footboard exercises for at least 5 minutes every waking hour and are encouraged to exercise more frequently if they can. Some physicians question whether patients will comply with this exercise program; we have found that patients will exercise regularly when the importance of these exercises is explained to them and encouragement is given after the operation. These calf exercises also help maintain muscle tone when several days of bed rest are necessary. We do not routinely use elastic antiphlebitic hose, pneumatic compressive boots, or low-dose heparin for patients who undergo vascular procedures. However, patients at higher risk for thromboembolism generally receive pneumatic compression devices on the lower extremities and/or some type of anticoagulant therapy, either with low-dose heparin or warfarin sodium (Coumadin).

B.   Hypercoagulability. Acute DVT is more likely to occur in patients with some abnormality of coagulation. Low levels of antithrombin III have been found in women taking oral contraceptives. Antithrombin III activity also diminishes with soft-tissue trauma and operative wounding. Increased platelet adhesiveness may be another problem that predisposes certain patients to recurrent DVT. Recurrent venous thromboembolism has also been correlated with congenital deficiencies of protein C and protein S, the presence of antiphospholipid antibodies (e.g., lupus anticoagulant and anticardiolipin antibodies), a single point mutation in factor V Leiden causing activated protein C resistance, and abnormal levels of fibrinogen and plasminogen. These findings of hypercoagulability support anticoagulation as another method of preventing DVT, especially when thromboembolism is most likely to complicate patient recovery.

Certain patients are at increased risk of DVT and PE. They usually are referred to as **high-risk patients** and include those who have experienced (a) previous venous thromboembolism; (b) lower-extremity trauma (e.g., hip fracture) and other orthopedic surgery of the hip, knee, or lower limb; (c) major pelvic operations (e.g., open prostatectomy or gynecologic operations); (d) prolonged bed rest or extremity immobility (e.g., stroke or back surgery); (e) acute myocardial infarction; (f) chronic congestive heart failure; and (g) malignancies (e.g., pancreatic cancer), as well as those on oral contraceptives. Prophylactic anticoagulation does offer these patients significant protection against venous thromboembolism. Several anticoagulative agents are available: low-molecular-weight (LMW) heparin, low-dose heparin, warfarin, dextrans, and antiplatelet drugs. Of course, a major hazard of anticoagulant therapy in surgical patients is bleeding, but major bleeding complications are rare if therapy is properly delivered and monitored and certain contraindications are observed. These contraindications include an active peptic ulcer, intracranial or visceral injury, hemorrhagic diathesis, gastrointestinal bleeding, severe hypertension, and gross hematuria or hemoptysis.

1.   Adjusted-dose warfarin can be an effective prophylaxis for thromboembolism. However, there is not widespread acceptance of warfarin for prophylaxis. The dosage may be difficult to regulate and an excessively prolonged prothrombin time (PT) is associated with increased bleeding complications. Still, we have found adjusted-dose warfarin to be effective and safe when PT is maintained at an international normalized ratio (INR) between 2.0 and 2.7.

To standardize the PT for oral anticoagulation, the World Health Organization (WHO) has developed an international reference thromboplastin from human brain tissue and has recommended that the PT be expressed as the INR. With the past conventional use of rabbit brain thromboplastin reagents, a PT ratio of 1.3 to 1.5 (16 to 20 seconds) corresponds to an INR of 2.0 to 3.0. Recent clinical trials support less intense oral warfarin therapy (INR of 2.0 to 3.0) for most clinical conditions.

Generally, warfarin anticoagulation should be reserved for patients with hip fractures, major hip surgery, open prostatectomy, and major gynecologic pelvic procedures. Low-dose heparin has not been uniformly effective in this group of high-risk patients. Patients who are chronic users of warfarin for prosthetic heart valves or who have had a past thromboembolism may remain on warfarin during other major operations, provided the PT or INR is adjusted to lower levels. Another alternative in such patients is discontinuance of warfarin and coverage with low-dose heparin (5,000 units q8h) during the perioperative period.

2. Low-dose unfractionated heparin has received widespread attention for its use in the prevention of fatal postoperative PE. A metaanalysis of 78 randomized trials with over 15,000 patients confirms its benefit. Compared to those who receive no prophylaxis, heparin-treated patients experience a 40% reduction in nonfatal and a 64% reduction in fatal PE. The usual dosage schedule has been a loading dose of 5,000 units given subcutaneously 2 hours before operation and then 5,000 units every 8 to 12 hours until the patient is fully ambulatory. This low-dose heparin enhances antithrombin III activity with minimal to no change in coagulation tests. However, bleeding and wound complications may be more common in patients on low-dose heparin, although the absolute excess in bleeding is only about 2% to 3%. Therefore, the use of low dose heparin probably should be reserved for those individuals at increased risk of thromboembolism, including patients with prior venous thromboembolism, those immobilized for long periods, and those subjected to major procedures involving extensive extremity or pelvic dissection or soft-tissue trauma.

3. LMW heparins have three potential advantages over unfractionated heparin: (a) effective prophylaxis with once-daily administration, (b) improved efficacy, and (c) a lower frequency of bleeding. The LMW heparins have higher bioavailability and extended half-life compared to unfractionated heparin. Several randomized clinical trials have demonstrated that LMW heparin is as effective and as safe as unfractionated heparin in the management of proximal DVT. In addition, it does not require monitoring or dose adjustment. A metaanalysis of the literature from has concluded that the relative risk of DVT with LMW heparin compared with standard heparin was 0.74, the risk of PE was 0.43, and the risk of major bleeding was essentially the same (0.98).

4. Dextrans and antiplatelet drugs appear to have some merit in thromboembolism prophylaxis, but the data are equivocal. **Low-molecular-weight dextran** (LMD) is a glucose polymer that impairs platelet function by causing decreased platelet aggregability. An effective dosage regimen for LMD is 500 mL of a 10% solution started as a 100-mL i.v. bolus in the operating room and continued at 20 mL/h until the patient is ambulatory. Bleeding complications of dextran therapy are similar to those of oral anticoagulants. Other potential problems include volume overload in patients with heart failure, allergic reactions, and renal tubular damage. Dextran also is more expensive than other anticoagulative agents. Its role in prophylaxis may be in treating patients who cannot receive heparin because of heparin-associated thrombocytopenia.

5. **Aspirin** inhibits platelet function and has proved effective only for males in thromboembolism prophylaxis after total hip replacement. The final place of aspirin in prophylactic therapy for other patients remains to be established. **Dipyridamole** appears to be ineffective in preventing venous thromboembolism. However, neither of these agents is currently a firstline choice in patients at high risk of venous thromboembolism.

6. Many questions about the **optimum methods of thromboembolism prophylaxis** remain unanswered. In our practice, we continue to limit warfarin or low-dose heparin prophylaxis ± pneumatic compression devices to high-risk patients. Other patients receive simple mechanical prophylaxis with leg elevation and footboard exercises. This approach has resulted in a low (1% to 2%) incidence of clinically apparent and significant venous thromboembolism in patients hospitalized with peripheral arterial or venous disease.

  C. **Vein injury.** During elective operations, meticulous attention must be given to the gentle dissection and handling of veins. Large-vein injuries should be repaired by fine lateral suture technique, and ligation should be avoided. The surgeon also must avoid prolonged compression of the vena cava or other large veins with retractors or packs. Experimental studies have also documented endothelial tears that occur in extremity veins remote from an elective operative site. These endothelial lesions may become the focus of DVT.

  II. Diagnosis. Patient history and physical examination frequently are unreliable in establishing an accurate diagnosis of either acute DVT or PE. In fact, about 75% of patients who are evaluated for suspected venous thrombosis or PE do not have these conditions. Since either condition requires systemic anticoagulation, with its potential complications, we recommend the following approach to ensure that an accurate diagnosis is established.

  A. **Superficial thrombophlebitis** generally is recognized by the physical findings of a tender superficial venous cord. Usually, there is no deep vein involvement. If the process extends to the groin, extension into the deep femoral system may be present. Duplex ultrasound is the best method to ascertain thrombotic involvement of the common femoral vein.

  B. **Deep venous thrombosis** is suggested by leg pain, swelling, and tenderness. Since these findings are not specific for venous thrombosis, treatment generally should not be started without further noninvasive studies or a venogram to confirm the diagnosis. If the patient has had no previous DVT, our initial diagnostic test is a duplex ultrasound examination in high-risk patients or venous plethysmography in low-risk patients (see Chap. 5). Compression ultrasonography is highly sensitive (sensitivity, >90%) for detecting proximal femoropopliteal vein thrombosis but is less sensitive (approximately 50%) for detecting calf-vein thrombosis.

Noninvasive studies, however, have definite limitations, especially in the pelvic veins, below the knee, and in the profunda femoris vein. Also, Doppler examination may be difficult to interpret if the patient has had previous DVT that has not recanalized. If the results of noninvasive tests are normal, other etiologies for the leg symptoms are investigated. Venography is reserved for patients with equivocal noninvasive results and an elevated clinical suspicion of DVT. Most experts now agree that positive noninvasive studies without a venogram are sufficient evidence to begin therapy in most patients.

C. Pulmonary embolism may present with chest pain, dyspnea, and occasionally hemoptysis. The source of the emboli is nearly always the leg or pelvic veins. Similar symptoms may occur with myocardial ischemia, bronchitis, pneumonia, or pleurisy, so PE must be confirmed by other tests.

1. Although hypoxia demonstrated on **arterial blood gas testing** is common with PE, a low arterial Po_2 is not diagnostic. Other laboratory tests may be abnormal but often are inconclusive also. Electrocardiographic abnormalities may include a rhythm disturbance and ST segment depression or T wave inversion, particularly in leads III, aVF, V1, V4, and V5. These findings are indicative of myocardial ischemia associated with acute PE. The electrocardiogram (ECG) can also rule out an acute myocardial infarction as the cause of chest pain. The chest radiograph may look normal. In seriously ill patients, the radiograph may show infiltrates from pneumonitis or atelectasis.

2. Plasma markers (D-Dimer test) can be used to supplement other tests. A normal plasma D-dimer, a fibrin-specific product, and a negative anatomic test for DVT or PE generally rule out significant thromboembolism.

3. Radioisotope lung perfusion scanning has become the primary screening test for PE. False-positive tests, however, may occur in many patients due to preexisting lung pathology such as asthma, emphysema, chronic bronchitis, pneumonitis, or neoplasm. Consequently, the chest radiograph should be checked before a lung scan to identify any disease process that may affect the scan. **In properly performed and interpreted scans, normal results essentially exclude a significant pulmonary embolus.** High-probability scans predict the presence of PE in about 90% of patients. If other alternative diagnoses appear unlikely, a positive ventilation–perfusion scan with a large V/Q mismatch or multiple moderate areas of V/Q mismatch is definitive. In cases of intermediate probability of PE, we recommend a rapid computed tomography (CT) chest scan or a pulmonary angiogram. In our recent experience, about 30% of patients can be treated after a lung scan alone, while the remainder need a CT scan or a pulmonary angiogram for definitive diagnosis and treatment.

4.   Pulmonary arteriography remains the definitive diagnostic test for pulmonary thromboembolism if lung scanning or rapid CT scan cannot define the diagnosis. One must remember that most pulmonary emboli resolve in days to several weeks, and consequently, a pulmonary arteriogram may look normal after a while.

D.   Recurrent pulmonary embolism from lower-extremity clots that occur while the patient is on adequate anticoagulation is indication for a vena cava filter. In addition, we consider a vena cava filter in patients with a documented extensive iliofemoral thrombosis or PE who cannot be safely anticoagulated (e.g., because of a recent brain tumor resection). Candidates for a vena cava filter usually have a rapid chest CT scan or a pulmonary arteriogram to establish the diagnosis and a venacavogram to define the anatomy. The surgeon and interventional radiologist must know whether the patient has any major vena cava anomalies and where the renal veins are located before attempting placement of a filter.

E.   Subclavian–axillary venous thrombosis is usually associated with thoracic outlet syndrome or central venous catheters. Acute diffuse upper limb swelling and a tight discomfort or pain are the most common manifestations. Thrombolytic drugs can recanalize the vein and quickly alleviate symptoms. Of course, definitive treatment requires surgical correction of the thoracic outlet compression. To prevent propagation of clot into the superior vena cava or retrograde into the arm, we favor removing all central venous lines that precipitate thrombosis. Anticoagulation with heparin is continued until acute symptoms resolve. Most patients are continued on coumarin anticoagulants for 2 to 3 months while the veins have a chance to recanalize and heal. Thoracic outlet surgical decompression is usually delayed for 2 to 3 months, although some surgeons favor early first rib resection. This delayed period of time generally allows the subclavian vein to recanalize in some patients and is associated with maximum development of collateral venous pathways that reduce edema.

III.   Treatment. In Chapter 2, we emphasize that the natural history of DVT and PE may be altered by anticoagulation. In certain situations, surgical intervention also may help the patient. Thrombolytic therapy has also added another important alternative to managing serious DVT and PE.

A.   Treatment of **superficial thrombophlebitis** depends on the extent of the phlebitis and the general health of the patient. Elastic support, local heat, and an antiinflammatory medication (e.g., aspirin or a nonsteroidal antiinflammatory agent) may relieve localized superficial phlebitis. Resolution may take 7 to 14 days. If the phlebitis involves most of the greater saphenous vein and the leg is swollen, rest and elevation may hasten recovery. Anticoagulation is reserved for patients in whom deep venous thrombophlebitis is documented or in whom the phlebitis extends to the saphenofemoral junction and deep venous extension seems likely. If the thrombophlebitis is confined to superficial veins and the patient is a good operative risk, excision of the thrombosed vein and ligation and stripping of the greater saphenous vein may be curative and may shorten the time of disability.

B. For **established DVT,** the patient is systemically heparinized with an intravenous bolus of 5,000 to 10,000 units, followed by a continuous infusion of 1,000 to 1,500 units/h.

1. Continuous heparin infusion has been associated with fewer bleeding complications than has intermittent intravenous therapy. A solution sufficient for 6 to 8 hours of therapy should be used to avoid accidental heparin overdose. Ideally, continuous heparin therapy should be administered by an infusion pump. Although the ideal method of monitoring heparin therapy is debatable, an activated partial thromboplastin time test (APTT) is the standard in most hospitals. Anticoagulation is considered adequate when these test values are at least 1.5 to 2.0 times the pretreatment values. There is a common misconception that an APTT greater than twice normal (usually >100 seconds) is associated with more bleeding complications. On the contrary, clinical trials demonstrate a lack of association between a supratherapeutic APTT (ratio of 2.5 or greater) and the risk of clinically important hemorrhage. Platelet counts should also be checked at least every other day, since heparin may induce thrombocytopenia, intravascular thrombosis, or hemorrhage. Heparin-induced thrombocytopenia generally is recognized at least 3 days after onset of therapy, appears more commonly in patients with prior heparin therapy, and may be reversed by stopping heparin. **Recent clinical trials indicate that the length of heparin therapy can be shortened to 5 days without loss of effectiveness or safety if oral anticoagulants are started on the first or second day of treatment for DVT or PE.**

2. Oral anticoagulants are started during heparin therapy and are continued for 3 to 6 months. During this period, the deep veins usually recanalize slowly. Since warfarin inhibits blood clotting by interference with liver synthesis of vitamin K–dependent clotting factors (II, VII, IX, X), adequate anticoagulation with oral agents requires several days of therapy. The appropriate dosages of the common anticoagulants are provided in Table 21.1. The safest method of instituting warfarin therapy is the nonloading technique, giving 10 to 15 mg orally each day until prothrombin time is in the therapeutic range. An INR of 2.0 to 3.0 is therapeutic. A more prolonged INR places the patient at increased risk of bleeding complications. Such doses are just as effective and less likely to cause bleeding complications than maintaining a higher dosage.

The target INR for warfarin should be **at least 2.0 to 3.0** for at least two days before stopping the heparin. When oral anticoagulation is started, the level of protein C falls quickly and may result in a thrombogenic potential. **To avoid this coagulation potential, one should give heparin for at least four days and not discontinue it until the INR has been in the therapeutic range for two consecutive days.**

Table 21.1. Anticoagulants used for thrombotic prophylaxis and disorders

Tradename	Generic	DVT prophylaxis	Treatment for acute DVT
Unfractionated heparin			
—	Heparin sulfate	2,500–5,000 U s.c. twice daily	40–80 U/kg i.v. bolus and 2–18 U/kg/h i.v. infusion
Low-molecular-weight heparins			
Fragmin (Pharmacia & Upjohn Co., Bridgewater, NJ)	Dalteparin	2,500–5,000 U (60–120 mg) s.c. before surgery then daily	120 U/kg s.c. q 12 h for 5 days
Lovenox (Rhône-Poulenc Rorer, Collegeville, PA)	Enoxaparin	30 mg s.c. q 12 h	1 mg/kg s.c. q 12 h
Normiflo (Wyeth-Ayerst, Philadelphia, PA)	Ardeparin	50 U/kg s.c. q 12 h	130 U/kg s.c. q 12 h
Orgaran[a] (Organon Inc., West Orange, NJ)	Danaparoid	750 U q 12 h s.c. with first dose 1–4 h before surgery. Postsurgery dose no sooner than 2 h after surgery.	—
Thrombin inhibitor			
Lepirudin[a] (Hoechst Marion Roussel, Kansas City, MO)	Hirudin	—	0.75 mg/kg subcutaneously twice daily × 5–7 days[a]
Antifibrin compound Arvin[a] (Knoll Pharmaceuticals, Mount Olive, NJ)	Ancrod	4 U/kg s.c. followed by 1 U/kg s.c. daily for 4 days	1 U/kg in 250 or 2 U/kg in 500 mL normal saline or D5W infused over 12 h. Maintenance 0.5 U/kg in 250 or 1 U/kg in 500 mL infused over 24 h

[a] In setting of heparin-induced thrombocytopenia and thrombobis (HITT) or DVT.
From Schiele F, Vuillemenot A, Krammarz P, et al. A pilot study of subcutaneous recombinant Hirudin (HBW023) in the treatment of deep venous thrombosis. *Thromb Haemost* 1994;71:558–562, with permission.

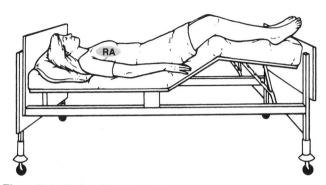

Figure 21.1.   Bed position for patients with lower-extremity venous thromboembolism. RA, right atrium.

Oral anticoagulation is usually continued for **at least 3 to 6 months.** It may be continued longer or indefinitely in patients with underlying risk factors for venous thromboembolism. For patients who cannot take warfarin (e.g., pregnant women), adjusted-dose heparin is an alternative. A subcutaneous dose of heparin is administered twice a day to maintain a prolonged APTT, which is initially regulated by measuring the APTT just prior to the next dose.

3.   Leg pain and swelling may be alleviated by bed rest, leg elevation, local heat, and analgesics. Figure 21.1 illustrates the proper bed position. Bed rest not only alleviates leg pain and edema but also allows the thrombus to organize and adhere to the vessel wall, a process that generally requires 24 to 72 hours. Bed rest is continued until leg swelling and tenderness resolve. For calf thrombosis, this usually takes 3 to 5 days. For iliofemoral thrombosis, 5 to 7 days may be required. When ambulation is begun, we have the patient use a below-the-knee elastic support (30 to 40 mm Hg) to reduce pain and swelling. This elastic support is continued for a minimum of 2 to 3 months. If the thrombosis involved the popliteal and femoral veins, we recommend that the patient wear lifelong 30 to 40 mm Hg below-the-knee compression hose to alleviate postphlebitic syndrome.

4.   The role of **thrombolytic therapy** in acute DVT is still debated despite clinical trials advocating it for proximal DVT of less than 72 hours in duration. Complete lysis of iliofemoral thrombosis with maintenance of value integrity has been accomplished with combined thrombolytic agents and heparin therapy. Thrombolytic therapy also may offer improved results in patients with extensive iliofemoral thrombosis and cutaneous gangrene (phlegmasia cerulea dolens). Thrombolytic therapy is expensive and may be associated with major bleeding complications or allergic reactions. It is contraindicated in patients with active internal bleeding and recent (within 2 months) cerebrovascular accidents or other active intracranial disease. It also may cause serious hemorrhage after recent (within about 10 days) major surgery, obstetric delivery, organ biopsy, and previous puncture of a noncompressible vessel. Therefore, thrombolytic therapy must be used only by physicians who are completely familiar with its dosage and contraindications and in a setting in which therapy can be continuously monitored (see Chap. 6).

5. Surgical therapy of acute DVT has had less than spectacular results over the years. Late evaluation indicates that one-third of patients undergoing iliofemoral venous thrombectomy have good to excellent results, another one-third are improved, and one-third are not changed by operation. However, more recent experience with venous thrombectomy with a temporary arteriovenous fistula demonstrated that less than 10% of anticoagulated patients with iliofemoral venous thrombosis were completely free of postthrombotic symptoms compared to 40% to 45% of operated patients. Late venography has shown a 60% to 65% patency rate. Venous thrombectomy plus temporary arteriovenous fistula may be recommended for young patients with acute iliofemoral venous thrombosis to avoid development of incapacitating postphlebitic syndrome. In our experience, however, the role of venous thrombectomy for acute DVT remains very limited.

C. Pulmonary embolism (Table 21.2) also requires systemic heparinization followed by long-term oral anticoagula-

Table 21.2. Classification of pulmonary thromboembolism

Class	Signs	Pulmonary artery occlusion (%)	Pulmonary pressure (mm Hg)	Management
I	None	<20	Normal	Anticoagulation
II	Tachypnea	20–30	<20	Anticoagulation
III	Collapse, hypoxemia	30–50	>20	Anticoagulation, thrombolytic therapy, vena cava filter
IV	Shock, hypoxemia	>50	>25–30	Pulmonary catheter embolectomy, vena cava filter
V	Cor pulmonale	>50	>40	Anticoagulation, vena cava filter

Adapted from Greenfield LJ. Pulmonary embolectomy and vena caval interruption. In: Bergan JJ, Yao JST, eds. *Vascular surgical emergencies*. Orlando: Grune and Stratton, 1987:453–460.

tion. The dosages, methods of administration, and duration of therapy are the same as those used for acute DVT (Table 21.1). Heparin and warfarin are intended to prevent further thromboembolism or clot propagation in the lung. They do little to resolve an existing thrombus. In contrast, thrombolytic therapy appears to allow more complete resolution of thromboemboli than do heparin and oral anticoagulants. Thrombolytic therapy also appears to improve capillary perfusion and diffusion, which may decrease the incidence of late pulmonary hypertension. Emergency pulmonary embolectomy, either by percutaneous suction catheter or surgery, is indicated for salvageable patients who have documented massive PE and persistent refractory hypotension despite maximum medical therapy. Chronic pulmonary embolectomy also may improve chronic hypoxia and respiratory disability in selected patients with recurrent PE and chronic organized pulmonary thrombi.

D. Recurrent pulmonary embolism after adequate anticoagulation or in situation where anticoagulation is contraindicated generally is considered an indication for a vena cava filter. Contraindications usually include gastrointestinal hemorrhage, recent stroke or neurosurgery, or hemorrhage requiring transfusion after anticoagulation was started. It must be remembered that small pulmonary emboli may continue during anticoagulation as lower-extremity or pelvic vein thrombi lyse. Such small emboli may go unrecognized or cause minimal physiologic problems and consequently would not be considered adequate indications for vena cava interruption.

Vena cava filtering prevents further PE in at least 90% of patients. Approximately 25% of patients who have a vena cava filter will develop chronic leg swelling. Vena cava filtering may be accomplished by a variety of percutaneously placed devices. Operative caval clipping or ligation is performed rarely anymore. Although the Greenfield filter has been the primary choice in recent years, other filters are available and applicable to most patients. All of them can be placed percutaneously via the jugular or femoral vein. A venous cutdown is seldom necessary anymore. We recommend that, before vena cava filtering is attempted, a rapid chest CT scan or a pulmonary arteriogram be done to document embolism and an inferior venacavogram be done to delineate the level of the renal veins and any anomalous venous patterns, such as a double vena cava.

Vena cava filters and associated caval thrombosis may cause acute leg swelling. Bed rest and leg elevation usually is helpful after the procedure. When ambulation resumes, below-the-knee elastic support hose (30 to 40 mm Hg) should be worn to prevent postphlebitic syndrome. A few patients will have edema to their groins and may be more comfortable with full-length pantyhose-type elastic support hose. If anticoagulation can be continued, it appears to improve the postphlebitic syndrome in about 80% of patients compared to only 50% of patients who have anticoagulation discontinued after filter placement.

SELECTED READING

Alastair JJ, Wood MD. Management of venous thromboembolism. *N Engl J Med* 1996;335:1816–1827.

Goldhaber SZ. Pulmonary embolism. *N Engl J Med* 1998;339:93–104.

Lofgren EP, Lofgren KA. The surgical treatment of superficial thrombophlebitis. *Surgery* 1981;90:49–54.

Plate G, Einarsson E, Ohlin P, et al. Thrombectomy with temporary arteriovenous fistula: the treatment of choice in acute iliofemoral venous thrombosis. *J Vasc Surg* 1984;1:867–876.

Schulman S, Granqvist S. The duration of oral anticoagulant therapy after a second episode of venous thromboembolism. *N Engl J Med* 1997;336:393–398.

Toglia MR, Weg JG. Venous thromboembolism during pregnancy. *N Engl J Med* 1996;335:108–114.

Wakefield TW. Treatment options for venous thrombosis. *J Vasc Surg* 2000;31:613–620.

Postphlebitic Syndrome and Chronic Venous Insufficiency

Most patients who have had femoropopliteal deep vein thrombosis will develop some degree of postphlebitic syndrome. However, in 20% to 50% of patients with symptoms and signs of chronic venous insufficiency, no history of deep venous thrombosis (DVT) is obtainable. The classic physical findings are a chronically indurated ankle, dark stasis pigmentation around the ankle, and skin ulceration in some patients. Postphlebitic syndrome or primary deep valvular incompetence can be especially disabling for active ambulatory workers, since leg dependency increases pain and swelling and impedes ulcer healing. Fortunately, proper elastic leg support, skin care, and, in some situations, surgery can alleviate chronic venous insufficiency enough that patients can remain comfortable and active.

Management of postphlebitic syndrome is based on our present understanding of its pathophysiology (see Chap. 2). Thrombophlebitis damages deep venous valves and often leaves them incompetent. The musculovenous pump can no longer reduce ambulatory venous pressures. Consequently, the patient has chronic venous hypertension in the lower leg when he or she stands. These high venous pressures are transmitted through communicating veins from the deep to superficial venous system. The exact means by which this chronic venous hypertension causes stasis skin changes and ulceration is still unclear. The most recent evidence suggests that local capillaries leak fibrinous protein that is not adequately removed by fibrinolysis. A liposclerosis occurs and local tissue oxygen diffusion may be impeded. The result is tissue necrosis and skin ulceration. **Skin ulceration seldom occurs unless the popliteal vein valves are incompetent.**

In patients with chronic iliofemoral venous obstruction, venous capacitance is increased at rest and cannot compensate during exercise. The result is severe thigh pain and sensation of tightness with vigorous exercise **(venous claudication).** Symptoms are apparently more common in patients with chronic venous obstruction than in those who have recanalized veins with incompetent valves. A surprising observation is that 5 to 10 years after lower-extremity DVT, 80% of patients will have symptoms of chronic venous insufficiency regardless of the initial site of the thrombosis.

In l996, an international consensus group under the auspices of the American Venous Forum published a classification and grading of chronic venous disease of the lower limbs. This CEAP classification defines clinical class (C) and the etiology (E), its anatomic (A) distribution in the veins, and the pathologic mechanism (P) of development (reflux or obstruction or both). This methodology facilitates standard reporting of diagnosis and treatment protocols. Table 22.1 presents a common modification of this system for clinical terminology and communication.

Table 22.1.   Clinical classification of chronic venous disease

Class	Definition
0	No signs of venous disease
1	Telangiectases or reticular veins
2	Varicose veins
3	Lower limb edema
4	Venous stasis changes (e.g., pigmentation, venous eczema, lipodermatosclerosis)
5	Venous stasis changes with healed ulcer
6	Venous stasis changes with an active ulcer

Adapted from the Consensus Group classification and grading of chronic venous disease in the lower limbs. *Vasc Surg* 1996;30:5.

I.   **Prevention.** Proper elastic leg support can alleviate the symptoms of leg pain and swelling. In addition, skin ulceration is less likely to occur in patients who routinely wear elastic leg support. To be effective, elastic leg support must be combined with a program of leg elevation at intervals throughout the day and proper skin care.

A.   In postphlebitic syndrome, ambulatory ankle venous pressures seldom drop more than 20% to 30% during leg exercise. Normally, ankle venous pressures would drop about 70% with exercise. The greatest venous pressure is found at the ankle, where most postphlebitic changes occur. This chronic venous hypertension **cannot be corrected by elastic leg support.** However, elastic leg support can prevent some of the leg edema caused by the elevated venous pressures.

Experience has demonstrated that the leg support should provide at least 30 to 40 mm Hg pressure at the ankle to prevent postphlebitic edema. This amount of pressure can be provided by either an elastic bandage or an elastic support hose. Commonly used 30 to 40 mm Hg support hose are the Jobst graduated pressure hose, the Futuro elastic hosiery, and the Sigvaris graduated compression support. We generally recommend that the support hose be fitted below the knee and not carried above the popliteal space. There are several reasons for recommending below-the-knee support only. First, postphlebitic problems nearly always occur below the knee, where venous pressures are highest. Thigh swelling seldom is a problem after acute DVT has resolved. Second, support hose that comes above the knee often binds or constricts the popliteal space, especially if the hose slip down the leg. Third, patients generally do not like a heavy support hose that covers the entire leg. Many patients who are given full-length or pantyhose-type heavy support hose will wear them only when visiting their physician for a check-up. However, some patients with vena cava occlusion and severe leg swelling to the waist will need full-leg heavy support hose and will wear them without complaint.

Several suggestions should be offered to the patient to ensure the proper and comfortable use of heavy support hose. First, the hose should be put on immediately on arising in the morning. Otherwise, early leg swelling may begin before the elastic support can control it. This routine usually requires that the patient bathe or shower before going to bed at night. Second, because heavy hose may be difficult to slide on the leg, the patient may need a special stocking application device. A preferable method is to wear a knee-length light nylon hose beneath the heavy support sock. Some companies provide a silky slipper that can be removed after the heavy support hose is in place.

Elastic support hose must be properly fitted, or the patient will not wear them. We encourage patients to contact the fitting shop for adjustments if their new hose do not fit satisfactorily. We also periodically recheck patients in the outpatient clinic to ensure that their hose fit properly. In general, most heavy elastic support hose will need to be replaced every 6 to 12 months.

B. Leg elevation remains a simple and effective method of alleviating ankle edema. patients with postphlebitic syndrome should elevate their legs above the level of the heart for 10 to 15 minutes every 2 to 4 hours while they are ambulatory. This recommendation may seem impractical for the working individual. However, most workers are allowed several breaks during their normal work hours, when this elevation can be done. Periodic leg elevation allows most patients to remain comfortable during work. An explanatory note from the physician to the patient's employer often avoids any problem that the patient may encounter by periodically sitting down on the job.

C. Skin care is important if dermatitis, local infections, and ulcerations are to be prevented. Scaly pruritic skin of the foot or ankle may indicate fungal infection, which is managed by a topical fungicide such as Desenex (Pharmacraft, Pennwalt Corporation, Rochester, NY, U.S.A) or clotrimazole 1% solution (Lotrimin, Schering Corporation, Kenilworth, NY, U.S.A). Eczematous stasis dermatitis may be alleviated by a topical steroid cream, such as hydrocortisone cream 1%. Routine leg washing should be done with warm water and a mild soap. We discourage soaking the leg, since this may macerate friable skin and increase swelling due to dependency of the extremity.

D. Diagnostic evaluation. The anatomy and hemodynamics of the postphlebitic lower limb can be defined by descending venography, duplex scanning, Doppler signal analysis, and various types of plethysmography (see Chap. 5). For initial evaluation, we generally perform the Doppler analysis to assess valvular incompetency and impedance plethysmography to determine obstruction. Photoplethysmography is a good method to non-invasively examine ambulatory venous pressure and venous recovery time. Recently, duplex ultrasound has become an excellent method to image superficial and deep veins for both patency and reflux.

II. Venous ulcers classically occur on the medial side of the ankle at either the upper internal ankle perforator or the middle internal ankle perforator (Fig. 22.1). Less commonly, they occur on the lateral or posterior calf at the site of the lateral ankle perforator or the mid-posterior calf perforator (Fig. 22.1). In our experience, ulcers may also present adjacent to the medial malleolus.

The oldest, most widely used, and most successful method of healing venous ulcers is use of a compression bandage. This ban-

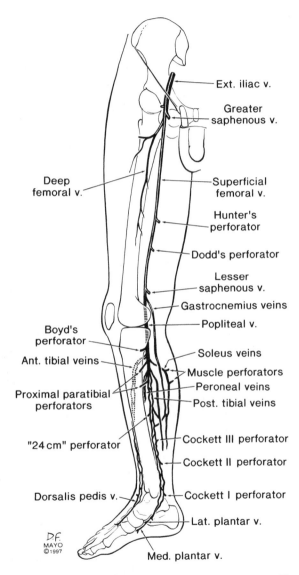

Ext. iliac v.

Greater
saphenous v.

Deep
femoral v.

Superficial
femoral v.

Hunter's
perforator

Dodd's perforator

Lesser
saphenous v.

Gastrocnemius veins

Popliteal v.

Boyd's
perforator

Ant. tibial veins

Soleus veins

Muscle perforators

Peroneal veins

Proximal paratibial
perforators

Post. tibial veins

"24 cm" perforator

Cockett III perforator

Cockett II perforator

Dorsalis pedis v.

Cockett I perforator

Lat. plantar v.

D.F.
MAYO
©1997

Med. plantar v.

Figure 22.1.   Location of major lower-leg venous perforators. The
perforating vein sites (numbered) on the medial leg, especially
Cockett I, II, and III, are common locations for postphlebitic
venous ulcers. Ulcers seldom occur at the posterior and lateral
venous perforators.

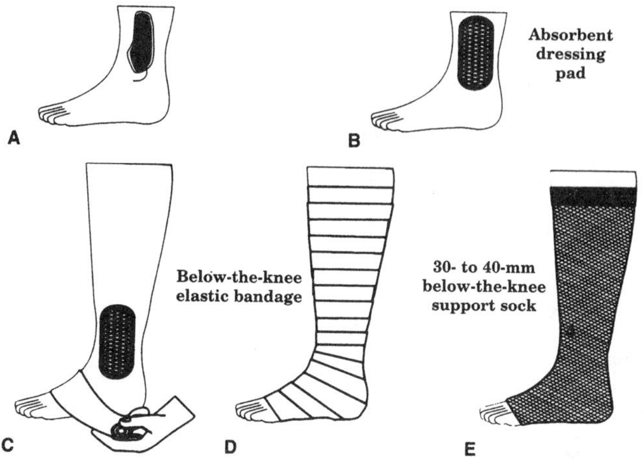

Figure 22.2. Application of a compressive bandage for a venous ulcer. A: The ulcer should be washed with warm water and a mild soap. In general, topical antibiotics should be avoided since they may cause topical allergic reactions. For grossly infected ulcers, the infection should be controlled before the bandage is applied. B: A soft absorbent pad should be placed over the ulcer. C,D,E: The leg from the foot to the knee is wrapped with a compressive dressing: an Unna's paste boot bandage, an Ace wrap, or a 30- to 40-mm below-the-knee support stocking.

dage simply controls local ankle edema until the ulcer heals. The same result could be obtained by putting the patient on strict bed rest; however, such treatment incapacitates active individuals and may be attended with recurrent DVT.

Adherence to certain principles of compression therapy for venous ulcers will ensure success.

A. Control infection. If the ulcer appears infected, a culture should be taken and the wound washed with soap and water. Local cellulitis usually responds to a 5- to 7-day course of an oral antibiotic, such as a cephalosporin, 250 to 500 mg q6h. Local infection should be controlled by leg elevation and antibiotics before a compression bandage is applied. In general, topical antibiotics should not be applied beneath an Unna's paste boot, since topical allergic reactions are common. Generally, a sterile petroleum jelly is adequate to prevent the adherence of bandages.

B. Apply compression. The compressive bandage must be strong enough to counteract the very high venous pressures (80 to 100 mg Hg) that cause these ulcers (Fig. 22.2). Such compression can be accomplished with removable elastic bandages or an Unna's paste boot covered with a firm elastic wrap from the level of the toes to below the knee. This bandage can be left in place for 7 to 10 days before being changed. The commercially available Unna's boot bandages usually contain zinc oxide.

III.   Recurrent or nonhealing venous ulcers. Proper elastic compression, leg elevation, and control of local infection will heal at least 85% of venous ulcers. A few patients will continue to have recurrent venous ulcers despite routine compression therapy. These patients often must stand for very long periods at work or do not routinely wear their support hose. When a suspected venous ulcer is not healing despite routine care, the physician must question whether some other factor is retarding healing. Other coexistent problems may be arterial ischemia, steroid-impaired healing, collagen vasculitis, or skin cancer.

If other etiologies have been excluded, several options are available for management of recurrent venous ulcerations. Some authors recommend continued nonoperative compressive therapy, sometimes with more leg elevation or bed rest. Certainly this approach eventually succeeds in many patients. Nonetheless, some active patients continue to have incapacitating leg swelling, pain, and recurrent ulceration. A surgical procedure may help such patients.

    A.   Subfascial ligation of perforating veins, or subfascial endoscopic perforating vein surgery (SEPS). In our experience, the healthy active patient with recurrent venous ulceration despite compression therapy is a candidate for a surgical approach to alleviating chronic venous hypertension. This operation may require stripping of the great and small saphenous veins in approximately 70% of patients as well as subfascial ligation of all incompetent perforating veins of the lower leg. Subfascial ligation of perforating veins can be performed through a variety of incisions and by using endoscopic instruments. In the 1990s, endoscopic imaging systems and instruments were introduced to minimize wound complications of the previous medial leg incision of the Linton procedure. SEPS has become the technique of choice for operative obliteration of incompetent perforating veins.

Although SEPS is successful initially in healing 80% of chronic venous ulcers, the long-term results indicate a higher recurrence rate. At 2 years, the ulcers recur in 30% to 45% of patients with postphlebitic limbs and in 20% of patients with primary valvular incompetence. Success with subfascial ligation requires **meticulous attention to the details of surgical technique and postoperative care.** Several principles of perforating vein ligation must be emphasized:

    1.   SEPS is indicated in patients with active (class 6) and healed (class 5) ulcers in the setting of chronic venous insufficiency. Invasive infection and wound necrosis should be under control before the procedure.

    2.   Before operation duplex ultrasonography is used to ascertain patency and incompetency of both the superficial and deep venous systems. Incompetent perforators are also localized and marked preoperatively with duplex imaging.

    3.   After surgery, the operated leg should be protected for a minimum of 7 to 14 days in a compressive bandage. Then, a 30 to 40 mm Hg below-knee compression stocking is prescribed.

    4.   The patient usually remains at bed rest until the initial bandage is changed. Bed rest presents leg edema that occurs with this procedure. Either low-dose heparin, 5,000 units s.q.

every 8 to 12 hours, or oral warfarin sodium (Coumadin) should be considered to prevent DVT.

5. If wound healing appears satisfactory at the first dressing change, a compressive elastic Ace wrap are reapplied from the toes to below the knee. This bandage is essential until the sutures are removed.

6. On the first postoperative day, the patient should begin to dangle the leg over the bedside for short periods of time (3 to 5 minutes). This routine allows the leg to become gradually accustomed to a dependent position again before full ambulation.

7. Depending on the extent of surgery and postoperative pain, ambulation begins the first postoperative days for 5 to 10 minutes every 2 to 4 hours. At first, the ankle may be stiff and crutches or a walker may be used to assist some patients. A normal walking pattern generally returns within 1 week to 10 days, depending on the preoperative leg condition and the extent of surgery.

8. Wound healing problems are best managed by bed rest and delayed ambulation. Skin grafting may be necessary.

9. Patients who undergo subfascial venous interruption must understand that they must continue to wear below-the-knee elastic support hose following operation, as the procedure does not correct the deep venous hypertension due to valvular incompetence and reflux.

B. Other operations. Direct transvenous repair of incompetent femoral vein valves has successfully alleviated severe chronic venous insufficiency in selected patients. Crossover femorofemoral or direct iliofemoral vein bypass grafts for iliofemoral venous occlusion can also relieve severe leg swelling, incapacitating venous claudication, and recurrent venous ulceration. However, these direct surgical attacks on the deep veins and valves can be technically difficult procedures, so there has not been widespread acceptance of direct venous reconstruction for most patients with postphlebitic syndrome or primary valvular incompetence.

SELECTED READING

Gloviczki P, Yao JST, eds. *Handbook of venous disorders*. 1st edition. London: Chapman & Hall Medical, 1996.

Gloviczki P, Bergan JJ, Menawat SS, et al. Safety, feasibility, and early efficacy of subfascial endoscopic perforator surgery: a preliminary report of the North American registry. *J Vasc Surg* 1997; 25:94–105.

Gloviczki P, Bergan JJ, Rhodes JM, et al. Mid-term results of endoscopic perforator vein interruption for chronic venous insufficiency: lessons learned from the North American Subfascial Endoscopic Perforator Surgery Registry. *J Vasc Surg* 1999;29:489–502.

Kistner RL. Definitive diagnosis and definitive treatment in chronic venous disease: a concept whose time has come. *J Vasc Surg* 1996;24:703–710.

Linton RR. John Homan's impact on diseases of the veins of the lower extremity, with special reference to deep thrombophlebitis and the post-thrombotic syndrome with ulceration. *Surgery* 1977;81:1–4.

Moore DJ, Himmel PD, Sumner DS. Distribution of venous valvular incompetence in patients with the postphlebitic syndrome. *J Vasc Surg* 1986;3:49–57.

O'Donnell TF. Lessons from the past guide the future: is history truly circular? American Venous Forum Presidential Address. *J Vasc Surg* 1999;30:775–786.

Raju S, Fredericks RK, Neglen PN, et al. Durability of venous valve reconstruction techniques for "primary" and postphlebitic reflux. *J Vasc Surg* 1996;23:357–367.

Miscellaneous Problems

Hemodialysis Access

In 1972, an amendment to the Social Security Act provided Medicare coverage for patients suffering from end-stage renal disease. This legislation opened the way for tens of thousands of patients to undergo hemodialysis. Although dialysis was initially denied to patients older than 45 years and patients with diabetes, these groups are no longer excluded. The magnitude of the current expenditure is impressive as $16 billion was spent on 300,000 patients with end-stage renal disease in 1998. More than 200,000 patients are dialysis-dependent.

Procedures for dialysis access are the most common vascular surgical procedure performed in the United States. In most medical centers, residents and fellows play a primary role in the placement of hemodialysis access. One of the most predictable aspects of chronic hemodialysis is the need for access revision. Access failure is especially common for prosthetic arteriovenous (AV) shunts. Consequently, this chapter focuses on essentials in the initial evaluation, placement, and revision of hemodialysis accesses.

INDICATIONS FOR DIALYSIS

Dialysis for acute or chronic renal failure is indicated when one or more of the following clinical problems are present.

I. Hyperkalemia (>6 mEq/L), especially when accompanied by electrocardiogram (ECG) or neuromuscular abnormalities, requires immediate dialysis. Dietary restriction and potassium-bonding resins may suffice for lower levels of hyperkalemia.

II. Fluid overload is another indication for both acute and chronic dialysis. This includes patients who have not responded satisfactorily to fluid restriction and diuretics.

III. Worsening acidosis results from the kidneys' inability to excrete hydrogen and resorb bicarbonate and represents an indication for hemodialysis.

IV. Drug overdose is a less common indication for hemodialysis but one that occasionally arises in an emergency room or critical care practice.

V. Uremic signs and symptoms are the most common indication for chronic dialysis. They become prominent as the blood-urea-nitrogen (BUN) and creatinine levels rise. Mortality and morbidity may be reduced if the BUN level is maintained below 100 mg/dL. Neurologic symptoms that require dialysis include lethargy, seizures, myoclonus, and peripheral polyneuropathies.

CHOICES OF ACCESS FOR HEMODIALYSIS

Several techniques can be used to establish dialysis (Fig. 23.1). Selection of the appropriate technique for an individual patient depends on several clinical factors. Does the patient need immediate dialysis or will dialysis will be started in a number of days or weeks? Does the patient need temporary or permanent access? Does the patient have satisfactory extremity arterial inflow and suitable venous outflow veins for construction of an access? If

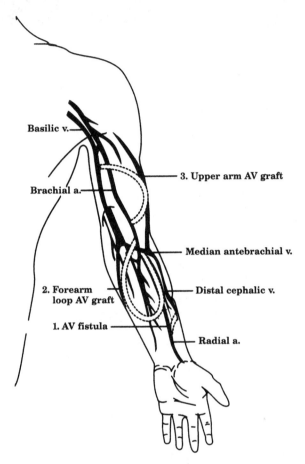

Figure 23.1. The three most common types of upper-extremity hemodialysis accesses include (1) a primary radiocephalic arteriovenous (AV) fistula, (2) a forearm polytetrafluorethylene AV shunt graft, or (3) an upper arm AV graft.

peritoneal dialysis is selected, is the patient's abdominal cavity suitable for such a technique?

    I. A variety of **dialysis catheters** are currently available for acute hemodialysis. These catheters provide quick access and are generally placed percutaneously or by surgical cutdown in the internal jugular or subclavian veins. They may be used for days to weeks. Infection or central venous thrombosis, however, are ever-present dangers for this form of hemodialysis.

    A. The most common dialysis catheters (Shiley, VasCath, or Quinton catheters) are **noncuffed, dual-lumen catheters** placed percutaneously using the Seldinger method.

B.   Cuffed dialysis catheters (PermCath or VasCath) are generally placed by a venous cutdown. These catheters are relatively soft and well-tolerated by patients and will often function for weeks or even a few months. Again, central venous thrombosis and catheter infection are the major complications and generally necessitate catheter removal.

II.   An **autologous AV fistula** of the upper extremity is the most durable and complication-free chronic dialysis access (Fig. 23.1). The most common type of primary AV fistula is constructed between the cephalic vein and the radial artery at the wrist **(Brescia–Cimino fistula).** The 3-year patency rate for an autologous AV fistula is 80% to 90%, compared to 60% to 70% for prosthetic AV grafts. A Cimino–Brescia fistula, however, takes about 6 to 8 weeks to mature. Consequently, it cannot be used as soon as a prosthetic AV shunt. Other types of autologous AV fistulae include an antecubital anastomosis between the basilic or cephalic veins and the brachial artery. Cephalic vein transposition to the distal radial artery in the forearm has also been used with success. **Clinical practice guidelines suggest that autologous AV dialysis fistulae should represent at least 50% of all dialysis access procedures in a busy vascular practice.**

III.   Synthetic AV grafts are the most common type of access for chronic dialysis. Our first choice is a loop polytetrafluoroethylene (PTFE) AV shunt placed in the nondominant forearm of the patient (Fig. 23.1). In our experience, this type of access has been preferable to a straight forearm graft in the radial artery to an antecubital vein. Such straight forearm grafts have a limited area for puncture, may be difficult to perform to heavily calcified radial artery and appear to have decreased patency rates compared to forearm loop grafts. Our second choice for an upper-extremity AV graft is an upper-arm loop graft between the brachial artery and the axillary vein. When the nondominant upper extremity has been expended for dialysis access, we then move to the opposite upper extremity. The lower extremity is used only when the upper extremities can no longer accept some type of hemodialysis access. Although grafts can be placed in the groin area, infection is a greater problem than it is in the upper extremity.

IV.   Chronic peritoneal dialysis is another alternative preferred by some patients. Peritoneal dialysis can be performed at home and generally at a lower cost than hemodialysis. The major long-term disadvantage is the possibility of recurrent peritonitis. For patients with difficult upper-extremity access for hemodialysis, chronic peritoneal dialysis becomes an important option.

PATIENT ASSESSMENT

History and physical examination provide critical information in determining the suitability and type of dialysis access. The following factors should be considered in each patient.

I.   One must ascertain whether the dialysis is intended to be **temporary** or **permanent.** If patients develop acute renal failure in the setting of previously normal renal function, many of them will recover from acute failure over a period of days to weeks. In contrast, patients who develop acute renal insufficiency in the setting of chronic renal failure are likely to need chronic dialysis.

II.   Several aspects of the **history** influence the type and outcome of dialysis access procedures. First, one must assess whether the patient has other medical comorbidities (e.g., poor cardiac function that may make hemodialysis more difficult.) In addition, diabetics have worse results with long-term dialysis and are particularly susceptible to hand ischemia due to vascular steal from their AV access. Second, one must ascertain whether the patient is right- or left-handed. Generally, access should be placed in the nondominant upper extremity. Third, any prior or current arterial or venous problems of the upper extremity (including prior arterial or central venous catheter placements) must be identified. Such abnormalities will often affect the suitability or placement of an AV access. Fourth, any prior hemodialysis access procedures must be identified, including their prior locations and any problems associated with the previous fistula. Likewise, prior abdominal operations may affect peritoneal dialysis. Finally, anticoagulation problems must be identified, including tendencies to both thrombosis or hemorrhage.

   III.   Physical examination is the primary determinant for the hemodialysis access site.

   A.   Skin condition must be checked for signs of infection or other dermatologic disorders that would impair healing.

   B.   The extremities should be examined for **swelling or edema** which would suggest subclavian or axillary vein thrombosis or lymphedema due to other operations (e.g., past mastectomy).

   C.   The **cephalic and basilic veins** should be inspected for patency and size. They should be palpated carefully for compressibility (normal vein) or firm cords (chronic thrombosis). Application of an upper arm tourniquet is helpful in delineating suitable veins in some patients.

   D.   The axillary brachial, radial, and ulnar **pulses** should be palpated and **blood pressure** recorded in both arms. Decreased pulses or a difference in blood pressure of more than 5 to 10 mm Hg indicates proximal arterial occlusive disease or local arterial thrombosis from prior procedures.

   E.   The proximal subclavian arteries in the area of the supraclavicular fossa should be auscultated. **Bruits** indicate underlying arterial stenosis. The proximal left subclavian artery is one of the sites most susceptible to atherosclerotic disease.

   F.   Perfusion of the hand should be checked with an **Allen's test.** With the patient's hand making a tight fist, the examiner should compress the radial and ulnar arteries. Separately, the radial and then the ulnar artery should be released as the examiner looks at the opened hand for return of capillary refill. The majority of hands are ulnar dominant. Documentation of this fact indicates that obliteration of the radial artery or diversion of flow from the radial artery into an AV fistula will not compromise perfusion to the hand.

   G.   The abdomen should be examined for prior **surgical scars.** Prior abdominal operations may compromise the placement of a chronic peritoneal catheter.

SELECTION OF ACCESS

   I.   The best access for **acute dialysis** is a subclavian or jugular vein percutaneous catheter. These catheters can be used immediately. Occasionally, one may need to construct an external Scribner AV shunt at the wrist or ankle.

II. The type of access for **chronic dialysis** depends on the timing for dialysis.

A. If dialysis is scheduled for the future (weeks to months), an autogenous AV fistula is the best choice. **Preoperative duplex ultrasound may be useful to identify and mark arteries and veins suitable for fistula formation.** Although it is not our routine, some studies have reported an overall increase in the use of autogenous fistulae using preoperative duplex. These same studies report higher patency rates of AV fistulae with the use of preoperative duplex.

B. Dialysis that is ongoing or will be needed in less than 1 month usually requires a prosthetic AV graft. Peritoneal dialysis is another option. Prosthetic grafts generally take 5 to 10 days to achieve good tissue incorporation. Puncturing the grafts prior to tissue incorporation can result in subcutaneous hematomas and poor healing of the graft. Quick-sealing prosthetic grafts may allow puncture of hemodialysis AV shunt grafts within 24 hours

PREOPERATIVE PREPARATION

I. The indication for dialysis, the type of dialysis, and potential complication should be discussed with the patient and any family members. In particular, infection, thrombosis, and ischemic steal syndrome of the hand should be explained.

II. Prophylactic antibiotics (e.g., cephazolin, 1 g) have may reduce the risk of infection.

INTRAOPERATIVE TECHNIQUE

The details of surgical construction of the hemodialysis access are beyond the scope of this handbook. However, a few technical concepts and tips should be mentioned.

I. Most extremity hemodialysis access procedures can be performed under **local anesthesia.** A supplemental axillary block may be helpful in some individuals.

II. Although **anticoagulation** is not mandatory, a small dose of heparin (e.g., 2,000 to 3,000 units) may alleviate early thrombosis in synthetic grafts where venous vasoconstriction may initially cause slower flow rates.

III. Skin incisions should be constructed so that the graft has good tissue coverage at the end of the procedure. Whenever possible, skin incisions should not be placed directly over the course of the synthetic graft.

IV. When the access has been completed, it is essential to check the **presence of pulses** at the wrist. In addition, it is helpful to auscultate flow in the palmar arch of the hand with a sterile continuous-wave Doppler. The loss or diminution of wrist pulses and the absence of Doppler flow in the palmar arch are harbingers of postoperative hand ischemia.

POSTOPERATIVE CARE

The period of greatest risk for postoperative thrombotic or ischemic complications is the first 12 to 24 hours.

I. The extremity with the new dialysis access should be placed at a **position of comfort.** Generally, it does not need to be elevated. In fact, elevation may exacerbate hand ischemia in patients who have marginal perfusion following placement of an AV shunt. Constrictive bandages should be avoided.

II.   The access should be checked for patency within 6 hours of placement. The two most reliable signs of patency are **palpable thrills** over the venous anastomosis and distal vein. In addition, a loud **machinery murmur** heard with the stethoscope is indicative of shunt or fistula patency.

III.   The hand must be checked for symptoms or signs of **ischemic steal syndrome.** The earliest symptom is numbness of the fingers. With severe ischemic steal, progressive paresis of the intrinsic muscles of the hands will evolve over 24 hours. An absent radial pulse that was previously present is the key physical finding in such patients. In addition, patients with a hand ischemia will have monophasic or no Doppler flow over the radial, ulnar, and palmar arteries. **If ischemic steal syndrome of the hand is present and progressive, the AV access must be revised immediately.** One technique is to decrease flow in the shunt by "banding," which involves narrowing the flow in the graft by a variety of techniques. One technique that has worked well for us has been reduction of a 6-mm graft to a 4-mm size by the lateral application of small Weck clips along the side of the proximal graft for approximately 1 cm. With adequate banding, the wrist pulses will usually increase and the Doppler signals of the wrist arteries and palmar arch will improve from monophasic to biphasic signals.

IV.   Generally, a synthetic AV graft can be punctured in 7 to 10 days. An autogenous AV fistula will need to mature for 6 to 8 weeks before use. Development of an autologous fistula is assisted in some patients by daily exercise of the hand (e.g., squeezing a soft, rubber ball).

LATE COMPLICATIONS

A variety of complications can occur any time with a hemodialysis access. The most important complications are thrombosis, infection, chronic hand ischemia, or pseudoaneurysms along the graft.

I.   **Infection** is uncommon with an autogenous AV fistula. Synthetic grafts are more susceptible. Generally, physical findings of erythema, induration, tenderness, and purulent drainage from incisional sites are pathognomonic. Occasionally, a patient will present with a fever of unknown origin and minimal signs of local graft infection. Positive blood cultures may be present and an Indium-labeled white blood cell scan may localize infection to the graft. An infected synthetic graft must be removed entirely. A localized infected graft segment can occasionally be resected with a new segmental bypass around the infected area.

II.   **Thrombosis** is more common with synthetic AV grafts. In fact, 30% to 40% of such grafts will have acute occlusion within 3 years. Most of these occlusions occur suddenly with no warning. However, a few grafts will begin to show a decreased flow rate on dialysis. A flow rate of less than 250 to 300 mL/min and a recirculation rate greater than 15% (or venous pressures in excess of 150 mm Hg) indicate a failing graft. **In such cases, a fistulogram or a duplex ultrasound may identify a site of stenosis.** Most synthetic grafts fail at the venous anastomosis where intimal hyperplasia occurs and should be revised before acute occlusion.

III.   Pseudoaneurysm is another relatively common problem of chronic synthetic AV grafts. These aneurysms usually occur at puncture sites where subcutaneous hematomas have formed. They can gradually erode through the skin and lead to serious hemorrhage and should be repaired by resection of the pseudoaneurysm site and grafting around the area.

SELECTED READING

Ascher E, Gade P, Hingorani A, et al. Changes in the practice of angioaccess surgery: impact of dialysis outcome and quality recommendations. *J Vasc Surg* 2000;31(Part 1):84–92.

Berman SS, Gentile AT, Glickman MH, et al. Distal revascularization-interval ligation for limb salvage and maintenance of dialysis access in ischemic steal syndrome. *J Vasc Surg* 1997;26:393–402.

Byrne C, Vernon P, Cohen JJ. Effects of age and diagnosis on survival of older patients beginning chronic dialysis. *JAMA* 1994;271:24.

Decaprio JD, Valentine RJ, Kakish HB, et al. Steal syndrome complicating hemodialysis access. *Cardiovasc Surg* 1997;5:648–653.

Hakaim AG, Nalbandian M, Scott T. Superior maturation and patency of primary brachiocephalic and transposed basilic vein arteriovenous fistulae in patients with diabetes. *J Vasc Surg* 1998; 27:154–157.

Martson WA, Criado E, Jaques PF, et al. Prospective randomized comparison of surgical versus endovascular management of thrombosed dialysis access grafts. *J Vasc Surg* 1997;26:373–380.

Silva MB Jr, Hobson RW II, Pappas PJ, et al. A strategy for increasing use of autogenous hemodialysis access procedures: the impact of preoperative noninvasive evaluation. *J Vasc Surg* 1998;27: 302–307.

Silva MB Jr, Pappas PJ, Padberg FT Jr, et al. Increasing use of autogenous fistulas: selection of dialysis access sites by duplex scanning and transpostion of forearm veins. In: Yao JST, Pearce WH, ed. *Practical vascular surgery.* Stamford: Appleton and Lange, 1999: 41–53.

Vascular Access Work Group. National Kidney Foundation–Dialysis Outcome and Quality Initiative (DOQI) clinical practice guidelines for vascular access. *Am J Kidney Dis* 1997;30(suppl 3):S150–S191.

Wolfe RA, Ashby VB, Milford EL, et al. Comparison of mortality in all patients on dialysis, patients on dialysis awaiting transplantation, and recipients of a first cadaveric transplant. *N Engl J Med* 1999; 341:1725–1730.

Vascular Trauma

Significant arterial and venous injuries are a relatively small problem in all types of trauma. However, when arterial or venous injuries are present, they become pivotal in mortality (i.e., exsanguinating hemorrhage) and morbidity (i.e., limb loss or stroke). Blood vessel injuries contribute to more than 100,000 accidental deaths that occur each year in the United States.

Much of what is known about the treatment of traumatic vascular injuries comes from military conflicts of the 20th Century. Currently, vascular trauma is most commonly the result of violent crimes, motor vehicle crashes, and interventional procedures. In busy emergency departments, gunshot wounds account for 55% of vascular injuries, knives 35% and blunt trauma the remaining 10%. The vast majority (75%) occur in an extremity. Neck wounds account for 15%, while arterial injuries of the visceral arteries (5%) and aorta (5%) are less frequent.

The scope of vascular trauma is so large that books have been written on the subject. This chapter, however, focuses on the initial recognition and management principles of arterial and venous injuries. It is primer and not a treatise.

MECHANISMS OF INJURY

Management of arterial and venous injuries is determined by the mechanism and severity of injury.

I. Penetrating wounds from knives and low-velocity missiles (i.e., pistol bullets) cause localized damage to blood vessels. In contrast, high-velocity bullets (1,500 to 3,000 ft/sec, e.g., hunting rifle) create a wide area of explosive **cavitation damage** around the missile tract. This damage zone extends for an area 30 to 40 times the size of the missile. The violence of the blast expansion disrupts surrounding muscle, may rupture blood vessels and nerves, and may fracture bone at distances removed from the missile path. As the blast cavity collapses, debris (i.e., clothing, dirt, skin) may be drawn into the wound. Likewise, close-range shotgun blasts scatter multiple pellets into the wound and often propel fragments of the shotgun wadding and clothing into the body.

II. Blunt trauma causes vascular injury by several mechanisms. **Bone fractures** may directly injure vessels, while **joint dislocations** may cause stretch injuries or contusions of arteries. The result is intimal and media disruption with thrombosis. Posterior dislocation of the knee is a notorious cause of popliteal artery trauma and thrombosis. Bilateral first rib fractures are commonly associated with subclavian artery injuries. Traumatic carotid **arterial dissection** is classically associated with a sudden hyperextension of the neck. Finally, a **blunt or crushing injury** can contuse or disrupt an artery such as the renal artery following a motor vehicle crash.

RECOGNITION

The early diagnosis and repair of a vascular injury is essential in preventing serious hemorrhage and preserving limb or organ function. In the setting of multiple trauma recognition of a vascular injury is difficult because more obvious head, chest, or abdominal injuries divert attention away from a detailed vascular exam. Poor extremity pulses may be attributed initially to hemorrhagic shock, hypothermic vasoconstriction, crush injury, or vasospasm.

The following symptoms and signs should raise suspicion of arterial or venous damage:

I. **External hemorrhage** from a penetrating wound, especially in proximity to a large artery or vein, is pathognomonic for a major vascular injury.

II. A pale, cool, and **pulseless extremity** may or may not be due to arterial injury. However, absent pulses mandate further observation and objective evaluation (i.e., continuous-wave Doppler ultrasound examination and possible arteriogram).

III. **A penetrating wound adjacent to a major vessel** requires attention to be certain that no underlying vascular injury is present.

IV. Likewise, signs of a **major nerve injury** (i.e., paralysis and analgesia), especially associated with a penetrating wound, should lead to a search for associated vascular trauma.

V. **Fractures or dislocations** (i.e., knee or elbow) are commonly associated with vascular injuries. **Moreover, presence of a distal pulse does not rule out a vascular injury.** An intimal tear or flap may have occurred, but distal pulses may remain present as long as the artery does not thrombose. An arteriogram or other imaging modality (e.g., ultrasound) may be required to settle the issue if diminished Doppler pressures are found on examination.

VI. A large-extremity, neck, or abdominal **hematoma** should raise suspicion of a major arterial or venous disruption.

VII. A **bruit** or **machinery murmur** at or near an injury site suggests disturbed blood flow from an arterial stenosis or arteriovenous fistula.

INITIAL CARE

When a vascular injury is suspected, certain principles should follow the primary survey of the patient or the A, B, C's (airway, breathing, and circulation). These principles apply to the secondary survey of the patient and the early phases of injury management (Fig. 24.1). One should remember that **time from vascular injury to repair is a critical in a successful outcome** and that irreversible damage from ischemia occurs within 6 to 8 hours after arterial disruption.

I. **With the primary and secondary surveys,** intravenous lines should be placed and crystalloid infusion initiated. The front and back of the patient should be exposed to look for entrance and exit wounds. External bleeding from penetrating wounds can usually be controlled with direct pressure while the exam is completed. In addition to the standard chest, cervical spine and pelvis radiographs, plane films should be taken to assess injured extremities

Preoperative   **Intraoperative**

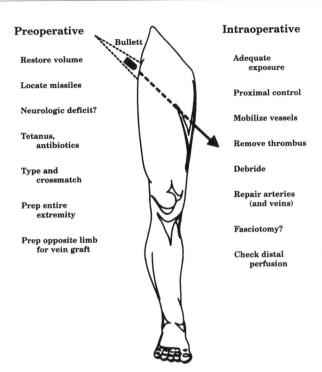

Restore volume   Adequate
                                                       exposure

Locate missiles   Proximal control

Neurologic deficit?   Mobilize vessels

Tetanus,   Remove thrombus
   antibiotics

Type and   Debride
   crossmatch

                                                    Repair arteries
                                                       (and veins)
Prep entire
   extremity   Fasciotomy?

Prep opposite limb   Check distal
   for vein graft   perfusion

Figure 24.1.   Principles of preoperative and intraoperative management of vascular injuries. (Adapted from Baker WH, Kang SS. Arterial injuries. In: Sabiston DC Jr, ed. *Textbook of surgery*. Philadelphia:
Saunders, 1997:1618.)

looking for foreign bodies or missiles. Blood should be typed and
cross-matched and tetanus prophylaxis and intravenous antibiotics given.

II.   Hypotension is a late sign of hypovolemic shock and
does not occur until a patient has lost more than 30% blood volume (Table 24.1). Blood should be transfused if the hypotensive
patient does not respond to initial boluses of crystalloid. **Systolic
blood pressure should be maintained at a level to support
mental status and urine output. Overresuscitation in an
attempt to achieve a "normal" systolic blood pressure may
actually worsen bleeding.**

III.   Continuous-wave Doppler exam of the extremity should
be performed as part of the secondary survey if there are concerns
for vascular injury. An **arterial pressure index** should be performed on any extremity in which a vascular injury is suspected.
This index is basically the same as the ankle-brachial index and
is calculated by dividing the systolic Doppler pressure in the
injured extremity by the pressure in an uninjured arm. Patients
with an arterial pressure index of 0.9 or greater in the extremity

Table 24.1. Classification of hemorrhagic shock

Class	Percentage of blood volume lost	Systolic blood pressure	Pulse pressure	Heart rate (bpm)	Capillary refill	Mental status
I	0–15% (<750 mL)	Normal	Normal	Normal	Normal	Normal
II	15–30% (750–1,500 mL)	Normal	Decreased	>100	Delayed	Anxious
III	30–40% (1,500–2,000 mL)	Decreased	Decreased	>120 (weak)	Delayed	Confused
IV	>40% (>2,000 mL)	Severely decreased	Severely decreased	>140 (nonpalpable)	Absent	Lethargic

Bpm, beats per minute.
Adapted from American College of Surgeons Committee on Trauma. *Advanced Trauma Life Support Program for Doctors: ATLS*, 6th ed. Chicago: American College of Sugeons, 1997.

of concern and no obvious signs of arterial injury may undergo close observation and serial examinations without arteriography.

IV.   Selective arteriography is recommended for patients in whom there is an abnormal arterial pressure index (<0.9). In addition, arteriography is recommended in patients with specific clinical presentations: first rib fractures (subclavian artery injury), deceleration chest injuries with sternal or rib fractures (torn thoracic aorta), posterior dislocations of the knee (popliteal artery injury) and high velocity gunshot wounds.

V.   Hard signs of arterial injury include external hemorrhage or expanding hematoma, or absence of distal pulses. In this setting, no specific diagnostic tests are needed and the patient should be taken to the operating room where arteriography can be performed. If a hematoma is present at the site of injury, **duplex ultrasound** may also help detect a false aneurysm or arteriovenous fistula.

VI.   Fractures should be splinted and dislocations reduced as soon as possible. It is important to document a neurologic and vascular exam of the extremity before and after fracture reduction or splinting as such manipulation may compromise distal nervous or blood supply.

OPERATIVE PRINCIPLES

Although the exact operative approach varies with the site of trauma, certain principles apply to the intraoperative management of all arterial or venous injuries.

I.   A wide operative field should be prepared. For a neck or upper-extremity wound, the prepped area should include the adjacent chest in case median sternotomy or thoracotomy is necessary. When the wound involves the abdomen, the patient should be prepped from the chin to the knees. Both lower extremities should be prepared when the wound involves one leg.

II.   An uninvolved lower extremity for access to a **saphenous vein** should be prepped. Saphenous vein remains the best arterial substitute for all but the largest injured arteries and veins.

III.   Proximal control of the artery should be gained before entering any traumatic hematomas. This may require an initial incision remote from the hematoma.

IV.   Damaged arteries and veins should be resected. Most injuries will involve a 1- to 2-cm segment of blood vessel. One must be certain that all of the damaged vessel has been removed before a reanastomosis or graft is placed.

V.   The distal circulation should be checked for accumulation of **thrombus.** Specifically, a Fogarty balloon catheter should be passed distally, gently inflated, and drawn back to retrieve distal thrombus.

VI.   In general, 1 to 2 cm of artery may be resected and reconstituted by a **primary anastomosis.** Larger areas of injury require a **graft.** Saphenous vein is appropriate for vessels measuring up to 6 mm. Larger vessels usually require a synthetic graft (i.e., Dacron or polytetrafluoroethylene).

VII.   Concomitant **venous injuries** should be repaired whenever possible. Ligation of major peripheral veins often results in long-term disabling venous stasis of the extremity. If the vein cannot be repaired by lateral suture, an autologous vein graft should be used. Patency for even 24 to 72 hours may be sufficient to allow the establishment of additional collateral venous return.

VIII. **All devitalized tissue** in the area of injury should be debrided. Such debridement is especially important in patients with high-velocity missile wounds. These wounds are generally associated with extensive, explosive cavitation destruction.

IX. After arterial repair, adequate **soft-tissue coverage** of the affected artery is imperative. An exposed arterial repair may dehisce due to desiccation or infection. Muscle is the preferable coverage and can often be secured by transposition of adjacent muscle. When extensive muscle and soft tissue have been destroyed by the injury, it may be necessary to use a **myocutaneous flap** for coverage.

X. **Displaced fractures** and **dislocations** must be stabilized to prevent tension on a vascular repair. Whether the fracture or dislocation should be managed first or after the vascular repair will vary from patient to patient. Because ischemia has often been prolonged, repair of damaged arteries or veins is often done first. External skeletal tractal or fixation is then performed. If a fracture or dislocation must be treated to allow adequate exposure for an arterial repair, a shunt can often be placed from the proximal injured artery to the distal injured artery to restore circulation while the fracture is being treated.

XI. **Concomitant nerve injuries** are usually identified and tagged with identifying sutures for delayed repair. Generally, disrupted nerves are not repaired at the time of the initial operation.

XII. Prolonged ischemia is often present with arterial injuries and muscle swelling, after reperfusion can create a **compartment syndrome.** Fasciotomy (Fig. 24.2) should be strongly considered at the time of initial arterial repair for (a) popliteal artery and vein injuries, (b) cases in which there has been a delay greater than 4 to 6 hours between injury, and (c) repair cases in which patient transport to another facility is necessary following vascular repair. If fasciotomies are not done at the initial operation, serial neurovascular exams must be performed looking for signs and symptoms of compartment syndrome.

XIII. Extremity **perfusion** must be assessed objectively in the operating room and during the early postoperative period. Return of a distal pulse is the best sign of success. An intraoperative arteriogram with 20 to 30 mL of contrast material is the standard means of imaging the site of reconstruction and distal run off. A sterile continuous-wave Doppler is also helpful in auscultating distal arterial signals. A sterile blood pressure cuff may also be used to monitor distal pulse volume recordings. If the arteriogram demonstrates distal arterial spasm, a direct intraarterial dose of papaverine (1 mL of papaverine mixed in 9 mL of normal saline) into the affected extremity will often alleviate the vasoconstriction.

XIV. **Anticoagulation** is avoided in patients with multiple systemic injuries. Small doses of regional heparinized saline can be instilled down the distal arterial tree during operation. However, doses in excess of 2,000 to 3,000 units of heparin may result in serious systemic anticoagulation and bleeding in other body sites (i.e., head or intraabdominal injuries).

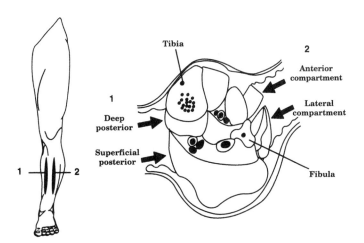

Figure 24.2.   Fasciotomy for compartment syndrome of the leg. The four compartments of the leg can be decompressed through two leg incisions. A longitudinal lateral leg incision (2) is made approximately halfway through the tibia and fibula. This incision allows decompression of the anterior and lateral fascial compartments. Care must be taken to avoid injury to the superficial peroneal nerve in the distal portion of this incision. The superficial and deep posterior fascial compartments are decompressed by a medial incision (1) made approximately one fingerbreadth medial to the tibia.

POSTOPERATIVE CARE

Since patients with arterial trauma often have injuries to other organ systems, they are generally observed in an intensive care unit. The following guidelines should ensure continued success of the vascular repair.

I.   Peripheral pulses should be monitored frequently for any sign of thrombosis. If one has difficulty ascertaining the presence of a peripheral pulse, continuous-wave Doppler should be used to auscultate arterial signals.

II. Continued surveillance for signs of **compartment syndrome** is critical, especially in the first 6 to 12 hours after operation. Muscles that were initially soft in the operating room may swell following reperfusion. The most common symptoms and signs of compartment syndrome are leg or forearm pain associated with tense, tender muscle groups. The patient may also complain of numbness in the extremity. Pulses may actually be present when significant compartment pressure has occurred. As pressure rises within a muscle compartment, tissue perfusion declines progressively and at a level of above 20 to 30 mm Hg becomes impaired. If clinical symptoms and signs cannot be assessed adequately, compartment pressure should be measured.

During **four-compartment fasciotomy** of the leg, the anterior and lateral compartments are decompressed through a lateral incision placed along the fibula. The superficial and deep posterior compartments can be decompressed by a medial leg incision (Fig. 24.2). One must be sure that the deep posterior compartment has been released by removing the gastrocnemius and soleus muscles from the tibia. This compartment contains the posterior tibial and peroneal vessels and failure to open it widely during leg fasciotomy can have devastating consequences.

III.   In the setting of extensive muscle injury the patient may develop **acute renal failure** from myoglobinuria. Myoglobin will cause a dark discoloration of the urine. When myoglobinuria is diagnosed hydration, diuresis (25 g of mannitol in 1 L of fluid) and alkalinization of the urine (with 50 mEq of sodium bicarbonate) are principles applied to prevent damage to the kidneys. **Persistent myoglobinuria usually indicates that further debridement of necrotic muscle is needed.**

RESULTS

Rapid transport of trauma patients by helicopter or ambulance to major surgical centers has decreased the average time from injury to treatment for most vascular injuries. The majority of patients currently arrive at trauma centers within 4 to 6 hours of initial injury. Most delays occur at the scene of the accident where the patient may not be discovered for a period of time, especially at night. Blunt trauma causes the most severe vascular injuries and accounts for most amputations (80% to 90%) and deaths (70% to 80%). Nearly all blunt trauma patients have serious associated injuries of other organs. Although blunt trauma counts for approximately 40% of vascular injuries, the remaining 60% are due to penetrating wounds. Penetrating vascular injuries account for approximately 10% of all amputations due to vascular trauma and result in 20% of the deaths related to arterial or venous injury.

The overall mortality rate for vascular trauma is in the 5% range. Blunt vascular trauma, however, carries a mortality risk of approximately 9% to 10%, while penetrating injuries are associated with a mortality rate of 1.5% to 3%. Currently, overall amputation rate for all vascular injuries is about 7% to 10%. Ligation of a major-extremity artery will result in a 50% amputation rate, which has been lowered significantly in the past 40 years with arterial repair. Injuries of the popliteal artery continue to reflect the highest amputation rate following arterial repair (20% to 30%). Although arterial and venous injuries can frequently be successfully repaired in an extremity, the limiting factor for many severely traumatized patients is associated major nerve disruption. Such patients often develop causalgia or reflex sympathetic dystrophy of the injured extremity.

SELECTED READING

American College of Surgeons, Committee on Trauma. Advanced Trauma Life Support Program for Doctors. Chicago, 1997.

Caps MT. The epidemiology of vascular trauma. *Semin Vasc Surg* 1998;11:227–231.

McIntyre WB, Ballard JL. Cervicothoracic vascular injuries. *Semin Vasc Surg* 1998;11:232–242.

Biffl W, Burch JM. Management of abdominal vascular injuries. *Semin Vasc Surg* 1998;11:243–254.

Hood DB, Weaver FA, Yellin AE. Changing perspecitves in the diagnosis of peripheral vascular trauma. *Semin Vasc Surg* 1998;11:255–260.

Johansen K, Watson J. Compartment syndrome: new insights. *Semin Vasc Surg* 1998;11:294–301.

Mattox KL. A new strategy in the resuscitation of trauma patients. In: Yao JS, Pearce WH, eds. *Practical vascular surgery*. Stamford: Appleton and Lange, 1999:375–389.

Perry MO, Bongard FS. Vascular trauma. In: Moore WS, ed. *Vascular surgery: a comprehensive review*, 5th ed. Philadelphia: Saunders, 1998:648–666.

Rich NW, Spencer FC. *Vascular trauma*. Philadelphia: Saunders, 1978.

Wind GG, Valentine RJ. *Anatomic exposures in vascular surgery*. Baltimore: Williams & Williams, 1991.

Coagulation Disorders

Preceding chapters of this handbook have addressed selected aspects of hypercoagulability (thrombophilia) and the management of thrombosis. This chapter provides a more comprehensive summary of hypercoagulable states and their management.

Hypercoagulable states in thrombogenesis were acknowledged in 1860 by Virchow, who recognized them as a part of the triad of factors contributing to thrombosis. It has been estimated that nearly 2 million persons in the United States die each year from arterial or venous thrombosis. Congenital disorders and/or acquired factors causing hypercoagulability are responsible for more than half of these events. Genetic factors are recognized as primary hypercoaguable states, while acquired disorders are considered secondary forms of hypercoagulability (Table 25.1).

I. Mechanisms. The coagulation cascade consists of the intrinsic and extrinsic pathways. The extrinsic pathway includes tissue factor, and factors VII, X, V, and II, and fibrin. The intrinsic pathway consists of factors, all of which are contained in blood—specifically, high-molecular-weight kininogen, prekallikrein, and factors XII, XI, IX, VIII, X, and V, as well as prothrombin and fibrinogen. The extrinsic pathway is viewed as the primary pathway of coagulation and is triggered by vascular damage and exposure of tissue factor to blood. Thrombin, created by the extrinsic pathway, activates factor XI of the intrinsic pathway in a positive feedback manner, assuring that clot will be formed independent of tissue factor.

Controls of this system exist to prevent excess thrombin formation and undesired thrombosis. Specifically, plasma proteins and endothelial receptors act as a counterbalance of the coagulation cascade. Antithrombin III acts as an inhibitor of thrombin and other coagulation factors to a lesser degree. The activity of antithrombin III is enhanced by heparin and heparin-like polysaccharides exposed on the vascular endothelium. Also exposed on the endothelial cell is the receptor thrombomodulin. Thrombin binds to thrombomodulin and loses its procoagulant potential. It then participates, with thrombomodulin, in the activation of the protein C system. Protein C is a proenzyme of a serine protease, which inactivates factor Va and VIIIa. Protein S is a cofactor to protein C and greatly accelerates its activity. As factor V is a central coagulation factor common to both the intrinsic and extrinsic pathways, its inactivation by protein C is especially important in controlling hypercoagulability.

II. Inherited hypercoagulability. Familial thrombophilia is present in nearly 40% of patients who are hypercoagulable. Discovery of antithrombin III deficiency and characterization of the protein C and protein S systems identified a small percentage of individuals and families affected by familial thrombosis. Protein C and S deficiency and antithrombin III deficiency are autosomal dominant forms of inherited hypercoagulability. However, antithrombin III, protein C, and protein S deficiencies are responsible for only 5% to 10% of cases of familial thrombosis (Table 25.1).

Table 25.1. Inherited thrombophilia

Disorder
Antithrombin III deficiency
Protein C deficiency
Protein S deficiency
Activated protein C resistance
Factor V R506Q (Leiden) mutation
Homocystinemia
Prothrombin gene variant (20210A)
Hypoplasminogenemia
Dysfibrinogenemia

In 1993, a point mutation in factor V of the coagulation pathway was identified as causing activated protein C resistance and associated hypercoagulability. This mutation at position 506 of the factor V polypeptide is called "factor V Leiden" and leads to an activated protein C resistance (APC resistance). Factor V Leiden is absent in certain ethnic groups but is present in up to 15% of some Caucasian populations. In contrast to the relative rarity of the protein deficiencies, APC resistance has been described in up to 60% of patients with familial thrombosis. Importantly, some individuals may be affected by more than one genetic disorder and usually present with thrombotic events at a young age.

A. Antithrombin III deficiency. Antithrombin III deficiency is an autosomal dominant disease, and its prevalence in the population is one in 2,000 to 5,000. Antithrombin III is synthesized by hepatocytes and inactivates thrombin as well as other coagulation factors. Its activity is greatly enhanced by heparin. Two types of antithrombin III deficiency exist, the most common resulting from decreased synthesis of a biologically normal molecule. These patients have functional levels of circulating antithrombin III which are only 50% of normal. The second type of antithrombin III deficiency is less frequent and results from a functional deficiency associated with specific molecular abnormalities in the molecule involving the heparin or thrombin-binding domains.

Antithrombin III deficiency is suspected when patients have recurrent, familial and/or juvenile deep vein or mesenteric venous thrombosis. This event frequently occurs in conjunction with another recognized predisposing event such as trauma, immobilization, pregnancy, or oral contraceptives. Deficiency may also be suspected by the inability to anticoagulate a person with intravenous heparin. Such patients may require large doses of heparin to achieve anticoagulation and may require treatment with fresh frozen plasma which contains antithrombin III or antithrombin concentrates to be anticoagulated.

Acquired antithrombin III deficiency may be seen with liver and kidney disease, sepsis, oral contraceptives, and some chemotherapeutic agents.

B. Deficiencies in protein C and S system. The protein C and S system is a major regulator of blood fluidity. Its actions are particularly important at the capillary level where there exists a relatively high concentration of thrombomodulin receptors on endothelial cells. These deficiencies are also inherited as autosomal dominant traits and are fortunately most frequently heterozygous. The prevalence of protein C deficiency is one in 200 to 300. Homozygous forms of protein C or S deficiency are associated with extreme, highly lethal forms of thrombosis in infancy termed **purpura fulminans.** Homozygous **and** heterozygous protein C or S deficiencies have also been associated with **warfarin-induced skin necrosis.** In this disorder, necrosis and skin infarction begin within days of beginning warfarin therapy. Its pathogenesis is related to a transient, severe hypercoagulable state related to an exaggerated protein C deficiency caused by warfarin. It is treated with heparin, vitamin K, and or plasma protein C concentrates.

Acquired protein C and S deficiencies occur with activation of inflammatory response syndromes. C4b binding protein (present in the activated complement system) binds and inactivates protein S creating a relative deficient state. Acquired deficiencies may also be present in liver disease, pregnancy, postoperative states and nephrotic syndrome.

C. Activated protein C resistance. The most recently described and the most prevalent hereditary hypercoagulable state is APC resistance. Also called "factor V Leiden," the prevalence of this hypercoagulable condition varies widely from one population to another but has been demonstrated in 40% to 60% of patients with familial thrombosis. A limitation in the testing of individuals for factor V Leiden is the limited ability to perform the test on patients who are anticoagulated. However, improved testing techniques now allow more accurate estimates of its prevalence.

Similar to protein C or protein S deficiencies, homozygosity for the factor V Leiden has a much higher risk of thrombosis than heterozygosity for the mutation. The most common manifestation of APC resistance is deep venous thrombosis. In contrast to those persons homozygous for protein C or protein S deficiency, **some** persons homozygous for factor V Leiden never experience thrombosis.

As with other inherited hypercoagulable conditions, the development of thrombosis in APC resistance is affected by the coexistence of other genetic or circumstantial risk factors. The most common risk factors affecting APC resistant individuals are oral contraceptive use, pregnancy, trauma and surgery. Women who are heterozygous for factor V Leiden and use oral contraceptives have a near 30-fold increase in venous thrombosis; and women who are homozygous have a several hundred-fold increase in similar events. Although our understanding of this hypercoagulable condition is relatively new, it does not appear to be associated with arterial thrombosis.

D. Hyperhomocystinemia. Abnormalities in the metabolism of homocysteine result in increased circulating levels of this sulphur-containing amino acid (>14 µmol/L). In addition, acquired hyperhomocystinemia may occur as a result of deficiencies of vitamin B_6, vitamin B_{12}, or folate. Hyperhomocystinemia is present in 5% of the population and is associated with early atherosclerosis and venous thrombosis. Elevated homocysteine levels act primarily by causing endothelial dysfunction and platelet activation. Because this condition can be altered favorably by B vitamin and folate supplementation, screening individuals who have premature atherosclerosis is recommended.

E.   Prothrombin gene variant (20210A). A genetic abnormality may exist on position 20210 of the prothrombin gene and is present in up to 20% of patients with familial venous thrombophilia. This genetic abnormality may also predispose to arterial thrombosis although the mechanisms for arterial or venous thrombophilia are not yet established.

F.   Other primary hypercoagulable states. Other more rare inheritable hypercoagulable syndromes exist and comprise mostly disorders of tissue plasmin synthesis or release. These patients have disorders in fibrinolysis and high rates of venous and arterial thrombosis.

III.   Acquired hypercoagulability (Table 25.2).

A.   Smoking. The nicotine and carbon monoxide in cigarette smoke cause endothelial dysfunction with increased platelet deposition and lipid accumulation. Smoking decreases the production of prostacyclin a potent vasodilator and inhibitor of platelet aggregation, and increases blood viscosity. These and other effects make smoking a common contributor to atherosclerosis and arterial thrombosis.

B.   Heparin-induced thrombocytopenia occurs in 2% to 3% of patients who undergo therapy with heparin. This acquired condition results from the formation of antiplatelet antibodies after exposure to heparin. Patients who have heparin-associated antiplatelet antibodies have extreme platelet aggregation and thrombosis (**heparin-induced thrombocytopenia and thrombosis; HITT)** when exposed to heparin. The development of antibodies is independent of patient age, gender or amount or route of heparin exposure. All forms of heparin, including low-molecular weight heparin, can result in antibody formation. Clinical presentation of heparin-induced thrombocytopenia and thrombosis include decreasing platelet count, resistance to anticoagulation with heparin and often severe thrombotic events. Management includes avoidance of all forms of heparin and inhibition of platelet function (Dextran 40) and use of the thrombin inhibitor lepirudin (Relfludan,

Table 25.2.   Causes of acquired hypercoagulable disorders

Cause
Cigarette smoking
Pregnancy
Oral contraceptives
Hormone replacement therapy
Heparin-induced thrombocytopenia
Antiphospholipid syndrome
Malignancy
Antineoplastic medications
Myeloproliferative syndromes
Hyperhomocystinemia
Inflammatory bowel disease

Hoechst Marion Roussel, Kansas City, MO, U.S.A.) if thrombosis has occurred.

C. Oral contraceptives/pregnancy. Exogenous estrogens are associated with an increased risk for venous thrombosis as well as coronary and cerebral arterial thrombotic events. Estrogens are associated with decreased antithrombin III and protein S activities and increases in activated factors VII and X. Estrogens have also been associated with decreased levels of thrombomodulin and a subsequent reduction in protein C activity. The combination of the factor V Leiden mutation plus the use of certain oral contraceptives places the patient at a nearly 30-fold increase for venous thrombosis.

Pregnancy is associated with an increase in nearly all of the clotting factors, an increased platelet count and a decrease in protein S activity. In addition, pregnancy is associated with decreased antithrombin. These factors combined with venous stasis from the uterus compressing venous drainage of the legs lead to at least a fivefold increase in venous thrombosis during pregnancy.

D. Antiphospholipid syndrome is present in 1% of the population and increases with age. Antiphospholipid syndrome is caused by circulating antibodies to negatively charged phospholipids and includes **anticardiolipin antibody** and **circulating lupus anticoagulant.** Different antibodies exist and are not present in all individuals. The assay for anticardiolipin is most sensitive and specific for the diagnosis. Circulating lupus anticoagulant may be independent of the underlying collagen vascular disorder or part of systemic lupus erythematosus. As many as one-half of individuals with lupus or lupus-like disorders have either circulating lupus anticoagulant or antiphospholipid antibody.

The pathogenesis of thrombosis in these individuals is not well understood. It has been suggested that autoantibodies inhibit endothelial cell prostacyclin production or interference of thrombomodulin-mediated protein C activation.

E. Malignancy. The association of malignancy and venous thrombosis is well recognized. Patients who develop deep venous thrombosis and have no other identifiable risk factors have a 10% chance of having an undiagnosed malignancy. The hypercoagulable state associated with malignancy is due to interaction of tumor cells and their products with host cells. This interaction leads to elimination of normal protective mechanisms that the host employs to prevent thrombosis.

Tumor cells may induce procoagulant properties such as secretion of tissue thromboplastin or proteases which activate clotting factors. Patients with malignant disease may also have increased levels of factors V, VIII, IX, and X. Cancer patients frequently have other risk factors that place them at risk for thrombosis such as chemotherapeutic treatment and indwelling central venous catheters.

F. Antineoplastic drugs. Chemotherapeutic agents have been associated with vascular abnormalities such as thrombotic thrombocytopenic purpura, Budd–Chiari syndrome, myocardial infarction and venous thrombosis. Thrombotic events are related to hypercoagulable states caused by the effect of these drugs or their metabolites on vascular endothelium.

G. Myeloproliferative syndromes. At least three myeloproliferative disorders have been associated with thrombosis and hypercoagulability likely secondary to increases in whole blood viscosity. The disorders, polycythemia vera, essential thrombocythemia and agnogenic myeloid metaplasia, may also affect platelet function either directly or indirectly. In addition to association with extremity venous thrombosis, the myeloproliferative disorders predispose individuals to mesenteric, hepatic or portal venous thrombosis. This type of hypercoagulable state rarely manifests as arterial thrombosis unless combined with another thrombotic risk factor.

IV. Management. The management of patients with identified hypercoagulable states is highly individualized and not yet defined by prospective studies. **Hypercoagulability is now viewed as a multigenic or multi–risk factor disease.** Except for a few rare inherited homozygous conditions, thrombophilia exists in patients with one or more additive risk factors. The decision to anticoagulate rests on the number of identified risk factors in a given patient and should involve a multidisciplinary approach (internists, hematologists, vascular medicine specialists and vascular surgeons). Generally, asymptomatic patients are not anticoagulated prophylactically unless additional risk factors such as surgery are anticipated.

Long-term prophylaxis with warfarin is considered when a patient has experienced two or more documented thrombotic events or a single life-threatening event. This general guideline may be changed in those patients with prosthetic grafts, heart valves or specifically identified hypercoagulable conditions. Immediate therapy for acute thrombosis consists of intravenous heparin and oral warfarin (see Chap. 21). Alternatively, high-dose low-molecular weight heparin given subcutaneously has proven effective and allowed outpatient anticoagulation in select cases. **Given the risk of warfarin-induced necrosis in patients with protein C or S deficiency, it is recommended to begin warfarin therapy with the patient anticoagulated on heparin.**

SELECTED READING

Cumming AM, Shiach CR. The investigation and management of inherited thrombophilia. *Clin Lab Haematol* 1999;21:77–92.

Falanga A, Rickles FR. Pathophysiology of the thrombotic state in the cancer patient. *Semin Thromb Hemost* 1999;25:173–182.

Hillarp A, Zoller B, Dahlback B. Activated protein C resistance as a basis for venous thrombosis. *Am J Med* 1996;101:534–540.

Miletich JP. Thrombophilia as a multigenic disorder. *Semin Thromb Hemost* 1998;24(suppl 1):13–20.

Selzman CH, Whitehill TA, Krupski WC. Thrombophilia and activated protein C resistance. *Ann Vasc Surg* 1998;12:601–604.

Silver D, Vouyouka A. The caput medusae of hypercoagulability. *J Vasc Surg* 2000;31:396–405.

Wakefield TW. Treatment options for venous thrombosis. *J Vasc Surg* 2000;31:613–620.

Subject Index

Subject Index

Numbers followed by the letter f indicate figures; numbers followed by the letter t indicate tables.